Mosby's Color Atlas and Text of

Neurology

Perkin

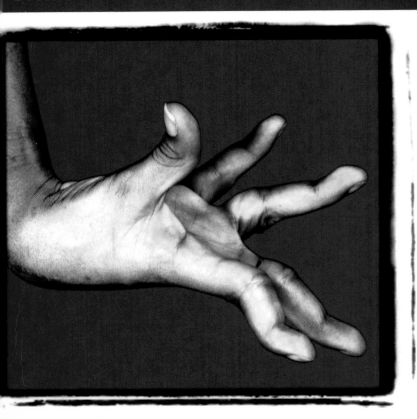

Mosby's Color Atlas and Text of
Neurology

G David Perkin BA MB FRCP
Consultant Neurologist
Charing Cross Hospital
London
UK

London Chicago Philadelphia St. Louis Sydney Tokyo

Project Manager	Jane Tozer
Development Editor	Sue Hodgson
Designer	Greg Smith
Layout Artist	Jenni Miller
Cover Design	Greg Smith
Illustration	Marion Tasker
Production	Gudrun Hughes
Index	Nina Boyd
Publisher	Fiona Foley

Published in 1998 by Mosby–Wolfe, an imprint of Mosby International (a division of Times Mirror International Publishers Limited).

Printed by Grafos SA, Arte sobre papel, Barcelona, Spain.

ISBN 0 7234 2497 7

For full details of all Times Mirror International Publishers Limited titles, please write to Times Mirror International Publishers Limited, Lynton House, 7–12 Tavistock Square, London WC1H 9LB, England.

A CIP catalogue record for this book is available from the British Library.

Library of Congress Cataloging-in-Publication Data applied for

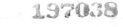

Contents

Contents

Preface and User Guide

This book aims to combine text and illustrations in such a way as to provide a coherent and easy to assimilate description of the common neurological disorders. It covers a basic neurological curriculum suitable for the medical student, but also includes sufficient detail to allow it to be used by graduates when preparing for higher examination and, in particular, the MRCP.

The text is divided into two main sections, the first dealing with common neurological symptoms, for example headache and altered consciousness, while the second deals with specific neurological disorders, for example multiple sclerosis.

Bullet points have been used throughout in order to reduce the overall volume of text without compromising the clarity of the information. Indeed, the aim has been to render the material into succinct accessible passages, enhanced by design features which help the student find their way around the text.

Each chapter contains a number of colour-coded sections to allow ready revision. Major definitions are boxed, as are the principal symptoms associated with particular conditions or syndromes. Throughout, summary boxes highlight the important messages within the text. Tables have been used liberally to provide a readily accessible review of data.

In addition, the book is profusely illustrated with clinical photographs, imaging and specially commissioned drawings, chosen to both complement and enhance understanding of the text.

It is a pleasure to record my indebtedness to Sue Hodgson, Development Editor, and to Jane Tozer, Project Manager, both of whom have provided stimulating challenges to my previous concepts of authorship! I am delighted to record my appreciation of Fiona Foley, Managing Director of Mosby International, who enthusiastically embraced my ideas for this book and helped refine them into the finished product. Finally, I thank my secretary, Irene Cassidy, who has shouldered the burden of typing the manuscript and has unfailingly and astonishingly transcribed my scribble into a coherent whole.

David Perkin

This book contains three different types of boxes:

> **Key points appear in yellow.**

> **Lists of symptoms appear in blue.**

> **Definitions appear in pink.**

chapter 1

Neurological History and Examination

HISTORY TAKING

History taking remains as critically important in the evaluation of a patient with neurological symptoms as it does in the general medical clinic, where over 80% of diagnoses are made on the basis of the history. As a result of its crucial role, the history is likely to take longer than the physical examination. The interview will use a judicious combination of open-ended and closed questions.

> **Definition of open-ended and closed questions**
>
> Open-ended questions deal with generalizations
> - How are you?
> - How are you feeling?
>
> Closed questions require a more specific response
> - Is your headache associated with photophobia?

A history confined to closed questions is rapidly completed but devoid of any personal element. Open-ended questions allow the patient much more licence but run the danger of introducing spurious material. The interview should include both with a tendency to move from open-ended to closed questions.

THE INTERVIEW

Initial approach

The interview should begin with a personal introduction. If you are a student, you should say so and be prepared for the patient to refuse further discussion. If you are seeing an in-patient, plan the timing of your interview around the ward schedule and the patient's own commitments. Although it is preferable to complete the physical examination at the same time as the history, the process may have to be divided into two sessions.

First questions

Initially, you need to determine whether the patient is capable of giving a history. If the patient is depressed, demented or dysphasic, the responses are likely to be unforthcoming or uninterpretable. Having established the patient's capability, ask the patient to outline the problem. If there are multiple complaints, establish their chronological order before exploring each in turn. By this means, your initial precis may be as follows:

F.T., aged 61 years. Accountant.
1. Ill-defined, right-sided headaches for 3 months
2. Some speech hesitancy for 6 weeks
3. Mild clumsiness of the right hand for 2 weeks

History of presenting complaint – Explore each of the patient's complaints in turn. If the patient describes a particular condition, for example, migraine, do not take it at face value but by assessing the nature of the patient's headache, decide whether that is the relevant diagnosis. For each complaint establish the following facts:

Time of onset – This is usually straightforward for recent events but more difficult for long-standing complaints. Very often the patient suggests a much shorter history than is apparent if the records are carefully examined.

Mode of onset – The speed of onset of a neurological symptom is of help in differential diagnosis, as is the pattern of its subsequent evolution. A histogram of level of symptoms against time helps to place the patient's problem in particular categories (**Fig. 1.1**).

Exacerbating and relieving factors – Patients will almost always want to explain their symptom on the basis of an environmental factor. A facial paralysis is attributed to exposure to a cold draught, a seizure to a sudden stress and a headache to the ingestion of a certain food. Although many of these beliefs carry no substance, some do, and they should be carefully recorded.

Pain assessment – For pain, the topics shown in **Figure 1.2** should be covered. If the patient is unable to specify the nature of the pain, give the patient a list to choose from, avoiding putting first the description you believe is most relevant to your working diagnosis. Assessment of pain severity is notoriously difficult. Sometimes it helps to compare the pain to a previous experience, for example, childbirth. The degree to which the pain interrupts everyday activities can be helpful but is influenced by the patient's personality. The total duration of a headache history is particularly valuable when deciding whether it is associated with a serious underlying pathology.

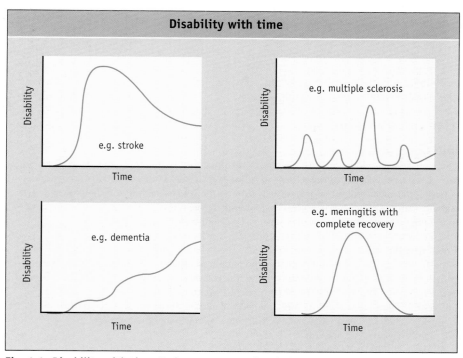

Fig. 1.1 *Disability with time.* *Various patterns and typical examples.*

Social history – Items to be covered include schooling, employment, drug history and consumption of tobacco and alcohol. An assessment of education gives some measure of premorbid intelligence. Employment history may be important if exposure to certain toxins could be relevant to the patient's symptoms or if the type of employment and its responsibilities may be beyond the patient's capabilities. Carefully detail all the drugs the patient is using, whether on prescription or over the counter. It will often be difficult to understand why certain drugs are being taken. You will find that many such drugs have been prescribed for years, the patient having long since forgotten the indication for their use. Frequently, some of the patient's symptoms can be related to adverse effects of the drug. When determining alcohol consumption, calculate the number of units consumed each week (**Fig. 1.3**). Many illicit drugs (e.g. Ecstasy, amphetamines and cocaine) can be associated with stroke. With foreign travel so common, enquiry about recent travel, the areas covered and malaria prophylaxis (if relevant) should be made. For many patients with neurological disease, their home situation and support is critically relevant when determining their capacity to be independent in the community.

Previous illness – Accounts of the patient's past illnesses often have to be supplemented by reference to hospital or general practice records. For each specific diagnosis that is given, determine the quality of information that was available to make it.

Family history – In addition to asking whether any family member has had a similar neurological illness, you need to determine the ages at death and the causes of death in close family members of previous generations. Where there is suspicion of a familial disorder, construction of a family tree can be helpful (**Fig. 1.4**). If autosomal recessive inheritance is suspected, enquire about parental consanguinity.

Assessment of pain

- Type
- Site
- Spread
- Periodicity
- Relieving factors
- Exacerbating factors
- Associated symptoms

Fig. 1.2 *Assessment of pain.*

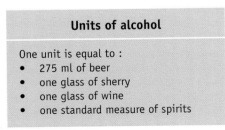

Units of alcohol

One unit is equal to :
- 275 ml of beer
- one glass of sherry
- one glass of wine
- one standard measure of spirits

Fig. 1.3 *Units of alcohol.*

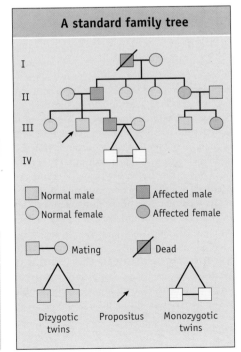

Fig. 1.4 *A standard family tree.*

3

- Making the patient aware of who you are is an important preliminary to history taking
- A judicious combination of open-ended and closed questions is appropriate when exploring the presenting complaints
- If patients use specific diagnoses in their history, explore in detail on what evidence the diagnosis was made

Systems review – Before embarking on the neurological system (although a full history will cover all the systems), some general enquiries are pertinent. Is there a disturbance of sleep pattern? Does the patient complain of tiredness (although the response is often positive, certainly for patients attending hospital)? Has there been weight loss, anorexia or episodic fever?

The nervous system

Headache – Almost all the population suffer from headache at some time. Follow the same enquiry that you would for other pain problems (see **Fig. 1.2**). Avoid attaching labels, for example, migraine, tension headache or, even worse, 'neuralgia'. Simply concentrate on obtaining as full a description as possible.

Loss of consciousness – Avoid using the term blackout or even letting the patient use it. If there have been episodes of loss of consciousness, determine whether warning symptoms occurred, in what situation and posture they happened and whether there were eyewitnesses. Was there incontinence, injury or a bitten tongue? Did the patient recover rapidly or only over several hours?

Dizziness and vertigo – Dizziness as a complaint seldom, if ever, provides a lead to a specific diagnosis. The term is used by different patients in different ways. Vertigo implies a sense of rotation, either of self or of the environment. The situation in which dizziness or vertigo occurs sometimes assists diagnosis. Hyperventilation attacks tend to occur in crowded places (e.g. supermarkets) and postural dizziness occurs particularly when getting out of bed in the morning, whereas benign positional vertigo typically occurs when the individual turns over in bed.

Speech and related functions – Ask about the patient's speech. Is there a problem of articulation or speech volume, or is the patient using the wrong words with or without a reduction in overall speech output? Note the patient's handedness (based on a number of skilled activities, not just writing). Does the patient appear to comprehend speech? Has there been any difficulty with writing or reading?

Memory – If the patient complains of memory loss (often patients deny it), determine if this refers to recent or more remote memory. Determine whether the problem is constant or fluctuant. Find out if there has been a prominent change in mood. Memory problems in younger patients are usually psychologically determined.

Symptoms relating to the cranial nerves

Vision – Are any visual symptoms negative (i.e. visual loss) or positive (in other words, scintillations or flashing lights)? Is the problem monocular or binocular (although patients seldom cover-test during attacks of visual disturbance)? Is the visual disturbance accompanied by headache?

Diplopia – If the patient complains of diplopia, ask whether the problem is relieved by covering one or other eye. Is the diplopia horizontal or oblique? Does it occur maximally in one position of gaze? Is it constant or fluctuant?

Facial numbness – Ask the patient to outline the extent of any facial numbness and whether it affects the tongue, gums or buccal mucosae.

Deafness – If deafness is apparent, is it unilateral or bilateral? Is there a family history of deafness or a history of exposure to noise? Is the problem progressive? Is the deafness more apparent when background noise is heightened? Is there accompanying tinnitus?

Dysphagia – Does any difficulty with swallowing affect solids, liquids or both? Does it relate to transferring food from the mouth or at a later stage of swallowing? Is there nasal regurgitation?

Limb motor or sensory symptoms – Is the problem confined to part or the whole of one limb, to one side of the body, to the lower limbs alone or to all four limbs? Does the patient describe numbness (i.e. a loss or reduction of sensation) or some distortion of sensation (e.g. a tight band around the limb)? Is any weakness intermittent or continuous and, if the latter, is it progressive? Does the weakness mainly affect the proximal or the distal part of the limb? Has the patient noticed muscle wasting or twitching? Is there muscle fatiguability?

Altered co-ordination – Patients with cerebellar incoordination tend to refer to the affected limb as being clumsy or even weak. When assessing upper limb co-ordination, ask about everyday tasks such as writing and dressing. Ask about the patient's sense of balance. Is the patient liable to stagger to one particular side or the other? Has he or she fallen?

- Many terms used in the neurological systems review are likely to be nebulous, for example, blackout, dizziness. Try to get the patient or their relative to describe the actual sensation experienced
- If patients refer to weakness, try to establish whether they mean loss of motor function or simply loss of co-ordination
- Make sure when you ask patients about a particular condition, for example, double vision, that they understand what the term means

EXAMINATION

HIGHER CORTICAL FUNCTION

Assessment of higher cortical function begins during history taking. The patient's mood, attention, speech content and insight will have already become apparent.

Orientation

Note the patient's sense of orientation in time and space.

Memory

For immediate recall, test digit repetition (five to seven digits forward and four to five in reverse are achievable) or 'serial sevens' (serially subtracting seven from 100).

For recent memory, ask about recent events, give the patient the names of four objects (and ask for them to be repeated after 10 min) and ask the patient to reproduce drawings 10 s after viewing them.

For remote memory, ask about schooling, childhood, work experience and family.

Intelligence

Give the patient a set list of questions.

Ask the patient to perform simple calculations.

Ask the patient to interpret proverbs of increasing complexity.

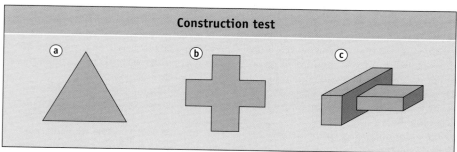

Fig. 1.5 *Drawings of increasing complexity to be reproduced by the patient.*

Ask the patient to copy designs of increasing complexity (**Fig. 1.5**).

Geographical orientation

Ask the patient to draw an outline of his or her native country and locate within it some of the principal cities.

SPEECH

Definition of speech defects

Dysarthria A defect of articulation without disturbance of language function
Dysphonia A defect of speech volume
Dysphasia A defect of language function in which there is either abnormal comprehension or production of speech or both. The language contains word substitutions, that is, paraphasias

To assess dysphasia, four basic functions are examined.

Fluency

Assess the amount of speech produced in a given period of time.

Ask the patient to name as many objects as possible in a particular category (e.g. fruits) in a set period of time.

Comprehension

Ask increasingly complex questions but restricted to those answerable by yes or no.

Repetition

Ask the patient to repeat simple words then increasingly complex sentences.

Naming

Point to a succession of dissimilar objects and ask the patient to name them.

When assessing reading, take account of the patient's educational background. Test writing by asking the patient to write first single words then sentences.

PRAXIS

Start by asking the patient to carry out a particular task. If the patient fails, get him or her to copy your own movement. If this also fails to elicit the movement, provide the object and

Mini Mental State Examination

Orientation
1. What is the year, season, date, month, day? One point for each correct answer.
2. Where are we? Country, county, town, hospital, floor? One point for each correct answer.

Registration
3. Name three objects, taking one second to say each. Then ask the patient all three once you have said them. One point for each correct answer. Repeat the question until the patient learns all three.

Attention & calculation
4. Serial sevens. One point for each correct answer. Stop after five answers. Alternative: spell WORLD backwards.

Recall
5. Ask for names of objects asked in Question 3. One point for each correct answer.

Language
6. Point to a pencil and a watch. Have the patient name them for you. One point for each correct answer.
7. Have the patient repeat "No ifs, ands, or buts." One point.
8. Have the patient follow a 3-stage command. "Take the paper in your right hand; fold the paper in half; put the paper on the floor." Three points.
9. Have the patient read and obey the following: CLOSE YOUR EYES. (Write this in large letters.) One point.
10. Have the patient write a sentence of his or her own choice. (The sentence must contain a subject and an object and make some sense.) Ignore spelling errors when scoring. One point.
11. Have the patient draw two intersecting pentagons with equal sides. Give one point if all the sides and angles are preserved, and if the intersecting sides form a quadrangle.

Maximum score = 30 points

Fig. 1.6 *Mini Mental State Examination.*

ask the patient to demonstrate its use. A more complex motor sequence is tested by asking the patient to go through a series of related movements.

RIGHT–LEFT ORIENTATION
Start with simple commands, then increase their complexity.

GNOSIS
In one form of visual agnosia, the problem with recognition is due to a failure of naming. In another, the failure to recognize can be overcome by asking the patient to handle the object, allowing its use to be demonstrated.

Screening tests have been devised to allow a rapid bedside assessment of cognitive function, for example, the Mini Mental State Examination (**Fig. 1.6**). Early dementia is probable with a score of 24–27.

PRIMITIVE REFLEXES

Primitive reflexes can sometimes be found in normal individuals. Their presence usually signifies a diffuse pathology, for example, dementia, but some are particularly sensitive to frontal lobe pathology and when unilateral, reflect contralateral damage.

The glabella tap

Performed by tapping repetitively with the index finger on the glabella. The blink response normally inhibits after three to four taps. The reflex occurs in Parkinson's disease and in dementia.

The palmo-mental reflex

Apply firm and fairly sharp pressure to the palm alongside the thenar eminence. Contraction of the ipsilateral mentalis causing puckering of the chin indicates a positive response.

Pout and suckling reflexes

A positive pout response consists of protrusion of the lips when they are lightly tapped by the index finger. A positive suckling reflex consists of a suckling movement of the lips when the angle of the mouth is stimulated.

Grasp reflex

Stroke the palmar surface of the patient's hand firmly from the radial to the ulnar aspect. A positive response results in the examiner's hand being gripped so tightly that release is difficult. A foot grasp reflex is elicited by stroking the sole of the foot towards the toes with the handle of a patella hammer. A positive response leads to plantar flexion of the toes (**Fig. 1.7**).

- When assessing for dysphasia, test fluency, comprehension, repetition and naming
- The Mini Mental State Examination is a useful, although flawed, bedside screening test for dementia
- Certain of the primitive reflexes, for example, the palmo-mental reflex, do not necessarily have pathological significance if they are bilateral

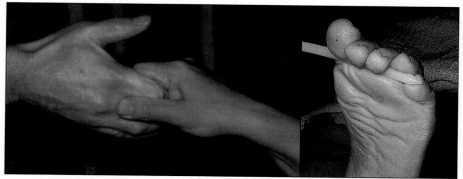

Fig. 1.7 *Hand and foot grasp reflexes.*

CRANIAL NERVE EXAMINATION

Olfactory (I)

If available, squeeze-bottles containing discriminant odours (e.g. ß-phenyl ethyl alcohol and isovaleric acid) are introduced into each nostril in turn. The patient is asked either to identify the odour or to describe it. If squeeze-bottles are not to hand, everyday odours that can be used include coffee, cinnamon and chocolate.

Optic (II)

Aspects of optic nerve function that are tested by the bedside include visual acuity, colour vision, visual fields and fundoscopy.

Visual acuity – For distance vision, use a Snellen chart. The patient sits or stands 6 m from the chart, which should be well illuminated. Each eye is tested in turn. Glasses, if normally worn, should be used. A visual acuity of 6/18 indicates that at 6 m, the patient can only read letters that a normal individual could read at 18 m. If acuity is less than 6/60, you can record vision as counting fingers, hand movements or perception of light. Refractive problems can be partly overcome by looking through a pinhole. Near vision is tested using test types produced by the UK Faculty of Ophthalmologists. Near and distance acuity do not necessarily correlate.

Colour vision – Colour vision is not tested routinely. For rapid screening, Ishihara colour plates are used. Although originally designed to detect colour blindness, they can give some information in acquired disease of the visual pathway (**Fig. 1.8**).

Visual fields – This is a critical part of the neurological examination that is frequently poorly performed. For bedside testing, sit approximately 1 m from the patient. The room should be well illuminated and the background white or at least plain, assuming that a red target is being used. The choice of target is partly dependent on the type of defect being looked for and the age and reliability of the patient. For peripheral defects, either finger movements or a 10 mm red pin can be used.

For testing the left visual field, ask the patient to cover or close the right eye while you close your left eye (**Fig. 1.9**). The limits of the peripheral field can be determined by bringing the pin or your moving fingers into the four quadrants of the field. Ask the patient if a red target appears red, rather than just whether he or she can see it.

For central field defects, a pin must be used. It helps to outline the blind spot first, both to establish that your technique is satisfactory and to confirm the patient's co-operation. Move the red pin along the horizontal meridian into the temporal field. Explain to the

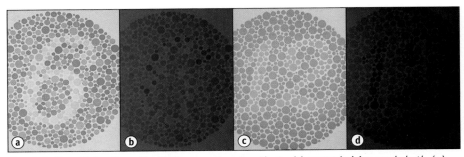

Fig. 1.8 *Two plates from the Ishihara series. A patient with normal vision reads both (a) and (c) without difficulty. A patient with red–green deficiency is unable to read (b) (number 6) but can read (d) (number 12).*

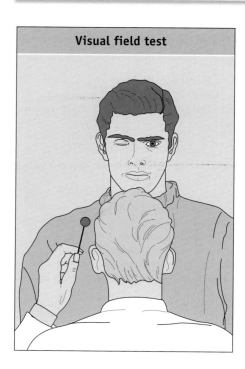

Visual field test

Fig. 1.9 *Testing visual fields by confrontation.*

patient that the pin will briefly disappear then reappear. Do not expect the blind spot necessarily to coincide with your own. Confrontational techniques are perfectly adequate to detect the field defects encountered in clinical practice (**Fig. 1.10**).

Definitions of visual field defects

Central scotoma	A defect centred on fixation
Altitudinal defect	A defect in the upper or lower half field
Bitemporal hemianopia	A defect in the temporal parts of both fields
Homonymous hemianopia	A defect in the temporal half of one field and the nasal half of the other. The defects may match (congruous) or differ (incongruous)

Finally, when assessing possible field defects caused by parietal lobe pathology, the fingers should be presented in the two half fields simultaneously (**Fig. 1.11**). In some patients with a parietal lesion, the target is seen in the contralateral half field when presented alone but is missed when a competing stimulus is presented in the ipsilateral half field (visual inattention or suppression).

Fundoscopy – Only rarely should the pupils be dilated for routine fundoscopy. If this is performed, record it in the notes and reverse the mydriasis at the end of the examination. If the patient is severely myopic, it sometimes helps to view through the patient's glasses. If necessary, take the patient into a dark room for the examination. Assess, in turn, the optic disc for its colour, the presence or absence of swelling and the presence or absence of venous pulsation, then assess the arteries, then the retinal veins. Examine the fundus for

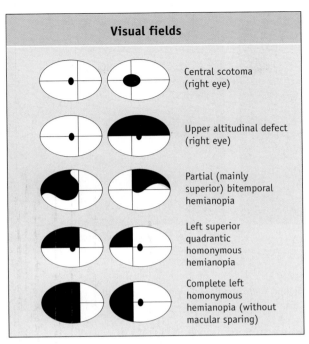

Visual fields

Central scotoma (right eye)

Upper altitudinal defect (right eye)

Partial (mainly superior) bitemporal hemianopia

Left superior quadrantic homonymous hemianopia

Complete left homonymous hemianopia (without macular sparing)

Fig. 1.10 *Common types of visual field defect.*

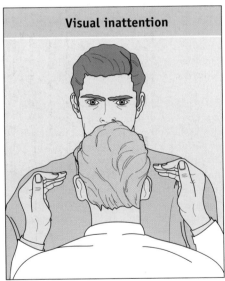

Visual inattention

Fig. 1.11 *Simultaneous presentation of finger movements in the two half fields.*

haemorrhages or exudates, describing their appearance and position using the disc as a clock face, for example, one blot haemorrhage at 6 o'clock, two disc diameters from the disc.

Early optic atrophy is difficult to detect. Slight temporal pallor occurs in normal individuals. Papilloedema is often unassociated with visual symptoms until it becomes chronic, although some patients have transient loss of vision triggered by movement (obscurations). One of the earliest signs of papilloedema is loss of retinal venous pulsation. Later, there is engorgement

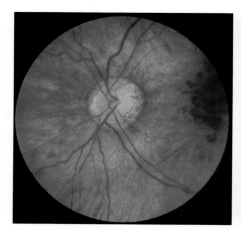

Fig. 1.12 *Optic atrophy.*

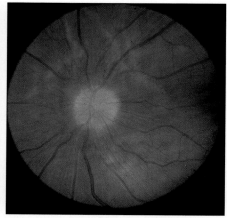

**Fig. 1.13 *Early papilloedema.* Dilated nerve
fibre bundles, superficial haemorrhages and
disc hyperaemia.**

of retinal veins, obscuration of the disc margins, flame haemorrhages and cotton wool spots
(retinal infarcts) (**Fig. 1.12 and 1.13**).

Oculomotor, trochlear and abducens nerves (III, IV, VI)

Begin by assessing the position of the eyelids. If there is a ptosis, is it bilateral or unilateral
and does it fatigue (on prolonged up-gaze)? Does one or other eye appear proptosed
(exophthalmos) or sunken (enophthalmos)? Next, examine the pupils, which should be
circular and symmetrical. A mild difference in pupil size of up to 2 mm is found in 20% of
the population (physiological anisocoria). If the pupils are irregular, ask about previous
trauma or ocular infection. If there is a marked difference in pupil size, check whether the
patient is using drops.

Pupillary light response – A pencil torch should be used and the background illumination
should be low. Ask the patient to fixate on a distant object. Conventionally, first the direct
and then consensual responses are assessed. Observing the consensual response in someone
with dark irises is next to impossible. Far better to perform a swinging light test in which the
torch is swung backwards and forwards from one eye to the other. Observe only the pupil
that is being illuminated. Normally, as the torch swings from the first eye to the second, the
pupil of the second eye briefly starts to dilate (having lost its consensual response) but then
constricts immediately as the torch reaches it. If there is a lesion of the optic nerve of the
second eye, then the pupil continues to dilate as the torch shines on it (relative afferent
pupillary defect) (**Fig. 1.14**).

Near reaction – The near reaction is not worth testing if the light response is intact. If the
light response is abnormal, test the near reaction by asking the patient to fixate on a target
as it approaches the eyes. If there is no immediate response, sustain convergence for a
minute or so to see if there is a delayed reaction.

Eye movements – Start by assessing whether the eyes are parallel. Ask the patient to look at
your forehead while you alternately cover one eye then the other (cover test) (**Fig. 1.15**). In a
non-paralytic squint (strabismus), covering the fixating eye produces a movement in the
squinting eye that allows it to take up fixation. If you suspect a paresis of one or more of the
ocular muscles, ask the patient to look in the six directions shown in **Figure 1.16** in order, as
far as possible, to test each muscle individually. If the patient has diplopia, certain rules may

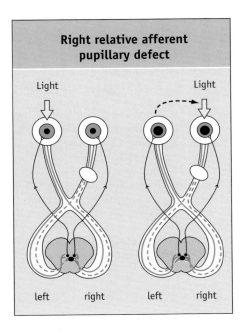

Right relative afferent pupillary defect

Fig. 1.14 *Right relative afferent pupillary defect.* Constriction of both pupils occurs when the light is shone in the left eye. As the torch is swung to the right eye, the pupil dilates because of loss of the consensual response.

left   right   left   right

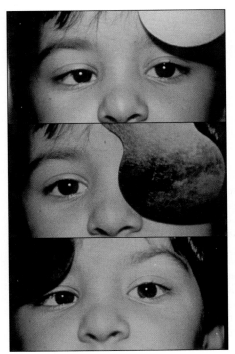

Fig. 1.15 *Cover testing. There is a right convergent squint (esotropia), which corrects temporarily when the left eye is covered.*

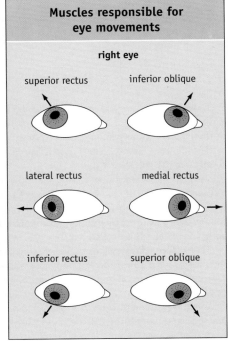

Muscles responsible for eye movements

right eye

superior rectus   inferior oblique

lateral rectus   medial rectus

inferior rectus   superior oblique

Fig. 1.16 *The muscles responsible for eye movements in particular directions.*

allow identification of the affected muscle:
- The diplopia increases in the direction of action of the paralysed muscle
- The false image is peripheral to the true image and belongs to the affected eye
- By cover testing, the eye responsible for the false image can be established

Finally, check whether the patient has an abnormal head tilt and whether it was present in old photographs.

Next, examine saccadic and pursuit movements in the horizontal and vertical planes. For the former, get the patient to refixate between two targets (say, two fingers). Saccades that overshoot are hypermetric and those that undershoot are hypometric. For pursuit, ask the patient to follow a slowly moving target (if the target moves too rapidly, saccades will intervene). Broken pursuit movements occur in both cerebellar and extrapyramidal disorders. If the eyes fail to respond to a saccadic or pursuit stimulus, perform the doll's head manoeuvre. Ask the patient to fixate on your eyes, grasp the patient's head and rotate it, first in the horizontal then in the vertical plane. An intact response (a measure of vestibular eye function) allows the patient's eyes to remain fixed on your own.

Finally, look for nystagmus that may be present in the primary position of gaze or only on deviation. Jerk nystagmus has fast and slow phases. Pendular nystagmus has phases of equal velocity.

Definition of degrees of jerk nystagmus to the right

1° Present on lateral gaze to right with fast phase to right
2° Present on forward gaze with fast phase to right
3° Present on lateral gaze to left with fast phase to right

Descriptive terms used include fine, medium or coarse, sustained or ill sustained, horizontal, vertical or rotatory. When looking for 1° nystagmus, do not abduct the eyes by more than 30°, otherwise end-point (physiological) nystagmus may supervene.

Trigeminal nerve (V)

For sensory examination, cotton wool (light touch) and pinprick (pain) should suffice, although occasionally temperature loss is the sole sensory abnormality. Details of sensory testing are given on pp26–28. Each division of the trigeminal nerve should be covered and the two sides of the face and scalp compared (**Fig. 1.17**). Avoid dragging the cotton wool across the skin. Non-organic sensory loss tends strictly to follow the confines of the face.

To test the corneal response, lightly touch the cornea with a wisp of cotton wool. Warn the patient what to expect. Patients who wear contact lenses will have dulled responses. Observe the ipsilateral and contralateral blink response and ask the patient to compare the two sides.

When testing motor function, first examine for any muscle wasting. Next, palpate the masseter and temporalis with the jaws clenched. Finally, ask the patient to open the jaw against resistance. In a unilateral trigeminal lesion, the jaw deviates to the paralysed side.

Finally, elicit the jaw jerk. With the mouth slightly open and the jaw relaxed, place your index finger on the apex of the jaw and tap it with the patella hammer. The response, a contraction of the pterygoid muscles, varies widely even in normal individuals.

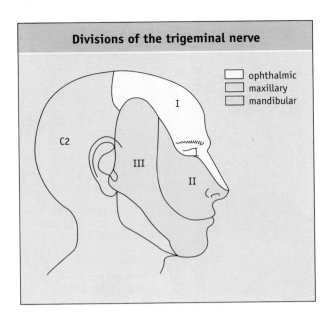

Divisions of the trigeminal nerve

- ophthalmic
- maxillary
- mandibular

I

C2

III

II

Fig. 1.17 *Cutaneous distribution of the three divisions of the trigeminal nerve.*

Facial nerve (VII)

Much information can be obtained when assessing facial nerve function by looking at the face at rest and during conversation. Is the face symmetrical? Do the eyes blink with an equal range of movement? Are there any involuntary movements of the face or movements of one part triggered by contraction of another? To test formally the muscles supplied by the nerve, ask the patient to elevate the eyebrows, close the eyes tightly, blow out cheeks, then purse the lips tightly together (**Fig. 1.18**). Emotional facial movements are sometimes spared when voluntary movement is affected. In an upper motor neuron facial weakness, the upper face is relatively spared (because of bilateral cortical representation). In a lower motor neuron weakness, all the muscles are affected equally unless the lesion is very distal. Sometimes, after a lower motor neuron weakness, misdirection of regenerating fibres leads to movement of one part of the face when another part contracts (aberrant re-innervation).

Testing taste by the bedside is unsatisfactory. The facial nerve supplies taste to the anterior two-thirds of the tongue. Sweet (sugar), salt, bitter (quinine) and sour (vinegar) solutions are applied in turn, the mouth being washed out with distilled water between testing. Although the facial nerve has a small cutaneous distribution (mainly around the ear), the overlap with adjacent nerves is such that testing this function is not feasible.

Acoustic nerve (VIII)

Auditory function – Each ear is tested separately. Ask the patient to occlude the ear not being tested by pressing on the tragus. Hearing sensitivity is tested either to a wristwatch (possible to approximately 0.75 m) or to a whispered sound (possible to approximately 0.8 m). Alternatively, generate a noise by rubbing the fingers together. The Rinne and Weber tests are used to distinguish nerve (perceptive) deafness (caused by cochlear damage or cochlear nerve damage) from conductive deafness (caused by an abnormality of the conducting system serving the cochlea).

Rinne test – Place a 512 Hz tuning fork on the mastoid process, then hold it adjacent to the pinna. In normal individuals and in patients with perceptive deafness, air conduction is

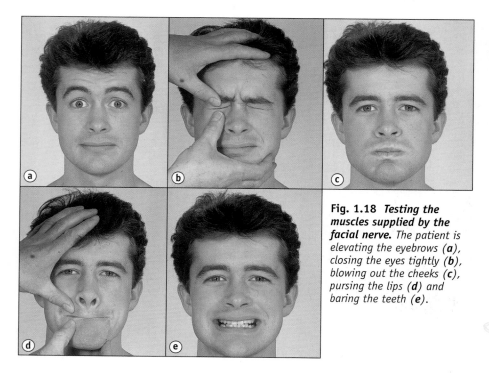

Fig. 1.18 *Testing the muscles supplied by the facial nerve. The patient is elevating the eyebrows (a), closing the eyes tightly (b), blowing out the cheeks (c), pursing the lips (d) and baring the teeth (e).*

better perceived than bone conduction (Rinne positive). In conductive deafness, the reverse applies (**Fig. 1.19**).

Weber's test – Place a 512 Hz tuning fork over the vertex or on the midline of the forehead. Normally, the sound is heard equally by the two ears. In perceptive deafness, it appears louder in the intact ear but louder in the deaf ear in conductive deafness (**Fig. 1.20**).

Vestibular function – There are no direct bedside methods for assessing vestibular function. In the presence of acute failure of the vestibular end organ or its nerve, certain physical signs appear:

- Unidirectional jerk nystagmus with the fast phase away from the lesion
- Past-pointing to a stationary object, with the eyes closed, to the side of the lesion
- Romberg fall or deviation on marching on the spot with the eyes closed (Unterberger's test) to the side of the lesion

The patient experiences vertigo in the direction of the fast component. If these requirements are not met, the problem is likely to be one affecting the central vestibular connections.

For patients with postural vertigo, it is necessary to assess the effect of head positioning (Barany manoeuvre). Position the patient at the edge of the couch, facing away from the edge. Rotate the head to one side then depress the head and trunk so that they are approximately 30° below the horizontal. If nystagmus appears, determine whether it begins immediately or after an interval, whether it persists or fatigues and whether it returns as the patient returns to the upright posture. Repeat the manoeuvre with the head rotated to the other side (**Fig. 1.21**).

Glossopharyngeal nerve (IX)

Examination of the glossopharyngeal nerve is difficult and seldom necessary. The nerve supplies the afferent arc of the gag reflex. Firmly press the end of an orange stick first

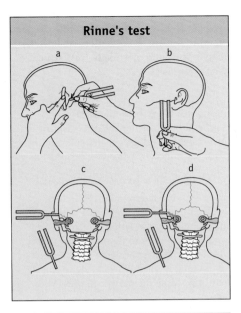

Rinne's test

Fig. 1.19 *Rinne test. Comparison of (a) bone conduction and (b) air conduction, (c) perceptive deafness and (d) conductive deafness.*

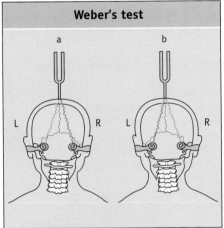

Weber's test

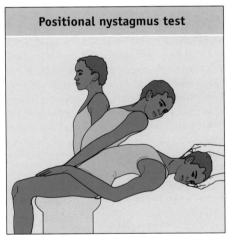

Positional nystagmus test

Fig. 1.20 *Weber's test. Left-sided perceptive deafness (a) and left-sided conductive deafness (b).*

Fig. 1.21 *Testing for positional nystagmus.*

into one tonsillar fossa, then the other. Ask for the subjective response and observe the reflex elevation of the palate, which should be in the midline. The nerve also supplies taste fibres to the posterior one-third of the tongue but this function is not testable in clinical practice.

Vagus nerve (X)

Bedside evaluation is confined to assessment of spontaneous and reflex movements of the uvula and posterior pharyngeal wall. Ask the patient to phonate (say 'aah'). The midline of the soft palate should rise centrally. A similar movement is provoked by performing the gag reflex. In a unilateral palatal palsy, the palate deviates to the intact side. Additional evidence for a vagal lesion may be forthcoming from listening to the patient's speech. Involvement of the recurrent laryngeal branch of the nerve results in hoarseness.

Accessory nerve (XI)

The accessory nerve is tested by assessing the sternomastoid and the upper fibres of trapezius (**Fig. 1.22**). For the sternomastoid, assess the bulk of the muscles then ask the patient to rotate the head against resistance. For the trapezius, observe the position of the shoulders then test elevation, first without, then with resistance.

Hypoglossal nerve (XII)

First inspect the tongue as it lies in the floor of the oral cavity; ignore minor twitching movements. Fasciculation imparts a shimmering motion to the surface. Decide whether the tongue is of normal bulk or wasted and, if the latter, whether the wasting is bilateral or unilateral. Now ask the patient to protrude the tongue. It deviates to the paralysed side in the presence of a unilateral hypoglossal paresis and slightly to the paralysed side in some cases of hemiplegia. Next, ask the patient to move the tongue quickly from side to side. Finally, you can assess tongue power, to some extent, by asking the patient to press your fingers with the tongue by pushing against the cheek.

- When testing visual acuity, make a note of whether the patient normally wears glasses and whether he or she is using them
- When assessing eye movements, decide initially whether the problem is likely to be supranuclear or infranuclear in origin
- The jaw jerk varies considerably in normal individuals
- Some degree of facial asymmetry is commonplace in the normal population
- Minor tongue movements at rest are unlikely to be significant

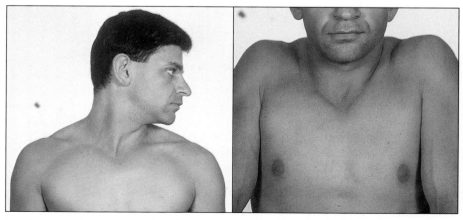

Fig. 1.22 *Testing head rotation (left) and shoulder elevation (right).*

MOTOR EXAMINATION

Inspection

Expose the relevant muscles, which may include the periscapular muscles and the glutei. Look for evidence of global or focal wasting: the former is often the consequence of cachexia and the latter frequently occurs in relation to joint injury. Formal measurement of limb diameter should be undertaken if there appears to be a discrepancy in size between the two limbs. Abnormal muscle bulk may also be pathological (**Fig. 1.23**). Look for fasciculation; the movements are erratic and therefore unpredictable. In a large muscle, the twitch-like contraction is usually obvious. In a small muscle, the movement may be very subtle. Patients should be relaxed and warm during the inspection.

Tone

Assessment of muscle tone is difficult. Most apparent hypertonia is caused by poor relaxation. Assess tone at several joints, making a comparison of flexors and extensors. A comparison of pronation and supination at the elbow is particularly valuable when looking for spasticity as is a comparison of quadriceps and hamstrings. Try the movement at differing velocities.

Definitions of muscle tone changes

Spasticity	Velocity dependent (may be absent with slow speed of displacement)
	Selective distribution (predominates in flexors of upper limbs and extensors of lower limbs and in pronators compared with supinators)
	Fades as stretch continues (clasp-knife effect)
Rigidity	Not velocity dependent
	More uniform distribution
	Activated by contraction of muscles in contralateral limb
	Uniform through range of displacement
Hypotonia	Difficult to detect. The limb is floppy and allows an excessive excursion of movement when displaced
Myotonia	Impaired relaxation of skeletal muscle after contraction. The abnormal contraction can sometimes be triggered by percussing the muscle

---

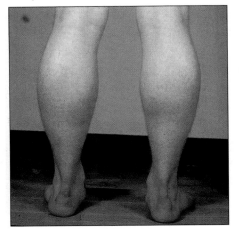

Fig. 1.23 *Pseudohypertrophy of the calf muscles.*

Power

Some weakness may be apparent during inspection, for example, a hemiplegic posture with flexion of the upper limb and extension of the lower. To go further, assess muscles using the UK Medical Research Council classification (**Fig. 1.24**). The muscles to be tested will be influenced by the patient's complaints. As a screen, assess the following: shoulder elevation, shoulder abduction, elbow flexion and extension, the first dorsal interosseous and abductor pollicis brevis. In the lower limbs, choose hip flexion and extension, knee flexion and extension and dorsiflexion and plantar flexion of the feet. You will be comparing one limb with the other, although in some cases of course, the weakness will be bilateral. Take account of sex, age, muscle development and pain when allotting grades.

Definitions of muscle power changes	
Paresis	Incomplete paralysis
Plegia	Total paralysis
Hemiplegia	Unilateral weakness of arm and leg
Monoplegia	Weakness of one limb
Paraplegia	Weakness of the lower limbs
Tetraplegia (Quadriplegia)	Weakness of all four limbs

Finally, test, if relevant, for muscle fatiguability by asking the patient to sustain contraction of the relevant muscle for 60 s before retesting.

Deep tendon reflexes

First position the patient in the supine position with the hands on the lower abdomen, the fingers extended but not touching. Each reflex is tabulated according to a recognized scale (**Fig. 1.25**).

UK Medical Research Council classification of muscle power	
Grade	Definition
0	Total paralysis
1	Flicker of contraction
2	Movement with gravity eliminated
3	Movement against gravity
4	Movement against resistance but incomplete
5	Normal power

Fig. 1.24 *UK Medical Research Council classification of muscle power.*

Grading reflexes	
Grade	Definition
0	Absent
±	Present only with reinforcement
+	Just present
++	Brisk normal
+++	Exaggerated response

Fig. 1.25 *Grading reflexes.*

The following reflexes (with their segment in brackets) are routinely tested (**Fig. 1.26**).

Biceps (C5/6) – Place the thumb or index finger on the right biceps tendon, then the thumb (with your left arm hyperpronated) on the left biceps tendon. Percuss the digit. If there is no response (and this applies when examining all the deep tendon reflexes) ask the patient to clench the teeth or grip the fingers of the arm not being tested (Jendrassik manoeuvre).

Supinator (C5/6) – Without changing the patient's position, strike the radial margin of the forearm approximately 5 cm above the wrist. If you wish, you can percuss through your index finger rather than directly. When the reflex is brisk, there may be associated flexion of the fingers. If such finger flexion occurs when the supinator reflex is depressed (and the same significance attaches to such an observation with the biceps reflex), the reflex is said to be inverted.

Triceps (C6/7) – Move first the right then the left arm across the abdomen so that the extensor aspect of the upper arm is fully exposed then strike the triceps tendon just above the elbow.

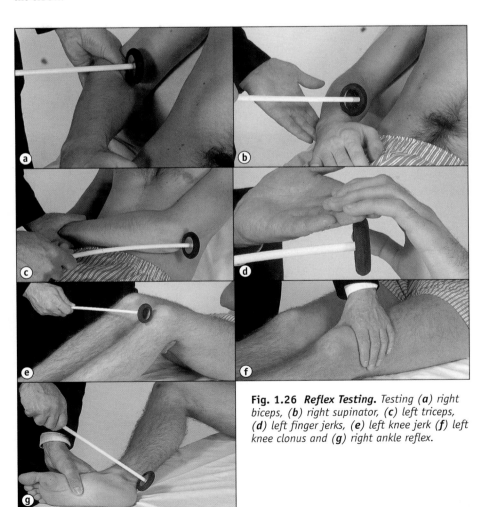

Fig. 1.26 *Reflex Testing.* *Testing (**a**) right biceps, (**b**) right supinator, (**c**) left triceps, (**d**) left finger jerks, (**e**) left knee jerk (**f**) left knee clonus and (**g**) right ankle reflex.*

Finger (C8) – This is not necessarily examined routinely. With the patient's arm pronated, exert slight pressure on the flexed fingers with the fingers of your left hand. Now strike the back of your own fingers with the hammer. A positive response leads to a brief flexion of the fingertips.

Knee (L2/3/4) – Insert your left arm underneath the patient's knees and flex them to approximately 60°, making sure that the legs are relaxed. Tap first the right patella tendon then the left. If the reflex is brisk, look for clonus by suddenly extending the patella tendon with the knee extended. Any clonus (even of two or three beats) is pathological and indicates an upper motor neuron disorder at that segmental level.

Ankle (S1) – Abduct and externally rotate the leg at the hip, then flex the knee (to approximately 60°) and the ankle (to approximately 90°). If hip abduction is limited, rest the leg on its fellow to allow access to the achilles tendon. If the reflex is brisk, look for clonus by forcibly dorsiflexing the ankle with the leg in the same position. Three to four beats of ankle clonus, providing it is symmetrical, is an acceptable finding in normal individuals.

Other reflexes

Abdominal – The abdominal responses are variable, decline with age and are liable to be depressed or absent in obese individuals or after child-bearing. The patient lies flat and must be relaxed. Draw a lollipop stick across the four segments of the abdomen around the umbilicus.

Cremasteric – Elicited by stroking the upper inner aspect of the thigh. Mediated through L1 and L2 and leads to retraction of the ipsilateral testicle.

Plantar response – The most important reflex in medicine. Elicited by applying firm pressure (with a lollipop stick) to the lateral aspect of the sole, moving from the heel towards the base of the fifth toe and then, if necessary, across the base of the toes (**Fig. 1.27**). The important movement to observe takes place at the metatarso-phalangeal joint of the big toe. Flexion indicates a normal response; extension (dorsiflexion) suggests a disorder of the upper motor neuron (positive Babinski). The movement will be absent if the toe is fused or if there is substantial loss of S1 cutaneous innervation.

Anal reflex – Assessed by pricking the skin at the anal margin. In normal individuals the anal sphincter contracts.

- Remember to look at the periscapular and gluteal muscles when assessing muscle bulk
- The most useful muscles for assessing tone in suspected spasticity are pronator teres and quadriceps
- Remember to relate patient's apparent muscle strength to his or her functional capacity
- Generally depressed reflexes with relative preservation of the ankle jerks are usually physiological

Other tests

Pronator sign – With the eyes closed, the patient holds the arms straight out with the palms upwards. A tendency for one or other arm to pronate and drift downwards is suggestive of an upper motor neuron lesion on that side.

Tinel's sign – Elicited by tapping over a peripheral nerve. If there is focal damage to the nerve at that side (e.g. entrapment or a neuroma) a shower of paraesthesiae are felt in the cutaneous distribution of the nerve.

Phalen's sign – Elicited by pressing the wrists together with the wrists fully flexed.

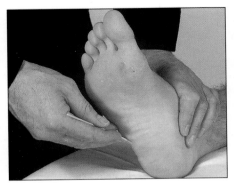

Fig. 1.27 *Testing the plantar response.*

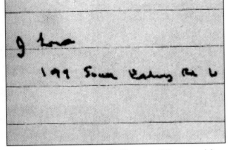

Fig. 1.28 *Parkinson's disease.* Micrographia.

Paraesthesiae appearing in the distribution of one or other median nerve suggests the diagnosis of carpal tunnel syndrome.

Neck stiffness – Elicited by flexing the patient's chin onto the sternum. Pain and resistance to flexion occurs with meningeal irritation (e.g. meningitis or subarachnoid haemorrhage) but can also be seen with cervical spondylosis and extrapyramidal conditions.

Kernig's sign – Elicited by extending the flexed knee while the hip is flexed. A positive sign (pain or resistance) occurs with meningeal irritation.

Straight-leg raising – The extended leg is flexed at the hip with the knee extended. Limitation of flexion (by pain) occurs with irritation of any of the roots contributing to the sciatic nerve (L4, L5, S1).

Femoral stretch – With the patient lying on his or her side, the leg is extended at the hip. Pain suggests irritation of any of the roots contributing to the femoral nerve (L2, L3, L4).

Lhermitte's sign – Elicited by flexing the neck. A positive sign consists of electric shock sensations in the spine, legs or (uncommonly) arms. The sensation is brief and fatigues with repetitive testing. It suggests a lesion of the dorsal columns of the cervical cord and is most commonly found in multiple sclerosis but also in cervical spondylosis, SACD, irradiation of the cord and after spinal trauma.

Movement disorders

Bradykinesia – Defined as a paucity of motor activity not attributable to muscle weakness or pain. May be in one or more limbs, in the face or in the trunk. In the face, look for facial expression, frequency of blinking and ability to express emotion. In the trunk, watch the patient's ability to get on and off a bed and the posture of the neck and trunk. In the upper limbs, test bradykinesia by asking the patient to polish, to perform the five finger exercise and to tap repetitively the index finger and thumb together. In the lower limb, ask the patient to tap repetitively your hand with his or her foot. Typically, with all these movements, the amplitude tends gradually to diminish. Recording serial specimens of writing is a particularly good way of assessing bradykinesia of the dominant hand (**Fig. 1.28**).

Involuntary movements – Begin by detailing the characteristics of the movement:

- Present at rest, with certain postures or during movement
- Frequency
- Distribution: one limb, one-half of the body or global. If in one limb, distal or proximal
- Short-lived or sufficiently sustained to produce an abnormal posture

Tremor – Rhythmic movement, usually confined to a single plane at a particular joint, can be classified as fine, moderate or coarse; resting, postural or with action; and also according to frequency.

Myoclonus – Rapid, recurring muscle jerks. Classified according to distribution. Some forms of myoclonus only appear when the limb is activated (action myoclonus).

Chorea – Brief, random movements that produce a 'fidgety' appearance. They may affect the face, lips, neck or the limbs. They can affect both distal and proximal muscles.

Athetosis – Slower than chorea. More prominent during voluntary activity and mainly distal. Often merges into or is associated with chorea (choreo-athetosis).

Hemiballismus – Violent swinging movements of one arm and the ipsilateral leg, maximal at the proximal joints. Usually caused by a lesion of the contralateral subthalamic nucleus.

Dystonia – Results in abnormal postures caused by the contraction of antagonistic muscle groups. Exacerbated by voluntary movement. May be generalized or localized.

Tics – Repetitive movements that appear, at least briefly, to be under voluntary control.

Dyskinesias – Brief, involuntary movements that often concentrate around the mouth (orofacial dyskinesias).

Myokymia – Confined to the eyelid is a normal phenomenon. More widespread facial myokymia is pathological. It produces a fine twitching motion of the face and can slightly distort the eye or angle of the mouth.

Asterixis – An abnormality of upper limb control found in certain metabolic disorders. With the arms extended and the fingers straight, a downward drift of the fingers and hands is interrupted by a sudden, upward, corrective jerk.

- Phalen's sign is more often positive than Tinel's sign in carpal tunnel syndrome
- The femoral stretch test is useful for assessing nerve root irritation at L2, L3 or L4
- Bradykinesia may be as much in evidence during everyday skilled activity as it is during formal examination
- When describing involuntary movements, note their distribution, whether they are proximal or distal and their duration

CEREBELLAR EXAMINATION

The examination of eye movements in patients suspected of having cerebellar disease is summarized on p14. Abnormal findings include hypometric or hypermetric saccades, broken pursuit movements and nystagmus and are influenced by the site of the pathology (**Fig. 1.29**).

Eye signs in cerebellar disease	
Location	**Sign**
Flocculus	Abnormal smooth pursuit gaze-evoked nystagmus
Flocculus/nodulus	Down-beat nystagmus
Vermis/fastigial nucleus	Ocular dysmetria
Lateral zones	Ocular dysmetria gaze-evoked nystagmus

Fig. 1.29 *Eye signs in cerebellar disease.*

Cerebellar dysarthria will have become evident during history taking. Speech volume and pitch are erratic with interruption of rhythm. When severe, staccato speech ensues.

LIMB EXAMINATION

Tone

The reduced limb tone in cerebellar disease is difficult to assess. If the patient holds his or her arms out with the wrists in the neutral position, the affected hand tends to sag below the horizontal.

Tremor

Rarely is a cerebellar tremor sufficiently severe to be present at rest. It may be present with a sustained posture but typically emerges during the finger–nose test. Ask the patient with first the right index finger and then the left to touch alternately his or her own nose and your outstretched index finger (**Fig. 1.30**). If the patient performs satisfactorily, move your target finger at random to increase the difficulty of the test. In cerebellar disease, the movement results in a tremor that is maximal as the target is approached. In addition, the patient's finger may overshoot (hypermetria) or undershoot (hypometria) the target. For the lower limb, ask the patient to perform the heel–knee–shin test (**Fig. 1.31**).

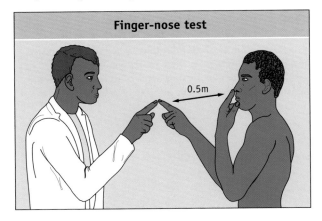

Finger-nose test

0.5m

Fig. 1.30 *The finger–nose test.*

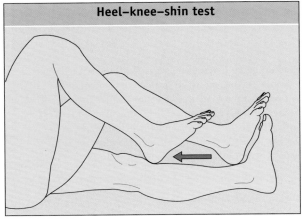

Heel–knee–shin test

Fig. 1.31 *Performing the heel–knee–shin test with the right leg.*

Posture control

In assessing upper limb cerebellar function, you can ask the patient to bring the outstretched arms rapidly upwards then stop them abruptly in the horizontal plane. In the presence of a cerebellar lesion, the affected arm fails to stop at the correct point and then oscillates about it.

Alternating movements

For the upper limb, ask the patient to tap first the dorsum then the palmar surface of one hand with the fingers of the other. In cerebellar disease, the movement breaks down, with loss of fluency and rhythm and erratic amplitude (disdiadochokinesis). For the lower limb, ask the patient to tap repetitively first with one foot and then the other. In cerebellar disease, the movement breaks down.

Gait

If truncal ataxia is severe, the patient shows truncal oscillations even when standing still. Be ready to support them. With midline cerebellar syndromes, the patient shows truncal instability when walking and uses a wide-based gait. In the presence of a unilateral cerebellar syndrome, the patient deviates to the affected side. When looking for more subtle disturbances of gait, you can get the patient to walk 'heel–toe', although performance varies widely in normal individuals.

SENSORY EXAMINATION

Much of the sensory examination depends on subjective responses by the patient. Consequently, the findings may be erratic and difficult to reproduce. The modalities tested are influenced by the nature of the patient's complaint. If there is an area of reduced cutaneous sensation, start testing within it before moving into areas of normal sensation. Certain terms used in describing sensory changes need to be accurately defined. Pinprick testing is best avoided in young children.

Definitions of sensory changes

Anaesthesia	Loss of light touch sense
Hypaesthesia	Reduction of light touch sense
Analgesia	Loss of pain sensitivity
Hypalgesia	Reduction of pain sensitivity
Hyperalgesia	Exaggerated response to pain at a normal threshold
Hyperpathia	Exaggerated response to pain with an altered threshold

---

Light touch

Use a wisp of cotton wool and avoid dragging it across the skin. With the patient's eyes closed, ask the patient to identify points of contact. Avoid testing areas of roughened skin. You may need to compare different parts of the same limb or comparable areas on the other limb, according to the problem. Sometimes it is necessary to test comparable areas on the two sides of the body simultaneously. In sensory suppression (extinction), the patient appreciates contact on either side when tested in isolation but ignores it on the side contralateral to a parietal lobe lesion when presented at the same time as a stimulus ipsilateral to the lesion.

Two-point discrimination

Using a pair of graded compasses, normal young individuals can perceive a separation of

Two-point discrimination test

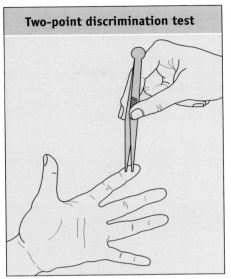

Fig. 1.32 *Testing-two point discrimination.*

Vibration sense

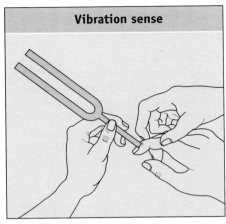

Fig. 1.33 *Testing vibration sense.*

approximately 3 mm on the finger tips, 1 cm on the palm and 3 cm on the sole of the foot (**Fig. 1.32**). The test is useful in that it provides a more objective assessment of sensory function.

Proprioception

The patient's eyes must remain closed during testing. Start at the most distal joint of the limb (an interphalangeal joint of the finger or toe). Grasp the digit or toe at the side and try to avoid moving more proximal joints. Normal individuals will correctly identify minute movements, particularly in the fingers. Record the approximate range of movement identified accurately (e.g. 10°) rather than writing JPS. Proprioception can be tested indirectly by asking the patient to maintain limb posture with the eyes closed. When proprioception is markedly impaired, the fingers move purposelessly with the eyes closed (pseudo-athetosis). Proprioception in the feet can be tested indirectly by performing Romberg's test. Loss of posture or swaying occurs when the patient stands with the feet together and closes the eyes.

Vibration sense

Tested with a 128 Hz tuning fork. The instrument can be applied either to a bony prominence or the pads of the fingers and toes. Start distally and work proximally (**Fig. 1.33**). Levels of vibration sense loss over the thorax are not assessable if the fork is applied to the ribs as the chest wall acts as a resonator. Semi-quantitative assessment can be achieved by waiting for perception of vibration to cease on one limb, then transferring the instrument to the other side.

Pain

Special sharps are provided for testing pinprick. Avoid using venepuncture needles because they are liable to puncture the skin. Dispose of the sharp after testing. Either the patient can be asked for a subjective response to the stimulus or the sharp and blunt ends of the pin can be presented at random with the patient's eyes closed. Use several stimuli at each site and avoid heavily calloused skin. For deep pain, you can either pinch the achilles tendon or squeeze a raised fold of the skin.

Temperature

Temperature sense is not tested routinely. For crude assessment of cold you can use a tuning fork. For detailed testing, tubes containing ice and hot water are used. Make sure that the hot tube is not liable to burn the skin. Rarely, either hot or cold sensitivity is selectively affected or the impairment applies to a fairly restricted range of temperature.

Weight, shape, size and texture

Certain sensory modalities are worth testing if a cortical lesion is suspected. For weight, ask the patient to compare the weight of an object first in one hand, then in the other. For shape recognition, ask the patient to name coins by manipulating them between the fingers while

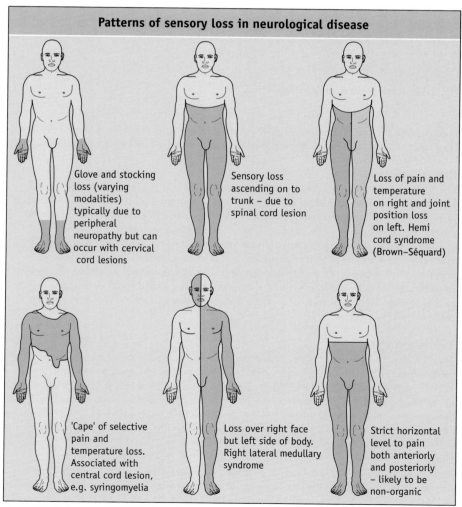

Patterns of sensory loss in neurological disease

Glove and stocking loss (varying modalities) typically due to peripheral neuropathy but can occur with cervical cord lesions

Sensory loss ascending on to trunk – due to spinal cord lesion

Loss of pain and temperature on right and joint position loss on left. Hemi cord syndrome (Brown–Séquard)

'Cape' of selective pain and temperature loss. Associated with central cord lesion, e.g. syringomyelia

Loss over right face but left side of body. Right lateral medullary syndrome

Strict horizontal level to pain both anteriorly and posteriorly – likely to be non-organic

Fig. 1.34 *Patterns of sensory loss in neurological disease.*

the eyes are closed. Remember to take account of any motor deficit in the hand and any speech difficulty. Use materials of different feel to assess appreciation of texture.

Particular findings

Certain patterns of sensory loss serve to identify the site of the underlying lesion (**Fig. 1.34**).

- Cerebellar tremor is typically absent at rest, appears during the holding of a posture but is particularly evident during a skilled movement
- Patients with a midline cerebellar syndrome will have substantial trunk and gait ataxia despite mild limb impairment
- Sensory testing requires a co-operative and alert patient
- Certain sensory modalities are particularly worth testing if a cortical lesion is suspected

THE UNCONSCIOUS PATIENT

GENERAL EXAMINATION

Before assessing the neurological system, other aspects need to be covered
- *Skin.* Evidence of injury, haemorrhage or drug abuse
- *Skeleton.* Evidence of fracture, abnormal posture or bleeding from the ear
- *Cardiovascular system.* Blood pressure, pulse, peripheral circulation, heart sounds
- *Respiratory system.* Assess the patient's respiratory rhythm and rate. Check for any fetor
- *Gastrointestinal system.* Palpate for abdominal masses
  The neurological assessment starts with documentation of the level of consciousness.

LEVEL OF CONSCIOUSNESS

Avoid terms such as stupor and coma. Record the best level of response, using the Glasgow Coma Scale (**Fig. 1.35**).

SIGNS OF MENINGEAL IRRITATION

Check for neck stiffness and a positive Kernig's sign, although with deepening levels of coma these signs disappear.

PUPILS

Assess the pupils for asymmetry or irregularity, then test the light response, using a bright pencil torch.

EYE MOVEMENTS

Note any spontaneous eye movements and whether the eyes are conjugate. Carry out the doll's head manoeuvre first in the vertical then the horizontal plane but only after ensuring there has been no neck trauma. If no movement occurs, caloric irrigation is performed with ice cold water. Into each ear in turn instil gently 50 ml, having checked that the external auditory meatus is patent and that there is no perforation of the tympanic membrane. If brainstem reflexes are intact, the eyes deviate tonically to the irrigated ear.

MOTOR RESPONSES

Assess posture and then any motor response to a noxious stimulus. First press over the sternum, then stimulate each limb in turn, squeezing the nail bed of an upper limb digit and

Glasgow Coma Scale		
	Patient's response	**Score**
Eye opening	Spontaneous	4
	To speech	3
	To pain	2
	None	1
Best verbal response	Oriented	5
	Confused	4
	Inappropriate	3
	Incomprehensible	2
	None	1
Best motor response	Obeying	6
	Localizing	5
	Withdrawing	4
	Flexing	3
	Extending	2
	None	1

Fig. 1.35 *Glasgow Coma Scale.*

the achilles tendon for upper limb and lower limb, respectively. All four limbs should be tested. The motor response may be purposive, decorticate, decerebrate or absent. In decorticate posturing, the upper limbs flex and adduct, the lower limbs extend and plantar flex. It typically occurs with an acute vascular event affecting the cerebral hemisphere or internal capsule. In decerebrate posturing, the upper limbs are extended, adducted and hyperpronated, with the lower limbs fully extended. This pattern is seen with pontine lesions but also in some forms of metabolic coma.

RESPIRATORY PATTERN

A number of differing respiratory patterns can be seen in coma. In Cheynes–Stokes respiration, the rate waxes and wanes with periods of apnoea. It is seen in metabolic coma and with deep bilateral hemisphere lesions. Central neurogenic hyperventilation occurs with lesions between the midbrain and pons. Apneustic breathing consists of recurrent episode of respiratory arrest in inspiration and is found with pontine lesions. Ataxic respiration is wholly erratic in rate and amplitude and occurs with medullary lesions.

Coma is either metabolic or structural in origin. Certain characteristics distinguish the two and are summarized in Chapter 3.

- The Glasgow Coma Scale is a useful, overall scale for quantifying a patient's conscious level
- The doll's head manoeuvre is an essential part of the assessment of brainstem function in the unconscious patient
- Motor responses seen in metabolic coma include decorticate and decerebrate posturing and hemiplegia
- Particular patterns of respiration in the unconscious patient point to the likely site of the pathological process

chapter 2

Headache and Facial Pain

Headache or facial pain is the only or predominant complaint in approximately 20% of new neurological out-patient referrals. Perhaps 60% of these patients will have either migraine or tension headache (**Fig. 2.1**). For the vast majority of these patients, a careful history taking suffices to establish the diagnosis.

MIGRAINE

Definition of migraine types

- Migraine without aura (common migraine)
- Migraine with aura (classic migraine)
- Other migrainous disorders

Distribution of the type of headache or facial pain among 1689 patients

Condition	Number of patients	Distribution (%)
Tension headache	596	35.2
Migraine	395	23.4
Headache (aetiology unknown)	267	15.8
Post-traumatic headache	117	
Facial pain (aetiology unknown)	90	
Depression	49	
Trigeminal neuralgia	58	
Migrainous neuralgia	34	2.0
Malignant tumour	29	2.8
Benign tumour	18	
Cranial arteritis	11	
Postherpetic neuralgia	9	
Benign intracranial hypertension	5	
Cough headache	7	
Subdural haematoma	2	
Sinus infection	1	
Glossopharyngeal neuralgia	1	

Fig. 2.1 *Distribution of the type of headache or facial pain among 1689 patients.*

Diagnostic criteria for migraine without aura

At least five attacks fulfilling the following criteria:
- Headache attacks lasting 4–72 h
- Headache has at least two of the
  following characteristics:
  Unilateral location
  Pulsating quality
  Moderate or severe intensity (inhibits or prohibits daily activities)
  Aggravated by walking, climbing stairs or similar routine physical activity
- During headache at least one of the following:
  Nausea or vomiting
  Photophobia and phonophobia

Fig. 2.2 *Diagnostic criteria for migraine without aura.*

Specific criteria have been established for the diagnosis of migraine with or without aura (**Fig. 2.2**).

PATHOPHYSIOLOGY

Mechanism for aura

This is probably the consequence of cortical spreading depression, perhaps, in turn, triggering alteration of blood flow in cerebral microvessels. The activation of N-methyl-D-aspartate receptors by glutamate occurs during cortical spreading depression.

Mechanism for pain

This is not clearly established and cannot be solely explained on the basis of vascular dilation. During a migraine attack, there is a fall in plasma 5-hydroxytryptamine (5-HT) levels. The trigeminovascular system (the connections of the trigeminal nerve to the cranial vessels) appears relevant. Synapses in this system are modulated by 5-HT and noradrenergic pathways. The 5-HT receptors in cerebral vessels are predominantly of the 5-HT1 type.

Activation of the system can increase cerebral blood flow, accompanied by release of vasoactive substances, including substance P and calcitonin gene-related peptide. Drugs that inhibit these changes in blood flow and peptide release are valuable in the treatment of migraine headache.

Epidemiology

- Prevalence figures vary. For a 1-year period, the figures are approximately 6% for men and 15% for women (overall 10%)
- An overall lifetime prevalence figure is 16%
- The female to male ratio is between 2:1 and 3:1 and applies whether or not there is an aura
- The most common age at onset is in the second and third decades
- Onset after 50 years is unusual
- The prevalence of migraine with aura is lower than the prevalence of migraine without aura. A 1-year prevalence figure is approximately 4%
- Migraine is possibly more prevalent in the less educated or low-income groups of the population

CLINICAL MANIFESTATION – SYMPTOMS

Symptoms of migraine without aura

- Headache
- Nausea and vomiting
- Photophobia
- Phonophobia

Additional symptoms of migraine with aura

- Visual
- Sensory
- Motor
- Speech

Migraine without aura

Headache – Most migraineurs have less than one attack each month. Perhaps one-third have more than four attacks each month. Although many attacks are brief, possibly 40% of patients describe the headache lasting beyond 24 h. Unilateral headache is more common than bilateral and the side of the headache may vary from attack to attack. The description of the headache often varies. Although sometimes throbbing or pulsating, other terms are used or the patient simply refers to the intensity of the pain, rather than its quality. Physical activity almost inevitably exacerbates the headache.

Nausea and vomiting – More than 90% of patients experience nausea and perhaps 50% experience vomiting, in at least some of the attacks.

Photophobia and phonophobia – These symptoms occur in the majority of patients who experience migraine without aura.

Diarrhoea – Approximately 10% of patients experience diarrhoea with migraine.

Migraine with aura

Comparable diagnostic criteria have been devised. A brief description is an idiopathic, recurring disorder manifesting with attacks of neurological symptoms unequivocally localizable to cerebral cortex or brainstem, usually gradually developing over 5–20 min and lasting less than 60 min. Headache, nausea and/or photophobia follow neurological aura symptoms directly or after an interval of less than 1 h. The headache usually lasts 4–72 h but may be completely absent.

Aura experiences include visual, sensory, motor, speech and other forms.

Visual – These are described as fortifications or teichopsia (seeing fortifications) (**Fig. 2.3**). They start at or near fixation and spread laterally with a binocular distribution. They are typically an uncoloured series of parallel zigzag lines and are associated with scotomatous defects.

Sensory – Most often in the ipsilateral arm and peri-oral region. Involvement of the tongue is common. The sensation typically marches from one area to the other.

Motor – Motor experiences, again, characteristically spread from area to area.

Speech – Speech problems usually manifest as dysphasia rather than dysarthria.

CLINICAL MANIFESTATIONS – SIGNS

Outside the migraine attack, physical examination is normal. Rarely, cerebral infarction occurs during the course of migraine, leading to persistent disability.

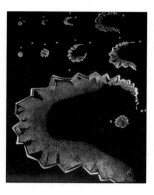

Fig. 2.3 *Typical pattern of scotoma development in migraine with aura.*

INVESTIGATION

Imaging is inappropriate in adults with an established pattern of migraine where there are no seizures and no focal signs outside an attack.

Focal slowing of the electroencephalogram has been reported during attacks of migraine with aura but the finding is of no value in terms of diagnosis or management.

An elevated protein concentration or pleocytosis has been found in the cerebrospinal fluid of some patients during attacks of hemiplegic migraine.

Studies of cerebral blood flow in attacks with aura show focal reduction of flow in the relevant arterial territory (**Fig. 2.4**).

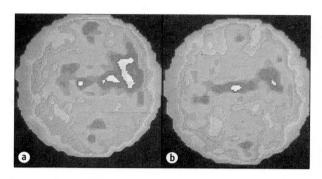

Fig. 2.4 *Positron emission tomography scan in migraine. (a) Reduced left hemisphere blood flow during attack. (b) Subsequently reverting to normal.*

MANAGEMENT

Avoiding triggers

Dietary factors operate in perhaps 10% of patients and include caffeine, chocolate, red wine, cheese, nuts and yoghurt.

Other possible triggering factors include stress, smoking, inadequate sleep and hunger.

Both deterioration and improvement have been described with the oral contraceptive or with hormone replacement therapy but most patients are unaffected. Worsening of attacks or a change in their nature should prompt withdrawal of oral contraception. Improvement may take up to 1 year to appear. It is possible that a progestrogen-only pill is less liable to induce migraine. Migraine also tends to improve during pregnancy.

Interval treatment

As an interval treatment (**Fig. 2.5**), many patients respond to aspirin, paracetamol or a combination of either with metoclopramide (which enhances analgesic absorption during a

Interval treatment for migraine	Prophylactic treatment for migraine
• Aspirin • Paracetamol • Other non-steroidal anti-inflammatory drugs • Ergotamine • Sumatriptan	• Pizotifen • β blockers • Calcium channel blockers • Amitriptyline • Methysergide • NA valproate

Fig. 2.5 *Interval treatment for migraine.*

Fig. 2.6 *Prophylactic treatment for migraine.*

migraine attack and also helps to suppress nausea).

Alternatively, another non-steroidal anti-inflammatory drug should be used. There is no firm evidence that one is innately superior to another. The drugs most often used are ibuprofen, ketoprofen, naproxen and diclofenac (these drugs are also effective prophylactic agents).

Ergotamine is effective in many patients who experience protracted aura. If the oral route is ineffective, the sublingual, inhaled or rectal routes should be tried. Side effects are common, including nausea, abdominal pain and leg cramps. The drug is contraindicated in patients with evidence of cardiovascular disease.

Sumatriptan is a specific 5-HT_1 agonist and causes vasoconstriction of the carotid arterial tree. Subcutaneous administration (in 6 mg doses) is more effective than oral (100 mg). Good control of both headache and nausea is achieved, although rebound headache within 24 h is common. Side effects include flushing, tingling, injection site reactions and tightness in the chest. Rarely, the chest pain appears to be caused by myocardial ischaemia. The drug is not given to patients with ischaemic heart disease, nor in association with ergotamine.

For nausea, if sumatriptan is not being used, helpful drugs include metoclopramide, prochlorperazine and domperidone.

Prophylactic treatment

Prophylactic treatment (**Fig. 2.6**) is considered for patients experiencing three or more disabling attacks each month. Some of the effective prophylactic agents act as 5-HT_2 receptor antagonists.

Pizotifen – This produces an improvement in 40–70% of patients at a dosage of 1.5–3mg/day. Side effects include drowsiness and weight gain.

β blockers – By blocking cranial vessel β receptors these agents inhibit vasodilation. The effective drugs are propranolol, metoprolol, timolol and atenolol. Side effects include fatigue, insomnia and vivid dreams.

Calcium channel blockers – Flunarizine, nimodipine and verapamil have all been reported to be effective.

Amitriptyline – This is an effective migraine prophylactic agent. Methysergide is also effective but induces side effects (including peripheral vasoconstriction, epigastric pain and fibrotic reactions) in approximately one-third of patients

Sodium valproate – An effective prophylactic agent but doses of up to 1.5 g/day may be needed.

There is no consensus as to how long prophylactic therapy should be maintained. If a good response is seen, cautious withdrawal of the agent after approximately 6 months is reasonable.

- Migraine without aura is more common than migraine with aura
- Investigation is not warranted in migraine patients unless there has been a change in the nature of the attacks or there are signs on neurological examination
- Simple analgesics, combined with metoclopramide, control the attacks in many patients
- Sumatriptan is the most effective agent for acute attacks
- Prophylactic therapy should be considered if there are more than three attacks each month

OTHER MIGRAINE TYPES

Ophthalmoplegic migraine

In ophthalmoplegic migraine (**Fig. 2.7**), most attacks begin before the age of 10 years.

This variant is more common in males and generally is not familial. It presents as a unilateral headache. The ophthalmoplegia follows the headache and may alternate between sides. The third nerve is usually affected with pupillary involvement, however, the sixth and fourth nerves are not immune from attacks. The oculomotor dysfunction can last for days to weeks and sometimes residual oculomotor dysfunction occurs. In older patients, the differential diagnosis includes a posterior communicating aneurysm.

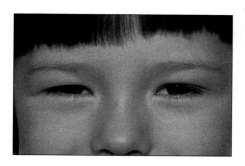

Fig. 2.7 Ophthalmoplegic migraine. *There is a right ptosis.*

Retinal migraine

This causes strictly monocular visual symptoms followed, although not inevitably, by headache.

Hemiplegic migraine

Defined as a migraine in which hemiparesis appears as an aura symptom and lasts from 1 h to 1 week. Imaging fails to reveal evidence of infarction. A familial form exists with an autosomal dominant pattern of inheritance

Menstrual migraine

If strictly defined as recurrent attacks during or shortly before menstruation, this form is relatively rare. Menstrual migraine appears related to falling levels of oestrogen and can be prevented by injections of oestradiol.

Basilar migraine

Basilar migraine tends to occur in childhood or adolescence. Accompanying features include visual disturbance, diplopia, nystagmus, ataxia and alteration of consciousness. Uncertainty exists as to the exact status of this entity and the origin of the symptoms and signs.

Migraine aura without headache

This typically produces isolated visual aura, is more common in males, may antedate or alternate with more typical attacks and becomes more common with increasing age.

TENSION HEADACHE

Definitions of tension headaches

- Episodic tension-type headache
  (muscle contraction, stress headache)
- Chronic tension-type headache
- Tension-type-like headache

Specific criteria have been established for the diagnosis of episodic and chronic tension-type headaches (**Fig. 2.8**).

Diagnostic criteria for episodic tension-type headache

At least 10 previous headache episodes fulfilling the following criteria (number of days with such headaches less than 180 each year):
- Headache lasting from 30 min to 7 days
- At least two of the following pain characteristics:
  Pressing or tightening (non-pulsating) quality
  Mild or moderate intensity
  Bilateral location
  No aggravation by walking, climbing stairs or
    similar routine physical activity
- Both of the following:
  No nausea or vomiting (anorexia may occur)
  Photophobia and phonophobia either both absent
    or only one present

Fig. 2.8 *Diagnostic criteria for episodic tension-type headache.*

PATHOPHYSIOLOGY

Chronic daily headaches sometime evolve in migraine patients and are then often linked with analgesic abuse. No firm evidence exists for abnormal scalp muscle contraction as the basis of most tension headache; indeed, some investigators believe that tension headache and migraine without aura share many biological mechanisms. In some patients, a depressive illness is responsible.

Epidemiology

- Few data are available. The condition appears to occur fairly uniformly in differing social groups
- The condition is more prevalent in women than men (1.5:1)
- Tension headache prevalence declines with age
- The commonest age at onset is during the second decade

CLINICAL MANIFESTATIONS – SYMPTOMS

Symptoms of tension headache

- A band-like, squeezing, tight or pressure sensation
- This sensation may be distributed diffusely through the scalp or concentrated in the temples and the occipital region
- There may be associated depression, anxiety or stress

Despite the frequency of the problem, most patients find that it does not interfere with their daily activities.

CLINICAL MANIFESTATIONS – SIGNS

No neurological abnormalities are found. Some patients have scalp tenderness, either diffusely or concentrated in certain areas, particularly over the temporalis and trapezius muscles.

MANAGEMENT

Treatment is often unsatisfactory. Some patients respond to simple analgesics but run the risk of analgesic abuse. Amitriptyline in low dose (10–50 mg/day) is the drug of choice. It appears to confer benefit irrespective of the presence or absence of depression. Other approaches include physiotherapy, relaxation therapy and treatment of any oromandibular joint dysfunction.

- Tension headache predominates in younger individuals
- The pathophysiological basis for the condition has not been established
- The neurological examination is normal
- Amitriptyline is the drug of choice

CLUSTER HEADACHE

Definition of cluster headache

Specific criteria have been devised for the diagnosis (**Fig. 2.9**)
Both episodic and chronic forms are recognized

Criteria for diagnosing cluster headache

At least five attacks fulfilling the following criteria:
• Severe unilateral orbital, supra-orbital and/or temporal pain lasting 15 – 180 min untreated
• Headache is associated with at least one of the following signs ipsilateral to the headache:
  Conjunctival injection
  Lacrimation
  Nasal congestion
  Rhinorrhoea
  Forehead and facial sweating
  Miosis
  Ptosis
  Eyelid oedema
• Frequency from every other day to eight each day

Fig. 2.9 *Criteria for diagnosing cluster headache.*

PATHOPHYSIOLOGY

The pain is believed to arise from retro-orbital structures, most likely the intracavernous portion of the internal carotid artery and the adjacent structures of the cavernous sinus. It has been suggested that the pathological process is vasculitic, causing interruption of venous outflow and disrupting the sympathetic fibres traversing the cavernous sinus. A variety of biochemical changes occur during the attacks, including depressed erythrocyte choline concentrations.

Epidemiology

- The condition is considerably less common than migraine, perhaps 50 times less, although not so in the author's own out-patient series
- Approximately 80% of patients are male
- A family history of the condition is rare
- Mean age of onset is in the late twenties
- Rarely, comparable cases have evolved in association with a structural brain lesion, often located around the cavernous sinus

CLINICAL MANIFESTATIONS – SYMPTOMS

Symptoms of cluster headache
• Unilateral pain • Continuous, characteristically intense • Attacks last from 15 to 180 min and usually occur once or twice a day • Alcohol can trigger the pain • Nausea may occur but vomiting is rare

The paroxysms typically occur at the same time of the day or night. The pain is always unilateral (although it may transfer sides in subsequent attacks) and is characteristically intense. It is orbital or peri-orbital but occasionally radiates ipsilaterally to the forehead, jaw or neck. The pain is not usually throbbing but more continuous.

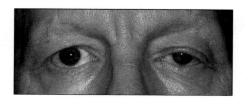

Fig. 2.10 *Horner's syndrome during an attack of cluster headache.*

CLINICAL MANIFESTATIONS – SIGNS

Various autonomic manifestations can occur during the attacks. They include the following:

- Lacrimation
- Conjunctival injection
- Rhinorrhoea or nasal obstruction
- Altered forehead sweating
- Horner's syndrome (which may persist) (**Fig. 2.10**)

Clinical course

Typically, bouts of pain last for a few weeks, then remit but return at intervals thereafter. Chronic cluster headache is defined as a headache phase persisting beyond 12 months.

MANAGEMENT

Prevention

The only preventative measures are avoidance of alcohol and any drug having a vasodilator effect.

Treatment of an attack

Ergotamine – Ergotamine can be effective by the oral, rectal or inhaled route. Cafergot® (Sandoz) suppositories are sometimes used to prevent nocturnal attacks. Careful control of intake is needed to avoid ergot intoxication.

Sumatriptan – Subcutaneous sumatriptan, in a dose of 6 mg, significantly reduces pain compared with placebo. Conjunctival injection where present is also reduced.

Oxygen – Inhalation of 100% oxygen relieves attacks within 10–15 min.

Prophylaxis

Ergotamine – This can be given on a regular basis, rather than just for individual attacks. The recommended oral dose is approximately 4 mg/day.

Lithium – Lithium has been used, mainly to treat chronic cluster headache. A dose of 900 mg/day is effective in at least 50% of patients.

Corticosteroids – These appear to be effective for the control of episodic cluster headache but are less valuable for the chronic form.

Other agents – Methysergide, pizotifen and verapamil are also used.

For patients who fail to respond to any medication, thermocoagulation of the gasserian ganglion can provide pain control.

- Cluster headache is strictly unilateral and concentrated round the eye
- Typically it is accompanied by a number of autonomic signs
- Ergotamine, oxygen and sumatriptan are effective for attacks
- Prophylactic agents used include ergotamine, lithium and corticosteroids

CHRONIC PAROXYSMAL HEMICRANIA

A rare condition, predominating in women, in which very frequent, short-lived attacks of pain occur of a type similar to cluster headache. Autonomic symptoms are common. Indomethacin, in a dose of approximately 150 mg/day, aborts the attacks within 48 h. In most patients, the attacks become chronic.

POST-TRAUMATIC HEADACHE

Post-traumatic headache usually lessens rapidly with time, although in a proportion of patients the problem persists for months or years. In some individuals, headache appears for the first time several weeks or months after the injury. There is no good correlation with the severity of the head trauma or with evidence of traumatic brain damage on imaging.

The headache is often accompanied by dizziness, altered mood and impaired concentration. Often, a similar headache occurs in individuals whose trauma did not involve the skull. The headaches are non-specific in quality. Psychological factors are considered to be important in the genesis of the problem.

Treatment is difficult and, unless there are migrainous components, is similar to that used for tension headache.

HEADACHE AS A SYMPTOM OF ORGANIC DISEASE

CEREBROVASCULAR DISEASE

Headache occurs in approximately 50% of patients with intracerebral haemorrhage and in approximately 25% of patients with cerebral infarction. If the headache is unilateral it tends to be ipsilateral to the lesion.

ARTERIAL DISSECTION

Headache is a prominent feature in carotid dissection and may be accompanied by facial or neck pain ipsilateral to the dissection. In vertebral dissection, the pain appears posteriorly or in the neck.

VASCULAR MALFORMATIONS

It remains uncertain whether there is a relationship between vascular malformation and episodic headache.

TUMOUR

Fewer than 10% of patients with brain tumour present with headache alone. Most patients with brain tumour who complain of headache do not give a history of pains with diurnal variation and associated vomiting.

SINUS DISEASE

Sinus disease of a chronic type is not a cause of headache. Acute sinusitis is readily identifiable from the presence of focal tenderness with purulent nasal discharge in the majority of patients.

NON-SPECIFIC HEADACHE

In some patients (16% in the out-patient series), the headache cannot be categorized. Patients with chronic headaches and normal neurological examination do not warrant investigation.

COUGH HEADACHE

Typically, coughing induces a severe bilateral headache usually subsiding within 60 s. The phenomenon can occur with lesions of the posterior fossa, including Chiari malformations, where it tends to follow the paroxysm of coughing after a short delay. The majority of cases are of unknown cause.

ORGASMIC HEADACHE

Typically appears at orgasm as a severe, often occipital, bilateral, throbbing pain. More common in men than women, some patients also have similar exertional headaches. A comparable headache is sometimes the consequence of subarachnoid haemorrhage.

CRANIAL ARTERITIS

Also known as temporal or giant cell arteritis.

PATHOPHYSIOLOGY

The responsible process is a granulomatous inflammation of the medium and large-sized arteries of the cranium and elsewhere. Within the cranium, the arteritis is confined to those arteries possessing an internal elastic lamina (**Fig. 2.11**).

The loss of vision is the consequence of involvement of the posterior ciliary artery leading to anterior ischaemic optic neuropathy.

Epidemiology

- The condition is rare under the age of 50 years
- The mean age at diagnosis is approximately 70 years
- The condition is slightly more common in women and almost confined to Caucasians

CLINICAL MANIFESTATIONS – SYMPTOMS

Symptoms of cranial arteritis

- Headache, usually localized
- Pain on chewing (jaw claudication)
- General malaise
- Proximal muscle stiffness and pain
- Visual loss

Headache occurs in the vast majority of patients. It particularly localizes to one or other temple but may be more generalized. It tends to be a constant, boring, intense pain, exacerbated by contact – for example, brushing the hair and also by exposure to cold. Pain on chewing occurs (jaw claudication).

Many patients feel generally unwell, with malaise, anorexia, weight loss and night sweats. Stiffness and pain in the shoulder and pelvic girdle muscles (polymyalgia rheumatica) may antedate or coincide with the headache or appear as a separate entity.

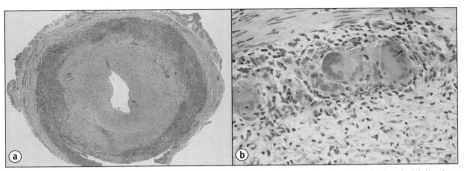

Fig. 2.11 Cranial arteritis. *Superficial temporal artery biopsy showing (a) intimal thickening and medial damage and (b) giant cells with inflammatory cell infiltration in the internal elastic lamina.*

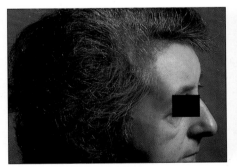

Fig. 2.12 Cranial arteritis. *Thickened superficial temporal artery.*

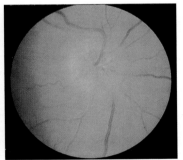

Fig. 2.13 Cranial arteritis. *Fundus photograph showing ischaemic optic neuropathy in the acute phase. Reproduced with permission from A Colour Atlas of Optic Disc Abnormalities, EE Kritzinger and HM Beaumont, Wolfe Medical Publications, London, 1987.*

Before persistent visual loss there may be amaurosis fugax. The visual loss may be altitudinal rather than total.

CLINICAL MANIFESTATIONS – SIGNS

The scalp vessels are tender and thickened. Pulsation is reduced more often than it is absent (**Fig. 2.12**). Scalp necrosis is rare. The optic disc is swollen and later pale (**Fig. 2.13**). Ophthalmoplegia is sometimes seen either as a sixth nerve or a pupil-sparing, third nerve palsy. Stroke incidence is low. Rarely, involvement of the aortic arch or of the mesenteric or limb vessels is symptomatic.

INVESTIGATION

Typically, the erythrocyte sedimentation rate is substantially elevated (over 70 mm in the first hour) but, rarely, is normal. Similarly, plasma viscosity is sometimes normal. Abnormal levels of serum alkaline phosphatase activity are found in both cranial arteritis and polymyalgia rheumatica. The pathological process is patchy. Long segment (2.5 cm) biopsies of the superficial temporal artery are taken and multiply sectioned.

MANAGEMENT

Corticosteroid therapy should be started immediately while biopsy is being arranged. There are advocates of both high-dose and low-dose regimes initially (e.g. 60 mg or 20 mg daily of prednisolone). Eventually, patients are maintained on 7.5–10 mg daily. The condition tends to resolve after 12–24 months, when treatment can be withdrawn.

- Cranial arteritis is an important condition to exclude in an elderly patient with a newly acquired headache
- The affected arteries are tender but usually still pulsatile
- The erythrocyte sedimentation rate is usually markedly elevated but rarely normal
- Corticosteroids are the drugs of choice

TRIGEMINAL NEURALGIA

Characterized by brief, intense lancinating pains, often recurring at frequent intervals and confined to one or more territories of the trigeminal nerve.

PATHOPHYSIOLOGY

The condition is usually triggered by cross-compression of the trigeminal nerve by arteries, vascular malformations or benign tumours, for example, epidermoids. Trigeminal neuralgia is also associated with intrinsic lesions of the brainstem. In some such patients, for example, individuals with multiple sclerosis, vascular cross-compression may still be the relevant pathology.

Epidemiology

- There is a female preponderance
- Mean age at onset is approximately 50 years
- Prevalence figures in women are approximately 20 per 100 000

CLINICAL MANIFESTATIONS – SYMPTOMS

Symptoms of trigeminal neuralgia

- Usually unilateral. Only 4% of patients complain of bilateral paroxysms
- The right side of the face is more often affected
- The third segment is more often affected than the second which, in turn, is more often affected than the first
- Brief paroxysms of intense, lancinating pain, seldom lasting longer than a minute are often triggered by cold, eating, speaking or touching the face (trigger zones) (**Fig. 2.14**)
- Typically, remission of pain occurs, lasting months or even years. Eventually, the pain becomes chronic

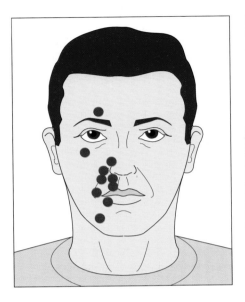

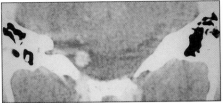

Fig. 2.14 _Trigeminal neuralgia._
Distribution of trigger zones.

Fig. 2.15 _Trigeminal neuralgia._
Postcontrast computerized tomography
showing an abnormal vascular loop in the
posterior fossa.

CLINICAL MANIFESTATIONS – SIGNS

By definition, there are no physical signs in this condition. The presence of sensory loss in the face suggests compression of the nerve by a mass lesion. In some patients, there is a concomitant hemifacial spasm (painful tic convulsif).

INVESTIGATION

Imaging is required to establish whether cross-compression of the nerve is present (**Fig. 2.15**).

MANAGEMENT

Drugs

Carbamazepine – The drug of choice. It is introduced gradually up to a maintenance dose that sometimes reaches 1.6 g/day but is more usually approximately 1 g/day. Side effects are common. Some patients tolerate the slow-release preparation better. A gradual withdrawal of medication is attempted if the patient appears to be in remission.

Phenytoin – Far less effective than carbamazepine and seldom effective if carbamazepine has failed. Doses of 300–400 mg/day are used.

Baclofen – An effective agent in doses that range from 50 to 60 mg/day. Sometimes it is worth combining the drug with carbamazepine. Side effects, including drowsiness, are again common.

Alcohol injection

The alcohol can be injected into the mandibular or maxillary divisions of the nerve or into the region of the gasserian ganglion. Many patients find the resulting facial numbness distressing and the procedure is now seldom practised.

Radio frequency gangliolysis

Often effective in controlling pain without causing a major disturbance of facial sensation. Relapses occur in some patients but can be treated by further procedures.

Microvascular decompression

Highly effective, with a low recurrence rate. The nerve is gently separated from the cross-compressing vessel, most often the superior cerebellar artery.

- Trigeminal neuralgia is a paroxysmal disorder that most commonly affects the mandibular division of the nerve
- Typically, paroxysms are induced by talking, eating or facial contact
- Carbamazepine is usually effective

GLOSSOPHARYNGEAL NEURALGIA

Consists of brief paroxysms of pain centred in the ear, throat or the base of the tongue. Typically triggered by swallowing or speaking, it is rare in comparison to trigeminal neuralgia. Occasionally, the condition is associated with cardiac complications, particularly bradycardia. Management is similar to that used for trigeminal neuralgia, although nerve section is used if the pain is intractable.

ATYPICAL FACIAL PAIN

Consists in an almost continuous unilateral facial pain sometimes extending to the neck. It is described as a deep, nagging, aching discomfort and predominates in women. Many patients are either anxious or depressed. Analgesics are of little benefit but some patients respond to tricyclic antidepressants or monoamine oxidase inhibitors.

POSTHERPETIC NEURALGIA

The first division of the trigeminal nerve is the one most commonly affected by herpes zoster. The pain is defined as persisting for more than 6 months after the original eruption. There is usually a combination of a deep gnawing pain with superimposed, more paroxysmal, sharp elements exacerbated by contact. The condition is more common in elderly people. It can be prevented, to some extent, by treating the acute phase with corticosteroids, acyclovir or amantidine. For postherpetic neuralgia, the drug of choice is amitriptyline, starting in small doses, perhaps 10 mg at night and increasing to tolerance.

TEMPOROMANDIBULAR JOINT DYSFUNCTION

Degenerative changes in the temporomandibular joint are associated with pain in the jaw, sometimes referred to the ear or temple. The pain is exacerbated by chewing. Pain in a similar distribution, without evidence of joint derangement, has been attributed to abnormal activity of the jaw muscles, either triggered by malocclusion of the jaw or the result of excessive jaw contraction in an anxious individual. Treatment is symptomatic.

chapter 3

Loss of Consciousness and Coma

EPILEPSY

Epilepsy is the consequence of focal or generalized epileptogenic discharges in the brain. Classification is based on a schema proposed by the International League Against Epilepsy and is summarized, in a simplified form, in **Figure 3.1**. The relative frequency of these seizure types is summarized in **Figure 3.2**.

A refinement of this classification has been produced, listing a number of closely defined epileptic syndromes, together with some less specific categories into which, theoretically, all generalized and partial epilepsies should fit. When such a classification is applied to patients seen in general practice, however, only one-third can be allotted into a particular category.

Fig. 3.1 *The International League Against Epilepsy scheme for the classification of epilepsy.*

Classification of Epilepsy

Partial (focal seizures)

A. Simple partial (consciousness preserved)
   1. Motor symptoms
   2. Somatosensory or special sensory symptoms
   3. Autonomic
   4. Psychic
   5. Mixed forms

B. Complex partial (consciousness impaired)
   1. Motor symptoms
   2. Somatosensory or special sensory symptoms
   3. Autonomic
   4. Psychic
   5. Mixed forms
   6. Impaired consciousness alone

C. Partial seizures with secondary generalization

Generalized seizures
   1. Absence attacks (petit mal)
   2. Myoclonic
   3. Clonic
   4. Tonic
   5. Tonic–clonic (grand mal)
   6. Atonic

Unclassified

Frequency of different epileptic types	
Complex partial and secondarily generalized	60 per cent
Primary generalized tonic–clonic	30 per cent
Absence and myoclonic forms	<5 per cent

Fig. 3.2 *Frequency of different epileptic types.*

Epilepsy can also be classified into symptomatic and idiopathic forms, the former the consequence of a defined structural or metabolic disorder, the latter being of unknown origin. The borderlands are, however, indistinct as evolving techniques of investigation may lead to reclassification of idiopathic into symptomatic seizures. Approximately two-thirds of all epilepsies have no defined cause. Symptomatic forms, in one study, included cerebrovascular disease (15%), tumour (6%), alcohol-related epilepsy (6%) and trauma (2%).

Genetic factors are important in epilepsy. A high degree of concordance is found for epilepsy in identical twins and the incidence of epilepsy in near relatives of a patient with the condition is substantially higher than in a control population. Inherited forms are estimated to account for at least 20% of all epilepsies.

Certain generalizations about the cause of epilepsy can be made according to the age of onset and the nature of the seizures.

- Any individual is capable of developing seizures if exposed to a sufficiently severe metabolic or structural insult
- Genetic factors in epilepsy are most relevant for patients presenting before the age of 20 years
- The likelihood of finding a structural lesion as the basis for the epilepsy is negligible for absence seizures but highly likely for patients with complex partial seizures

PATHOLOGY AND PATHOPHYSIOLOGY

The pathological and pathophysiological mechanisms of epilepsy differ according to the type of seizure.

Generalized (absence) seizures

Absence attacks are associated with a reverberating electrical discharge within the thalamus and cortex manifesting as 3–3.5 Hz spike and wave discharges on the electroencephalogram (EEG).

Complex partial seizures

These seizures usually originate in the mesial temporal lobe. Spread into adjacent structures, for example, the amygdala or the hippocampus, is associated with differing patterns of symptoms.

Focal motor seizures

Typically, these seizures originate in the primary motor cortex but may also begin in the supplementary motor area. Secondary generalization is likely to involve brainstem structures.

The proposed pathophysiological mechanisms contributing to an epileptic discharge include a membrane defect leading to an instability of the resting potential, abnormalities of potassium conductance or calcium channels, defects of the γ aminobutyric acid inhibitory system or an abnormality in excitatory neurotransmission.

Experimental animal studies suggest that a deficiency of γ aminobutyric acid-mediated neurotransmission could be relevant in the genesis of generalized seizures and that enhancement of excitatory amino acid receptor function, particularly of the N-methyl-D-aspartate type, occurs in human epileptogenic brain tissue.

Epidemiology

- Incidence rates lie between 20 and 70 per 100 000 of the population each year
- Point prevalence rates lie between four and 10 per 1000
- There is a slight male predominance
- Probably 70% of patients with epilepsy go into remission, either with or without treatment
- About one-half of the patients who go into remission do so within a year of diagnosis
- Perhaps three-quarters of patients with a single seizure develop further seizures (i.e. develop epilepsy)
- Poor prognosis, in terms of seizure recurrence, correlates with evidence of an underlying cerebral disorder, early onset and certain severe epileptic syndromes (e.g. Lennox–Gestaut syndrome)

- A simplified system of epilepsy classification distinguishes generalized, focal and focal with secondary generalization forms
- The chances of finding a structural basis for a patient's epilepsy are influenced both by the type of epilepsy and by the age of onset
- Perhaps three-quarters of patients who have had a single seizure progress to develop epilepsy

CLINICAL MANIFESTATIONS

Tonic–clonic seizures

Loss of consciousness occurs without warning. In the initial, tonic phase, respiration ceases and the patient becomes cyanosed. Within a few seconds the clonic phase supervenes with rhythmic jerking of all four limbs, seldom lasting more than a few minutes. Tongue biting sometimes occurs, typically along the lateral margin. There may be incontinence. The patient is then liable to enter a deep sleep. Headache is common after the attacks, as is diffuse bodily aching and stiffness. A brief warning (aura) or unilateral movement during the attack or unilateral signs after it indicate a focal origin.

Myoclonic epilepsy

Describes brief shock-like contractions of the limbs, usually the arms, sometimes culminating in a generalized seizure. They tend to occur in children and young adults. Juvenile myoclonic epilepsy starts around puberty. The condition is idiopathic and strongly genetic. In addition to myoclonus and tonic–clonic seizures (both usually in the mornings) there may be absences. Sleep deprivation and alcohol are potent triggering factors.

Absences (petit mal)

These are virtually confined to childhood, most beginning before the age of 10 years. It is uncommon for them to persist into adult life. Brief absences occur without loss of posture. The child is unaware of them. Long absences may be accompanied by automatisms, for example, lip smacking, chewing or fumbling hand movements. Approximately 50% of children with absence attacks develop tonic–clonic seizures in adult life.

Frontal lobe epilepsy

Features of frontal lobe seizures are those of simple or complex partial seizures, with or without secondary generalization. There are often adversive movements of the head and prominent lower limb motor activity. The attacks are often brief, frequently recurring but associated with little post-ictal confusion.

Focal motor seizures

Focal motor seizures usually begin at the corner of the mouth, in the thumb or in the foot, spreading to the rest of the limb or the whole half of the body. Secondary generalization may occur. After a focal motor seizure, limb weakness is usual, lasting from 24 to 48 h (Todd's paralysis). Seizures of this type are associated with lesions of the contralateral motor cortex. A sensory equivalent, with a similar spread of symptoms, is rare.

Benign rolandic epilepsy

Begins between the ages of 3 and 13 years. It produces simple partial seizures (typically with sensory and motor symptoms originating in the throat) often with secondary generalization. The attacks are usually nocturnal. EEG shows a centrotemporal spike focus but despite this, the condition is idiopathic with a strong genetic component.

Complex and simple partial seizures (temporal lobe epilepsy)

Assessment of the patient's awareness in these attacks is often difficult. Typically, patients describe altered tastes or smells, with epigastric sensations rising into the throat. According to the spread of the discharge there may be auditory or visual hallucinations, vertigo or dizziness and a variety of psychic symptoms including a sense of intense reality (*déjà vu*) or unreality (*jamais vu*) or feelings of intense fear or pleasure. Speech output becomes dysphasic if the dominant hemisphere is affected. Lip smacking is seen, along with purposeless movements of the limbs. After attacks, patients may carry out semi-automatic activities of which they are unaware.

> **Symptoms of complex partial seizures**
> - Altered taste or smell
> - Epigastric sensations radiating to the throat
> - Auditory or visual hallucinations
> - Vertigo
> - Intense familiarity (*déjà vu*) or unreality (*jamais vu*)

Other forms of epilepsy

Atonic (astatic) seizures – These occur in infants and children. Sudden loss of muscle tone leads to falls and consequent head injury.

Occipital epilepsy – Occipital epilepsy produces elementary visual hallucinations or loss of vision, sometimes with sensations of eyelid or eye movement or head or eye deviation. Spread to the temporal lobe can lead to altered awareness or automatisms.

INVESTIGATIONS

Seizures are commonplace in patients with metabolic disorders but only rarely are they the presenting feature of such disorders. Factors liable to trigger seizures include uraemia, hepatic failure, hypocalcaemia, hypercalcaemia, hypomagnesemia and hypoglycaemia.

Serological tests for syphilis are often performed in newly diagnosed patients with epilepsy. Certain blood and cerebrospinal fluid changes may follow generalized seizures.

Blood changes include rises in creatine kinase and prolactin concentrations; cerebrospinal fluid changes include an elevated protein concentration and (after prolonged seizures) a pleocytosis.

Electroencephalogram

In one large series of patients with epilepsy (excluding symptomatic patients), the EEG was abnormal or borderline in 56%. The yield of abnormal recordings is dependent on the type of epilepsy and whether any activation procedure has been used.

Abnormal recordings are virtually inevitable in absence seizures, consisting of generalized paroxysms of 3–3.5 Hz spike and wave discharges. Abnormal routine EEGs have been reported in up to 90% of patients with complex partial seizures (**Fig. 3.3**).

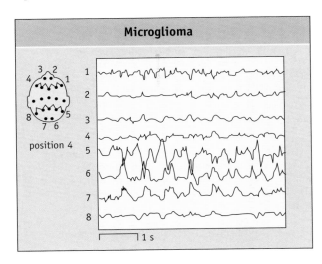

Fig. 3.3
Electroencephalogram showing right posterior temporal sharp activity in a patient with a microglioma.

The yield increases with sleep recordings or with metrazol activation. Nasopharyngeal electrodes are more likely than sphenoidal electrodes to add further information.

Prolonged EEG monitoring with video analysis is of value when uncertainty remains about the nature of the attacks. If, however, these occur at monthly intervals or less, ambulatory recordings add nothing to routine studies.

Depth electrodes are positioned stereotactically at sites determined clinically and by surface EEG criteria. When a localized focus on scalp EEG cannot be confirmed by depth studies, the outcome from surgery is poor. If surgery is confined to individuals whose depth recordings confirm the surface study, then outcome is improved.

Magnetoencephalography

Magnetoencephalography attempts to localize focal epileptic discharges by measuring the changes in the extracranial magnetic fields that the discharges generate. There is, in general, a good correlation between foci identified by magnetoencephalography and those discovered with depth electrodes (**Fig. 3.4**).

Computerized tomography

Opinions vary as to which patients with seizures should be scanned. There is no logic in scanning patients with absence seizures but scanning is mandatory in adults with focal seizures. For patients with a single, generalized, seizure and a normal neurological

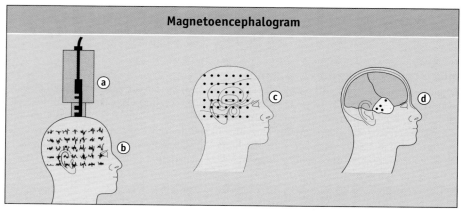

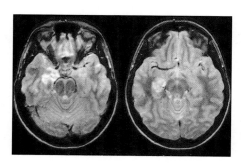

Fig. 3.4 *Magnetoencephalogram.* *The magnetometer (**a**) is positioned close to the head. In this patient, magnetic spikes were measured at more than 20 sites (**b**). An isofield contour map can then be derived (**c**) producing evidence of four different spike types in the temporal tip (**d**)*

Fig. 3.5 *Magentic resonance imaging* *showing an abnormal signal area (probably a dysembryoplastic neuroepithelial tumour) in the left mesial temporal region in a patient with epilepsy.*

examination, computerized tomography is probably only relevant for individuals above 30 years of age. Perhaps one-half of the adults with a single seizure have abnormal computerized tomography scans but many of these patients have atrophy alone. Focal seizures may reflect a metabolic insult rather than a structural process. Onset of refractory partial seizures after the age of 30 years is very often due to an underlying neoplasm.

Magnetic resonance imaging

Magnetic resonance imaging is of much greater value than computerized tomography in identifying pathological changes, particularly in patients with intractable focal seizures (Fig. 3.5). Volumetric analysis of the amygdala, hippocampus and anterior temporal lobe correlates well (in terms of unilateral atrophy) with EEG lateralization.

Positron emission tomography

Hypometabolism in the relevant temporal lobe has been found by positron emission tomography studies in 60–90% of patients with intractable complex partial seizures.

- Aura before a generalized seizure or focal signs after it imply a lateralized focus for the attack
- Psychic symptoms can be prominent in complex partial seizures and may obscure the diagnosis
- Magnetic resonance imaging is the imaging technique of choice for patients with epilepsy and is particularly valuable for patients with intractable focal seizures

TREATMENT

- Single seizures are usually not treated, although perhaps three-quarters of patients with a single generalized seizure will progress to epilepsy
- Absence seizures are treated with sodium valproate or ethosuximide
- First-line drugs for the focal epilepsies (and for tonic–clonic seizures) are sodium valproate, carbamazepine, phenytoin, phenobarbitone, primidone and lamotrigine (**Fig. 3.6**)

Fig. 3.6 *Drugs used for focal and tonic–clonic seizures.*

Drugs used for focal and tonic-clonic seizures		
Drug	**Dosage range (mg/day)**	**Therapeutic level (μ/ml)**
Phenobarbitone	30–200	20–40
Primidone	250–1500	20–40
Phenytoin	150–500	10–20
Carbamazepine	300–1600	5–10
Sodium valproate	600–2400	?80–150
Ethosuximide	500–1500	40–120
Clonazepam	1–8	(not established)

- Slow-release preparations allow carbamazepine and sodium valproate to be given twice daily
- Phenobarbitone, phenytoin and lamotrigine can be given once daily
- Side effects common to almost all these drugs include drowsiness, altered concentration and ataxia in high doses. Many of the drugs induce liver microsomal enzymes, with enhanced metabolism of folate and vitamin D
- Side effects associated more specifically with the drugs include

Phenobarbitone	Irritability in children
Primidone	Severe sedation
Phenytoin	Gum hypertrophy (**Fig. 3.7**)
Carbamazepine	Rash. Rarely, bone marrow depression
Sodium valproate	Transient hair loss, tremor, weight gain
Clonazepam	Severe sedation

A number of new drugs have been licensed as add-on therapy, particularly for patients with complex partial seizures.

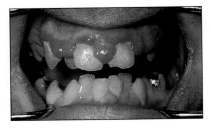

Fig. 3.7 *Gum hypertrophy secondary to phenytoin therapy.*

Gabapentin – Dosage 900–2400 mg/day. Generally well tolerated and does not interact with other drugs.

Vigabatrin – Dosage 1–3 g/day. Can be sedative and associated with behavioural changes in some patients and with visual disturbances.

Topiramate – Dosage 200–600 mg/day. Can cause sedation and renal stones.

Particular issues about therapy

Any drug should be introduced gradually and the dose then increased according to need. If the patient is intolerant of or fails to respond to the first drug, it should be withdrawn while the second drug is introduced. Polypharmacy is best avoided.

Many of the anticonvulsants (not gabapentin, valproate, lamotrigine or vigabatrin) lessen the efficacy of the combined oral contraceptive pill. A high-oestrogen content pill is then needed.

Clonazepam is principally used in the treatment of myoclonic epilepsy. Clobazam is useful for patients with catamenial (menstrual) epilepsy.

Checking of drug levels in the blood is performed far too often. Phenytoin levels rise exponentially with dosage and regular checking of blood levels is sensible. For drugs such as carbamazepine and phenobarbitone, levels are generally predictable from the dosage. Levels are useful in checking patients' compliance.

If patients become fit-free, withdrawal of anticonvulsants (which should be gradual) can be attempted after approximately 2–3 years. (Absence seizures tend to cease spontaneously after approximately the age of 15 years.) Perhaps 30% of patients will have a recurrence on drug withdrawal in these circumstances. Recurrence is most likely during the withdrawal period or the first 6 months thereafter. The role of an abnormal EEG in predicting recurrence is uncertain. Relapse is more likely if the epilepsy has been protracted or the seizures have been frequent before remission.

- Slow-release preparations of carbamazepine and sodium valproate improve compliance
- Phenobarbitone, phenytoin and lamotrigine can be given once daily
- Some of the anticonvulsants diminish the effectiveness of the oral contraceptive
- Withdrawal of anticonvulsants should be carried out slowly

PARTICULAR ISSUES

The role of surgery

Surgical procedures to control epilepsy aim either to remove the epileptogenic focus directly or to inhibit the spread of the discharge by interrupting relevant fibre pathways. Approximately 80% of all surgical resections involve part of the temporal or the frontal lobe. Investigators suggest that approximately two-thirds of the patients having temporal lobe resections became fit-free. Patients with mesial temporal lobe epilepsy, associated with hippocampal sclerosis, achieve a 70% remission with mesial temporal resection. Corpus callosum transection has been used in children with atonic and tonic–clonic seizures.

Epilepsy in pregnancy

Epilepsy sometimes worsens during pregnancy. Anticonvulsant levels tend to fall because of enhanced hepatic metabolism. Congenital malformations occur in approximately 6% of pregnancies in patients with epilepsy compared with 2–3% in the normal population. The features vary according to the drug:

- Phenytoin   Cleft palate, hare lip, digital abnormalities. Rarely, congenital heart disease
- Valproate   Neural tube defects
- Phenobarbitone and primidone   Cleft palate, hare lip and cardiac abnormalities
- Carbamazapine   Craniofacial defects, neural tube defects

The effect is usually established by the end of the first trimester. For detection of neural tube defects, maternal α foetoprotein is measured and ultrasound performed at the beginning of the second trimester. Lamotrigine and gabapentin are said not to be teratogenic.

Breast feeding

There is insufficient secretion in breast milk in the vast majority of patients to cause any symptoms in the infant.

Driving

The law regarding driving has been recently changed in the UK, largely with the hope of improving compliance. Patients with one or more daytime seizures, of any type, are requested to surrender their licence to the Driving Vehicle Licensing Authority until one year without seizures has elapsed. Patients with nocturnal seizures alone who have established that pattern for 3 years can then drive even if the nocturnal seizures persist. The Driving Vehicle Licensing Authority prefers patients not to drive during periods of drug withdrawal.

Pseudo-seizures

It has been estimated that up to 20% of patients referred to specialist centres because of intractable epilepsy have non-epileptic attacks. Seizures and pseudo-seizures often co-exist. Typically, patients with pseudo-seizures have their attacks only when onlookers are present. The movements are often violent and attempts to restrain the limbs or open the eyes are resisted. Incontinence is unusual and tongue biting decidedly uncommon. Self-injury, however, is encountered. The EEG can seldom be recorded or interpreted during an attack in which there are conspicuous movements but typically it reverts to normal soon after a pseudo-seizure. Prolactin levels rise conspicuously after tonic–clonic seizures, and so a normal value 20 min after an apparent tonic–clonic seizure suggests it was non-epileptic. Management of pseudo-seizures is fraught with difficulty and often unsuccessful.

Status epilepticus

> **Definition of status epilepticus**
>
> Recurrent seizures without recovery of consciousness in-between, or a single seizure lasting more than 30 min.

Seizures can occur in the form of tonic–clonic status, absence status or partial status (epilepsia partialis continuans). Status epilepticus may be the first manifestation of epilepsy or may occur in known individuals with epilepsy who have stopped their drugs or abused alcohol. Immediate protection of the patient's airway is essential together with intravenous access. A full biochemical screen is initiated and O_2 administered.

The immediate drug of choice is intravenous diazepam (10 mg injected rapidly), although some advocate intravenous lorazepam because of its longer action. If the patient is already on an anticonvulsant then that should be commenced. Both phenytoin and sodium valproate can be given intravenously (the former over 30 min, the latter as an infusion), pending the patient being able to take oral medication. Alternative drugs to consider for resistant status include intravenous chlormethiazole or an infusion of diluted paraldehyde. Respiratory depression is a recognized hazard of these regimes. Rarely, the patient has to be anaesthetized with thiopentone, paralysed and ventilated.

The stigma of epilepsy

Patients still encounter prejudice from friends, relatives and employers. The British Epilepsy Association provides valuable support and educational material.

- Patients whose epilepsy is secondary to mesial temporal sclerosis achieve a 70% remission with mesial temporal resection
- Congenital malformations are approximately twice as common in the offspring of mothers who have taken anticonvulsants in pregnancy compared with control individuals
- Pseudo-seizures and epilepsy often coincide

VASO-VAGAL ATTACKS

During simple faints, peripheral pooling of blood, secondary to dilatation of muscle arteries, coincides with bradycardia and a consequent reduction of cardiac output.

The phenomenon predominates in young females. The onset is most common during the second decade of life. Typical features include:

- Prodromal nausea, sweating and malaise, associated with pallor
- Onset of attacks while standing, typically in hot, enclosed environments, when witnessing unpleasant events or when undergoing venepuncture
- A gradual loss of posture with less likelihood of injury than occurs with epilepsy
- Rapid recovery of consciousness if the patient is recumbent

Symptoms of vaso-vagal attacks

- Prodromal nausea, sweating and malaise
- Gradual as opposed to abrupt loss of posture
- Rapid recovery

Less commonly, the patient may have a brief tonic contraction of the limbs or, rarely, a few clonic jerks. If the sufferer is kept upright, a typical tonic–clonic seizure may ensue. Urinary incontinence is unusual. Tongue biting does not occur. The patient should be advised to sit or lie down when warning symptoms appear. Attacks seldom persist beyond the age of 30 years.

MICTURITION SYNCOPE

This condition predominates in men of any age. Typically, attacks occur at night, often after an evening of alcohol ingestion. The attacks are probably the result of a vaso-depressor reflex triggered by a sudden reduction in bladder pressure. Attacks can be avoided by micturating in the sitting position.

COUGH SYNCOPE

This is rare. Paroxysmal coughing results in a modified Valsalva manoeuvre with faintness or brief loss of consciousness. The condition is prevented by dealing with the underlying respiratory disorder.

CARDIAC SYNCOPE

A cardiac disorder is a relatively common cause of faintness in older people. Abnormalities underlying such attacks include complete heart block and the sick sinus syndrome. In other individuals, drug-induced postural hypotension is responsible, caused, for example, by a diuretic, a tricyclic antidepressant or a phenothiazine. Many patients with cardiac syncope have a history of palpitations in association with their attacks or have an abnormal pulse on examination. The diagnosis is established if typical attacks occur during periods of arrhythmia recorded by 24 h electrocardiogram monitoring.

CAROTID SINUS SYNCOPE

Patients with this condition usually present either with vertigo or with syncopal attacks. The syncopal episodes are preceded by faintness and often coincide with pallor followed by flushing. They are sometimes triggered by neck rotation or pressure.

In most patients, the attacks are caused by asystole or atrioventricular block. In a small proportion, a pure vasodilator reaction occurs. In the former types, denervation of the relevant carotid sinus is curative; in the latter, some form of atrioventricular pacing is required.

DROP ATTACKS

Drop attacks mainly occur in older women. The patient falls forward, without warning, often injuring the knees or face. Any loss of consciousness is brief. In most patients, the cause is unknown and is not a manifestation of hindbrain ischaemia. There is no treatment.

NARCOLEPSY

In Europe and the USA, the prevalence of narcolepsy lies between 1 per 1000 and 1 per 10 000. The sexes are affected equally. The condition usually begins between the ages of 15 and 35 years. The cardinal features of the narcolepsy syndrome comprise narcolepsy, cataplexy, sleep paralysis and hypnagogic hallucinations.

Narcolepsy results in excessive sleepiness associated with brief periods of daytime sleep. Cataplexy produces brief periods of muscle weakness, sparing the muscles of respiration, typically triggered by emotion or sudden excitement. Laughter is the commonest precipitant. In sleep paralysis, brief periods of paralysis occur at the time of going to sleep or on awakening. The attacks can last as long as 10 min. Hypnagogic hallucinations are intense hallucinatory experiences that arise as the individual is about to sleep and occur in approximately 60% of patients with narcolepsy.

The condition has a strong familial component and approximately 98% of patients possess the histocompatibility antigens DR2 and DQwl. The inheritance is probably dominant with incomplete penetrance. EEG shows rapid eye movement sleep within 10 min of sleep onset. A routine EEG is insufficient for diagnosis because rapid eye movement sleep is recorded in less than one-half of the patients. Treatment generally uses either methylphenidate or dexamphetamine. Selegiline is a possible alternative. Tricyclic antidepressants are the treatment of choice for cataplexy and sleep paralysis.

OBSTRUCTIVE SLEEP APNOEA

Obstructive sleep apnoea affects approximately 2–4% of middle-aged men and approximately 1–2% of middle-aged women. It leads to increased daytime drowsiness and carries an increased risk of various cardiovascular complications. The vast majority of apnoeas are caused by collapse of the pharyngeal airway. Almost all sufferers are habitual snorers. An apnoea is defined as one in which breathing has ceased for over 10 s. In obstructive apnoea, continued respiratory effort occurs during the period of absent airflow. In central sleep apnoea, respiratory effort ceases along with the cessation of airflow. Additional clinical features include excessive daytime drowsiness, disturbed sleep and secondary polycythaemia.

Definition of obstructive sleep apnoea

- Occurrence of at least 15 apnoeas or hypopnoeas per hour of sleep.
- Two or more of the following: excessive daytime sleepiness, loud snoring, disturbed sleep and 2° polycythaemia or ankle swelling of unknown cause.

Various anatomical factors predispose to the condition, including obesity, narrowed airways, enlarged tongue and a greater tendency for airway collapse.

The diagnosis is best established by performing overnight studies in a sleep laboratory. As a screening test, overnight oximetry has been used. If the percentage of sleep time during which the oxygen saturation is less than 90% is under 1%, then sleep apnoea is effectively excluded.

Treatment includes weight control, avoidance of alcohol and nasal continuous positive airway pressure. The treatment has to continue long term and only approximately two-thirds of patients remain compliant. In some patients, surgical techniques, including tonsillectomy, adenoidectomy and uvulopalatopharyngoplasty are employed. Most recently, a combined mandibular and maxillary osteotomy has been proposed as treatment.

- Simple faints can lead to a generalized seizure if the patient is kept upright
- Cardiac syncope should be considered as a possible mechanism for 'funny turns' occurring in older individuals
- Narcolepsy is very strongly linked with certain HLA determinants
- Obstructive sleep apnoea is said to affect approximately 2% of the population

---

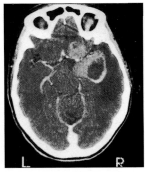

Fig. 3.8 *Computerized tomography scan showing herniation of a right temporal mass with distortion of the upper brainstem.*

Glasgow Coma Scale		
	Patient's response	**Score**
Eye opening	Spontaneous	4
	To speech	3
	To pain	2
	None	1
Best verbal response	Oriented	5
	Confused	4
	Inappropriate	3
	Incomprehensible	2
	None	1
Best motor response	Obeying	6
	Localizing	5
	Withdrawing	4
	Flexing	3
	Extending	2
	None	1

Fig. 3.9 *Glasgow Coma Scale.*

COMA

Coma due to structural disease is the consequence either of extensive bilateral hemispheric disease, a unilateral hemisphere mass lesion causing shift or a more discrete pathology confined to certain parts of the brainstem. Mass lesions in one hemisphere affect the conscious level by causing downward herniation of brain tissue through the tentorial notch, with secondary compression of the brainstem (**Fig. 3.8**). A vast array of metabolic disorders and many drugs are capable of altering the conscious level. Coma assessment is performed using a semi-quantitative scale that allows early identification of improvement or deterioration in the patient's status (**Fig. 3.9**).

STRUCTURAL CAUSES OF COMA
Supratentorial lesions causing coma do so through producing either central or uncal herniation of brain tissue. The features are summarized in **Figure 3.10**.

METABOLIC CAUSES OF COMA
Certain features help to distinguish metabolic from structural coma, whereas other features are shared.
- The pupils remain reactive until the late stages
- The eyes remain central, although reflex movements may eventually be lost
- The visual axes usually remain parallel
- Hemiplegia, as well as decorticate and decerebrate posturing, are encountered
- Either generalized or focal seizures may occur
- Myoclonic jerks occur in uraemia and in hypercapnoea
- Asterixis (a flapping hand tremor observed in the phase before coma) occurs in both renal and liver failure

Features of uncal and central herniation		
	Uncal	**Central**
Early	Dilatation of pupil of ipsilateral eye	Impairment of reflex upward gaze
	Contralateral hemiplegia. May be ipsilateral hemiplegia due to compression of contralateral cerebral peduncle against the tentorial notch	Contralateral hemiplegia Cheyne–Stokes respiration
Late	Loss of reflex movements in contralateral eye	Increasing loss of reflex horizontal eye movements
	Bilateral decerebrate posturing	Decorticate then decerebrate posturing of the unaffected limb
	Central neurogenic hyperventilation	Central neurogenic hyperventilation

Fig. 3.10 *Features of uncal and central herniation.*

HEPATIC ENCEPHALOPATHY

Usually appears in patients with chronic liver disease with portal hypertension. The encephalopathy is episodic, with ataxia, tremor, asterixis and confusion. Extensor plantar responses are seen and, rarely, a spinal cord syndrome occurs in association with portal hypertension. The EEG shows an evolving pattern culminating in diffuse bilateral delta activity. Treatment combines lactulose with institution of a low-protein or protein-free diet.

URAEMIC ENCEPHALOPATHY

There are no specific features of uraemic encephalopathy, although myoclonus is more common than in other metabolic encephalopathies. Seizures occur in up to one-third of patients. Treatment is by haemodialysis.

HYPOGLYCAEMIC ENCEPHALOPATHY

Most commonly occurs with insulin therapy but can occur in patients on oral therapy.

An acutely evolving hypoglycaemia results in hunger, agitation, sweating and malaise. Progression to coma and seizures can lead to irreversible impairment of brain function. Focal neurological deficit, for example, hemiplegia, can be a manifestation of hypoglycaemia.

Neurological symptoms are the usual presenting features of an insulinoma. Many patients develop symptoms after an overnight fast, the consequent hypoglycaemia being accompanied by inappropriately high insulin levels. The tumour is best localized by coeliac axis angiography. Distal pancreatectomy is performed if the tumour is in the tail of the gland (**Fig. 3.11**).

POSTANOXIC ENCEPHALOPATHY

Most cases of anoxic encephalopathy are triggered by cardiopulmonary arrest. Survival correlates with the duration of coma. If pupillary light responses or corneal responses are absent at 6 h after the arrest, there is little prospect for survival. Patients with a good prognosis have pupillary responses and spontaneous eye movements at the first examination, withdraw from pain at 24 h and obey commands within a week.

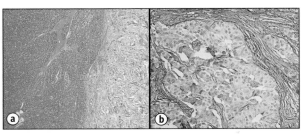

Fig. 3.11 *Insulinoma.* (a) *Haematoxylin and eosin.*
(b) *Reticulin stain.*

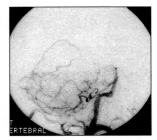

Fig. 3.12 *Basilar occlusion consequent to a left vertebral dissection.*

HYPERCALCAEMIC AND HYPOCALCAEMIC COMA

Coma can occur with either hypercalcaemia or hypocalcaemia. In hypocalcaemia, additional features include paraesthesiae, tetany and seizures. Chronic hypocalcaemia is associated with raised intracranial pressure, extrapyramidal manifestations and cataracts.

THE LOCKED-IN SYNDROME

Locked-in patients are alert and aware of their environment. They are tetraplegic because of an ischaemia affecting descending corticospinal and corticobulbar pathways in the ventral pons. Communication is achieved by vertical eye movements. Vertebral dissection is one of the causes of the condition. A similar state can be seen with other pathological processes (**Fig. 3.12**).

VEGETATIVE STATE

Definition of vegetative state

A clinical condition of unawareness of self and the environment in which the patient breathes spontaneously, has a stable circulation and shows cycles of eye closure and eye opening which may simulate sleep and waking.

The term continuing vegetative stage is applied to patients with coma persistence beyond 4 weeks and permanent vegetative state to patients for whom irreversibility can be confidently established. Patients in the vegetative state have no purposeful motor movement. Irreversibility is considered likely if the state has persisted for more than 12 months after a head injury or for more than 6 months after some other form of brain insult.

BRAINSTEM DEATH

The end point of many structural and metabolic insults to the brain is a state in which a deeply comatose patient maintains circulation but requires respiratory support. If brainstem function can be shown to have ceased in such patients, there is no prospect of recovery. The criteria for brainstem death are set out in **Figure 3.13**.

When applying the criteria, various precautions are essential:
• A metabolic or drug-induced state must be excluded
• A neuromuscular blocking agent must be excluded as the cause of the patient's loss of motor function

- Retesting of brainstem reflexes should be repeated after a 24 h interval
- Hypothermia must be controlled so that the patient's temperature is above 35°C when testing is performed
- A specific cause for the coma should be identified
- Certain spinal reflexes may still be present even in the presence of brainstem death. They include stretch reflexes, plantar responses and flexion of the upper or lower limb triggered by neck flexion

- Recognized features of metabolic coma include focal motor deficits and focal seizures
- The pupils remain reactive until the late stages of metabolic coma
- If pupillary responses or corneal responses are absent beyond 6 h after a cardiac arrest, there is little prospect for survival
- A vegetative state can be considered irreversible after head injury if it has persisted for over 12 months

Criteria for brainstem death

1. **Pupillary response**
    Use a bright torch (not an ophthalmoscope) to confirm that the pupils fail to respond.

2. **Corneal response**
    Gently apply a wisp of cotton wool to the cornea. There should be no response. Note that repeated testing can readily traumatize the cornea.

3. **Vestibulo-ocular reflex**
    Inspect the tympanic membrane to ensure that it is intact and not obscured by impacted wax. Insert a soft rubber catheter into the external auditory meatus and slowly inject approximately 50 ml of ice-cold water. Repeat the test in the other ear. There should be no ocular deviation.

4. **Motor response in cranial nerve distribution**
    This is most readily assessed by applying a painful stimulus to the glabella. The patient fails to respond.

5. **Gag or tracheal response**
    Either stimulate the palate or pass a suction catheter into the trachea. The patient fails to respond.

6. **Respiratory reaction to hypercapnoea**
    First administer a combination of 95 per cent O_2 and 5 per cent CO_2 via the respirator until the pCO_2 has risen above 40 mmHg (6.0 kPa). Disconnect the respirator, but administer 100 per cent oxygen through a tracheal catheter at around 6 l/min. Observe if any respiratory response occurs when the pCO_2 exceeds 50 mmHg (6.7 kPa).

Fig. 3.13 *Criteria for diagnosing brainstem death.*

chapter 4

Cranial Nerve Dysfunction

THE FIRST CRANIAL NERVE (OLFACTORY)

Disorders confined to the first cranial nerve are rare. Patients with olfactory nerve dysfunction typically complain of altered taste as well as altered smell. Conditions affecting the olfactory nerve include:
- Upper respiratory tract infection
- Closed head injury
- Subfrontal meningioma
- Dementia
    Olfactory hallucinations occur in simple and complex partial seizures. Terms related to first cranial nerve dysfunction are listed in **Figure 4.1**.

Definitions related to olfactory nerve dysfunction	
Anosmia	Total loss of smell
Hyposmia	Partial loss of smell
Hyperosmia	Exaggerated sense of smell
Dysomia	Distorted sense of smell

Fig. 4.1 *Definitions related to olfactory nerve dysfunction.*

THE SECOND CRANIAL NERVE (OPTIC)

The optic nerve is the sole part of the nervous system that is visible to the naked eye. Fundoscopy is therefore an essential part of the assessment of optic nerve dysfunction. Abnormalities of the optic nerve typically result in:
- A field defect that predominates centrally (**Fig. 4.2**), the result of the particular susceptibility of the macular fibres to the effect of compression or inflammation

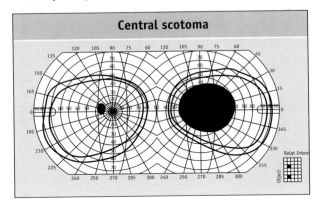

Fig. 4.2 *Central scotoma.*

Central scotoma

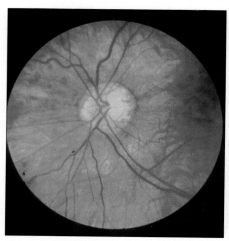

Fig. 4.3 *Optic atrophy.*

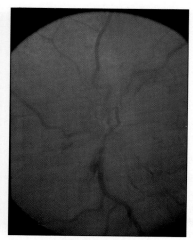

Fig. 4.4 *Fundus appearance in acute ischaemic optic neuropathy.*

- A disorder of colour vision
- An afferent pupillary defect
- Optic atrophy (**Fig. 4.3**)

The diagnosis of optic disc pallor is highly subjective. Avoid describing the disc as showing temporal pallor simply because of a knowledge of the presence of multiple sclerosis.

ISCHAEMIC OPTIC NEUROPATHY

Ischaemia of the anterior optic nerve (**Fig. 4.4**) is usually arteriosclerotic or arteritic but seldom embolic. The condition predominates in elderly people. Manifestations include:

- Sudden, painless visual loss
- Disc swelling followed by pallor
- Arcuate field defects
- A tendency to bilateral involvement

Unless arteritic, there is no specific treatment for this condition.

OPTIC NEURITIS

Optic neuritis is characterized by an inflammatory process either in the optic nerve head (papillitis) or the retrobulbar portion (retrobulbar neuritis). The condition is particularly characteristic of multiple sclerosis. Clinical features include:

- Preliminary ocular pain, particularly on movement
- Central visual loss
- Either a swollen (papillitis) or normal disc (retrobulbar neuritis)
- An afferent pupillary defect

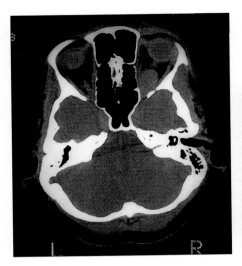

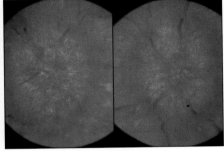

Fig. 4.5 *Computerized tomography scan of meningioma at the right orbital apex.*

Fig. 4.6 *Bilateral papilloedema.*

Perhaps 50% of patients with optic neuritis (the figure varies from author to author) develop multiple sclerosis.

OPTIC NERVE COMPRESSION

Optic nerve compression is seldom seen in clinical practice. The clinical features are similar to those of optic neuritis, except that progression is gradual and pain usually lacking. Proptosis declares the presence of a space-occupying lesion within the orbit (**Fig. 4.5**).

OPTIC NEUROPATHIES

Many other conditions can affect the optic nerve:

- Syphilis can produce slowly progressive bilateral failure or acute loss of vision
- Vitamin B_{12} deficiency may lead to progressive visual failure with bilateral central or centrocaecal scotoma (a field defect extending from fixation towards the blind spot)
- Drugs, for example, ethambutol
- Inherited disorders: Leber's hereditary optic atrophy predominates in men. The condition is determined by point mutations at several sites in the mitochondrial DNA

PAPILLOEDEMA

Papilloedema is a manifestation of raised intracranial pressure. Although sometimes asymmetrical, it is almost always bilateral (**Fig. 4.6**). Transmission of the raised pressure along the subarachnoid space of the optic nerve impairs venous return and axoplasmic flow.

Visual complaints are typically absent in the early stages. Later, the patient complains of greying-out of vision, typically induced by posture change. Other features of papilloedema include:

- Absent retinal venous pulsation
- Visual field defects. Initially, enlarged blind spots or inferonasal defects. Later, peripheral field constriction or central field loss

65

- The most important tests for optic nerve function are the swinging light test, assessment of the central field and fundoscopy
- Loss of retinal venous pulsation is an early sign of raised intracranial pressure

THE THIRD, FOURTH AND SIXTH CRANIAL NERVES (INCLUDING PUPILLARY ABNORMALITIES) (OCULOMOTOR, TROCHLEAR AND ABDUCENS)

Disorders of the oculomotor nerves are characterized by diplopia. Analysis of image separation, the direction of gaze triggering the diplopia and associated signs may serve to identify the responsible nerve.

Disorders of the pupil result either from interruption of its sympathetic or parasympathetic innervation or from disruption of the afferent component of the light reflex pathway (afferent pupillary defect).

IRIDOPLEGIA

In acute iridoplegia (**Fig. 4.7**), the pupil dilates and becomes fixed to all stimuli. The condition may appear spontaneously or after orbital trauma. A similar picture results from accidental or deliberate instillation of mydriatic drops.

THE TONIC PUPIL SYNDROME

Synonyms for the tonic pupil syndrome (**Fig. 4.8**) include the Holmes–Adie syndrome and the myotonic pupil. In some patients, it is accompanied by depression of the stretch reflexes. Characteristic features include:

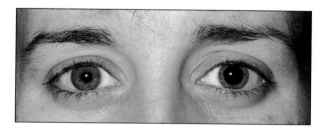

Fig. 4.7 *Acute iridoplegia.*

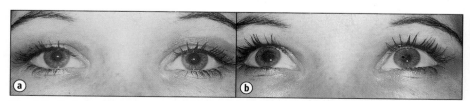

Fig. 4.8 *Tonic pupil syndrome. (a) The affected, left, pupil is larger than the right. **(b)** Immediately after release of the near effort (sustained for 60 s), the affected pupil is now smaller.*

- Female predominance
- Unilateral involvement
- A dilated pupil (becomes smaller over the years)
- Absent or depressed light reaction
- Delayed onset and release of the near reaction
- Delayed release of accommodation (vision blurs after switching from a near to distant object)
- Hypersensitivity to dilute parasympathomimetics (0.125% pilocarpine)

The condition is usually idiopathic but may follow orbital trauma or an acute iridoplegia. If the patient complains of photophobia, the pupil can be constricted with drops.

HORNER'S SYNDROME

Horner's syndrome results from interruption of the sympathetic fibres to the eye at any part of their course (**Fig. 4.9**). Features include:

- Ptosis, usually slight
- Miosis
- Anhidrosis over the face. The distribution depends on the site of the lesion (rarely detectable on routine examination)
- Enophthalmos (apparent rather than real)

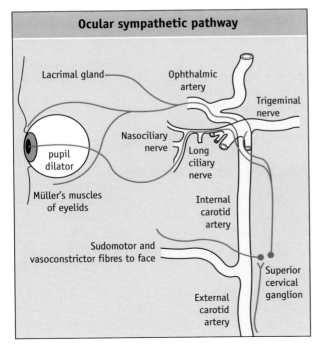

Ocular sympathetic pathway

Lacrimal gland

Ophthalmic artery

Trigeminal nerve

Nasociliary nerve

Long ciliary nerve

pupil dilator

Müller's muscles of eyelids

Internal carotid artery

Sudomotor and vasoconstrictor fibres to face

Superior cervical ganglion

External carotid artery

Fig. 4.9 *The ocular sympathetic pathway.*

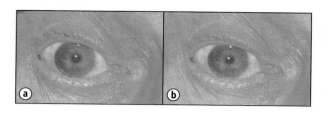

Fig. 4.10 *Horner's syndrome. Before (**a**) and after (**b**) instillation of cocaine.*

If there is uncertainty about the diagnosis, 4% cocaine should be instilled in the eye. A normal pupil dilates, a Horner's pupil remains constricted (**Fig. 4.10**). The use of other agents to determine whether the lesion is preganglionic or postganglionic tends to produce unreliable results. If the patient has an isolated Horner's syndrome and is otherwise well, only a chest radiograph is needed for investigation (to exclude an apical lung tumour: Pancoast's syndrome).

ARGYLL ROBERTSON PUPIL

An Argyll Robertson pupil (**Fig. 4.11**) is almost always associated with tertiary syphilis. Features include:

- Irregular, miosed pupil
- Depressed or absent light reaction
- Intact near reaction
- Iris atrophy
- Usually bilateral

The responsible lesion is probably prenuclear, close to the third nerve nucleus in the last part of the afferent portion of the pupillary light reflex.

- In a suspected tonic pupil syndrome, the tonic nature of the near reaction may take minutes to evolve
- In an isolated Horner's syndrome, investigation should be limited to a chest radiograph

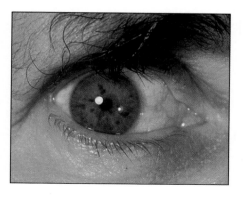

Fig. 4.11 *Argyll Robertson pupil.*

OCULOMOTOR NERVE DISORDERS

SIXTH NERVE PALSY

A sixth nerve palsy (**Fig. 4.12**) leads to an isolated weakness of the lateral rectus muscle. It results from a lesion in the central or peripheral course of the nerve (a nuclear lesion produces a gaze paresis due to involvement of the lateral gaze centre). Causes include:

- Diabetes
- Arteriosclerosis
- Multiple sclerosis
- Raised intracranial pressure (usually produces bilateral sixth nerve palsies)

FOURTH NERVE PALSY

This leads to an isolated weakness of the superior oblique muscle (**Fig. 4.13**). The patient has difficulty looking down and in. Causes include:

- Arteriosclerosis
- Head injury

THIRD NERVE PALSY

Lesions of the third nerve can occur at the nucleus, during its course within the midbrain or in the periphery.

- Nuclear lesions, if complete, also result in a contralateral superior rectus palsy
- Fascicular lesions (within the midbrain) may be accompanied by long-tract signs
  Contralateral hemiplegia (Weber's syndrome)
  Contralateral ataxia and intention tremor (Benedikt's syndrome) (**Fig 4.14**)
- Peripheral lesions, either partial or complete, the latter with or without pupillary involvement

Causes of a third nerve palsy include:

- Diabetes. Usually painful and pupil-sparing in 50% of patients
- Compressive, for example an aneurysm (**Fig. 4.15**), virtually always pupil-involving if the paresis is complete

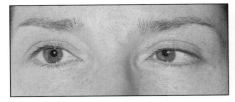

Fig. 4.12 *Right sixth nerve palsy.*

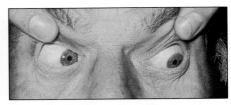

Fig. 4.13 *Right superior oblique palsy.*

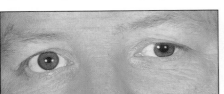

Fig. 4.14 *Benedikt's syndrome.*

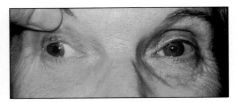

Fig. 4.15 *Third nerve palsy secondary to a posterior communicating aneurysm.*

Aberrant re-innervation may follow recovery of a third nerve palsy. Misdirection of fibres can lead to adduction on attempted up-gaze or lid retraction on attempted medial or down-gaze.

COMBINED PALSIES

Orbital lesions

Usually produce proptosis and may affect the optic nerve. Any ophthalmoplegia that occurs is as liable to result from direct muscle involvement as from nerve compression. Optic disc swelling can occur with abnormal shunt vessels on the disc, the consequence of impedance of venous drainage.

Superior orbital fissure lesions

May affect the first division of the trigeminal nerve as well as the oculomotor nerves. In the Tolosa–Hunt syndrome, an inflammatory condition around this site causes ophthalmoplegia, ocular pain and forehead numbness.

Cavernous lesions

Cavernous lesions (Fig. 4.16) can affect all the oculomotor nerves, along with the first and second divisions of the trigeminal nerve and the oculosympathetic fibres. Responsible pathologies include:
- Cavernous aneurysm
- Carotico-cavernous fistula
- Expanding pituitary tumour

- Compressive third nerve palsies almost always involve the pupil
- For any eye movement disorder sparing the pupil, consider myasthenia and dysthyroid eye disease

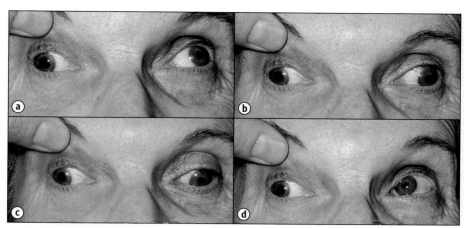

Fig. 4.16 *Cavernous aneurysm and its associated ophthalmoplegia.*

OTHER EYE MOVEMENT DISORDERS

Dorsal midbrain (Parinaud's) syndrome

Clinical features include:

- Impaired up-gaze
- Light-fixed, midposition pupils
- Convergence-retractory nystagmus on attempted up-gaze

The cause is usually a pinealoma, although, occasionally, it can be due to brainstem vascular disease, multiple sclerosis or other tumours.

Skew deviation

- Vertical imbalance of visual axes

The cause is virtually any intrinsic brainstem lesion (**Fig. 4.17**).

Internuclear ophthalmoplegia

This results from interruption of the medial longitudinal fasciculus. The side of the lesion is designated by the side of the impaired adduction (see **Fig. 10.8**).

Features include:
- Defective adduction
- Nystagmus in the abducting eye
- Vertical nystagmus and abnormal vertical pursuit if the lesion is bilateral

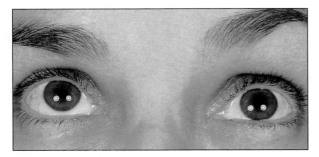

Fig. 4.17 *Skew deviation.*

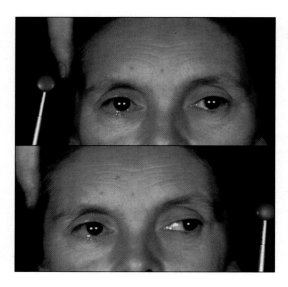

Fig. 4.18 *One-and-a-half syndrome.*

Causes:
- In younger patients, often multiple sclerosis
- In older patients, often cerebrovascular disease
- Unilateral internuclear ophthalmoplegia seen with many other pathologies and occasionally in drug-induced coma

One-and-a-half syndrome

This results from a lesion of the medial longitudinal fasciculus extending into the adjacent paramedian pontine reticular formation (**Fig. 4.18**).

Features include (for a right-sided lesion):
- Horizontal gaze paresis to the right
- Right internuclear ophthalmoplegia
- Only abduction of the left eye preserved as a consequence
- Vertical gaze preserved

Causes are vascular or demyelinating disease.

Horizontal gaze paresis

Horizontal gaze paresis may involve saccadic or pursuit movement or both.

Frontal lesions

Produce a contralateral saccadic palsy which recovers.

Pontine lesions

Pontine lesions produce an ipsilateral gaze palsy for saccades and pursuit.

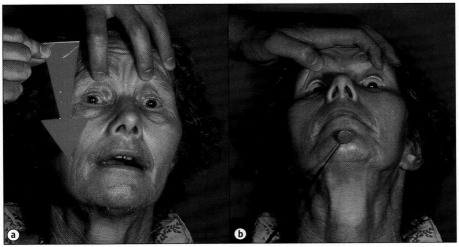

Fig. 4.19 *Progressive supranuclear palsy.* Failure of down-gaze (*a*) is improved by the doll's head manoeuvre (*b*).

Parieto-occipital lesions
These produce an ipsilateral pursuit paresis with contralateral homonymous hemianopia.

Vertical gaze paresis
Supranuclear ophthalmoplegia (**Fig. 4.19**) (Steele–Richardson–Olszewski syndrome) results in a vertical gaze palsy, initially for down-gaze, with preserved doll's head movements. Later, upward and horizontal gaze is affected (see p. 149).

Nystagmus

> **Definition of nystagmus**
>
> A to-and-fro motion of the eyes of equal velocity (pendular nystagmus) or differing velocity (jerk nystagmus).

Pendular nystagmus
- Usually congenital but also seen with multiple sclerosis and vascular disease

Vestibular nystagmus
- Caused by disease of the labyrinth or its connections
- When labyrinthine: there are often horizontal and rotary components. Slow phase to the side of the lesion
- When caused by central connections: more variable; it may be rotary, horizontal, vertical or a combination

Gaze-evoked nystagmus
Causes:
- Disease of brainstem or cerebellum
- Drugs, for example, phenytoin
- Vertical component (implies central pathology)

Down-beat nystagmus
When occuring on down-and-out-gaze suggests a lesion at the foramen magnum (e.g. Chiari malformation)

End-point nystagmus
- Physiological. Avoid eliciting it by assessing nystagmus at 30° of lateral gaze rather than beyond

Optokinetic nystagmus
Assessed using a drum with painted vertical lines. If the drum is rotated to the patient's right, there is a pursuit movement to the right followed by a saccade to the left. The movements are generated by the hemisphere towards which the drum is rotating.
- Deep parietal lesions lead to defective optokinetic nystagmus responses when the drum is rotated towards the affected hemisphere

- Avoid moving the eyes to the extremes when assessing nystagmus
- Vertical nystagmus implies a lesion of the central nervous system

THE FIFTH CRANIAL NERVE (TRIGEMINAL)

Isolated lesions of the trigeminal nerve are uncommon and are likely to reflect a pathological process affecting the peripheral course of the nerve.
Causes include:
- Trigeminal neurinoma. This produces a combined motor and sensory dysfunction
- Malignant invasion may occur as part of a neoplastic meningitis. Typically, there is severe facial pain leading to facial sensory loss with wasting of masseter and temporalis. The jaw deviates to the paralysed side on opening (**Fig. 4.20**)

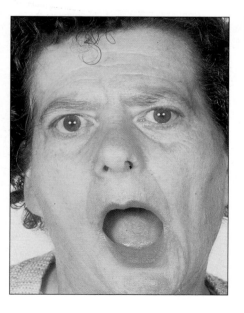

Fig. 4.20 *Trigeminal lesion.* *Deviation of the jaw to the left.*

- Isolated trigeminal neuropathy. A condition of unknown aetiology producing loss of sensation in one or more divisions of the trigeminal nerve. Motor function is usually spared. There is an association with collagen vascular disease and Sjögren's syndrome. The sensory loss is sometimes so profound that tissue necrosis occurs (**Fig. 4.21**)

Central lesions of the trigeminal nerve are more common and generally accompanied by other cranial nerve signs, together with long-tract manifestations.
Causes include:
- Cerebrovascular disease; for example, ipsilateral facial sensory loss to pain and temperature occurs in the lateral medullary syndrome
- Multiple sclerosis. Isolated facial sensory loss is a rare feature of this condition. Perhaps 3% of patients with trigeminal neuralgia have multiple sclerosis

TRIGEMINAL NEURALGIA
See p. 44.

THE SEVENTH CRANIAL NERVE (FACIAL)

UPPER MOTOR NEURON FACIAL WEAKNESS
This results from interruption of descending fibres passing from the contralateral motor cortex to the ipsilateral facial nerve nucleus. Involvement of the upper face is relatively mild (frontalis receives innervation from both hemispheres) but weakness of the lower face is substantial (**Fig. 4.22**).
Causes:
- Cerebrovascular disease
- Tumour
- Trauma

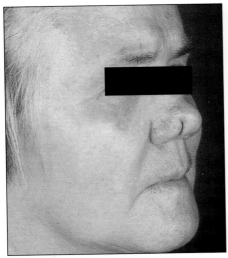

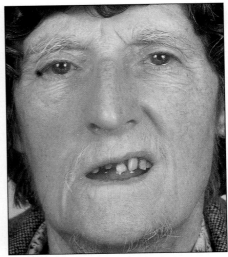

Fig. 4.21 *Neuropathic tissue loss from the nose.*

Fig. 4.22 *Upper motor neuron facial weakness.*

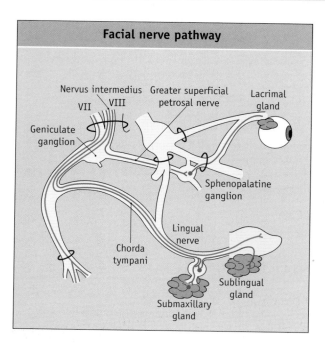

Facial nerve pathway

Fig. 4.23 *Course of seventh nerve.*

LOWER MOTOR NEURON FACIAL WEAKNESS

This results from damage to the facial nerve nucleus or any part of its intrapontine or peripheral course (**Fig. 4.23**). All the muscles supplied by the nerve are affected unless the lesion is very distal. Additional symptoms suggest a particular level.

Symptoms of lower motor neuron facial weakness

- Loss of taste over anterior two-thirds of tongue (proximal to origin of chorda tympani)
- Hyperacusis (proximal to origin of fibres to stapedius)
- Loss of lacrimation (proximal to geniculate ganglion)

Causes:

Bell's palsy

An acute lower motor neuron facial weakness of uncertain cause (**Fig. 4.24**)

Features include:
- Involvement at any age
- Prodromal aural pain in 50% of patients
- Complete recovery in approximately 80% of patients
- Occasionally, a positive family history
- Recurrence in approximately 10% of patients

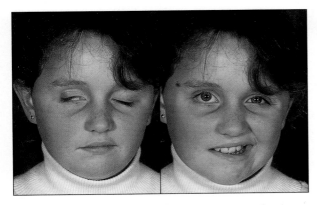

Fig. 4.24 *Right Bell's palsy in a girl of 11 years.*

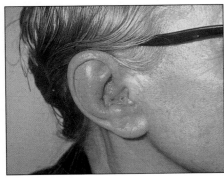

Fig. 4.25 *Vesicular eruption in the Ramsay–Hunt syndrome.*

Investigations

- Electromyogram analysis of facial muscles serves little purpose in the acute stages. If fibrillation potentials are found (only after approximately 2 weeks) then a confident statement of denervation can be made, with a higher likelihood of incomplete recovery
- An increased tongue threshold to galvanic stimulation, measured early, correlates well with subsequent evidence of denervation

Treatment

- Perhaps justifiable to give steroids if the condition is seen within 2 days of onset. Say, 40 mg prednisolone daily, decreasing by 5 mg every day

Ramsay–Hunt syndrome

- The consequence of herpetic involvement of the geniculate ganglion. The patient may have a vesicular eruption (**Fig. 4.25**) in the throat or over the pinna. The prognosis is similar to that of Bell's palsy
- Other causes include mumps, leprosy, parotid gland infection or tumour, leukaemia and sarcoidosis. Multiple sclerosis can cause a lower motor neuron facial weakness caused by a plaque within the pons

BILATERAL LOWER MOTOR NEURON FACIAL WEAKNESS

Difficult to recognize because there may be no asymmetry. The face sags and loses expressivity (**Fig. 4.26**).

Causes include Guillain–Barré syndrome, Miller–Fisher syndrome and sarcoidosis.

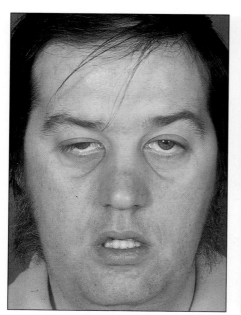

Fig. 4.26 *Bilateral facial weakness.*

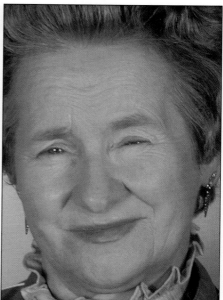

Fig. 4.27 *A paroxysm of left-sided hemifacial spasm.*

FACIAL MOVEMENT DISORDERS

- Fasciculation is virtually confined to patients with motor neuron disease
- Myokymia is irrelevant if confined to the lower lid. Pathological myokymia is more extensive. It produces a very fine shimmering motion in the affected muscle, caused, almost always, by a lesion around the seventh nerve nucleus. Multiple sclerosis is the most common cause
- Hemifacial spasm (**Fig. 4.27**) produces a haphazard contraction of facial muscles on one side. It usually begins around the eye but can spread to the half-face. It results eventually in mild facial weakness. Often caused by cross-compression of the facial nerve by an aberrant vessel near the pons, it can be treated by microvascular surgery
- Blepharospasm (see p. 154)
- Orofacial dyskinesia is an involuntary, semi-repetitive contraction of muscles around the mouth, often coupled with tongue movements. It can occur spontaneously in elderly people but can be triggered by phenothiazines and is also seen with dopa
- Facial tics are repetitive facial movements, partly under voluntary control

- The upper part of the face is relatively spared in an upper motor neuron facial weakness
- Bell's palsy, the most common cause of a lower motor neuron facial weakness, is associated with aural pain in one-half of the patients

THE EIGHTH CRANIAL NERVE (AUDITORY)

DEAFNESS

Classification of deafness

Can be divided into conductive forms (in which there is interference with sound transmission to the inner ear) and perceptive (sensori-neural) forms in which the end organ or the auditory nerve is affected.

Conductive deafness
- Bone conduction better perceived than air conduction (Rinne negative)
- With Weber's test, the sound is heard better by the deaf ear
  Causes include wax, otosclerosis and middle ear disease

Perceptive deafness
- Air conduction better perceived than bone conduction (Rinne positive)
- With Weber's test, the sound is heard better by the intact ear
  Causes include Meniéré's disease, acoustic neurinoma and vascular accident affecting the inner ear.
  Lesions of the central nervous system affecting either the cochlear nucleus, the ascending auditory pathway or the auditory cortex can also cause deafness. For example, unilateral or bilateral deafness are recognized features of multiple sclerosis.

TINNITUS

Consists of an abnormal sound in one or both ears. The sound may be continuous or intermittent and can be pulsatile, hissing or whistling in quality. The symptom can occur with inner ear disease and with arteriovenous malformations of the brain. Often the aetiology is unknown.

VERTIGO

Defined as a sense of rotation of the individual or the environment.

Peripheral vertigo

Considered to be secondary to some process affecting the labyrinth or the vestibular component of the acoustic nerve, for example:
- Meniéré's disease produces paroxysms of vertigo together with persistent tinnitus and progressive sensori-neural deafness
- Acute vestibular neuronitis. A description given to patients with acute vertigo often with vomiting, ataxia and malaise, on the assumption of an acute, perhaps viral, process affecting the labyrinth or the vestibular nerve
- Benign positional vertigo. Patients complain of attacks of vertigo triggered by sudden movement, particularly lying down in bed at night. Attacks can be reproduced by appropriate head positioning (see p. 16) causing a fatiguing rotary nystagmus to be elicited. The condition is self-limiting but can be shortened in duration by the patient deliberately inducing attacks by appropriate head positioning

Central vertigo

Liable to be more persistent than peripheral forms. When posture induced, the vertigo tends to be triggered immediately, showing less fatigue and more variability in terms of its precipitation than the peripheral form. Causes include cerebrovascular disease, multiple sclerosis and tumour.

THE NINTH CRANIAL NERVE (GLOSSOPHARYNGEAL)

Isolated lesions of this nerve are rare. Usually, therefore, a glossopharyngeal palsy is part of a more widespread neurological process. This includes:
- Jugular foramen syndrome. Results in a palsy of the ninth, tenth and eleventh cranial nerves. Causes include nasopharyngeal carcinoma and glomus tumours
- Chiari malformation. Downward stretching of the ninth nerve leads to unilateral or bilateral depression of the gag reflex. Other lower cranial nerves are disturbed and long-tract signs are likely (see p. 90)

THE TENTH CRANIAL NERVE (VAGUS)

Bilateral lesions of the supranuclear projections to the vagal nucleus form part of a pseudo-bulbar palsy. Vagal damage can occur within the brainstem or along its peripheral course. A unilateral vagal palsy (**Fig. 4.28**) leads to palatal deviation, hoarseness and dysphagia. Bilateral vagal palsies lead to total palatal paralysis, with dysarthria and severe dysphagia. The vocal cords are immobile and rest in an intermediate position, producing stridor on

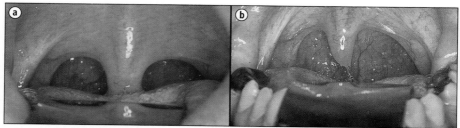

Fig. 4.28 Left vagus palsy. *The palate deviates to the right on phonation (b).*

deep inspiration. Recurrent laryngeal palsies, as a result of the retained innervation of the cricothyroid muscle, produce some residual adductor activity of the cords and consequently a greater degree of stridor.

Causes include:
- Nuclear vagal lesions caused by polio or brainstem vascular disease
- Peripheral vagal lesions (rare)
- Recurrent laryngeal palsies (usually left) caused by aortic aneurysm, thyroid surgery or malignant invasion

Palatal myoclonus is a rhythmic movement disorder at approximately 2–3 Hz. The face, larynx and diaphragm may also be affected. The patient may complain of a clicking noise, the consequence of pharyngeal contraction affecting the Eustachian tube. Causes of palatal myoclonus include brainstem vascular disease and head injury.

THE ELEVENTH CRANIAL NERVE (ACCESSORY)

The cranial component of the nerve cannot be separated, in terms of its clinical function, from the vagus. Involvement of the spinal accessory results in weakness of trapezius and sternomastoid. Isolated lesions (**Fig. 4.29**) of the nerve are rare.
Causes include:
- Upper cervical cord lesions
- Posterior fossa tumours
- Jugular foramen syndrome
- Trauma

    In some of these situations, other signs co-exist.

    Spasmodic torticollis (**Fig. 4.30**) is a focal dystonia affecting the neck muscles, including sternomastoid. Recurrent or persistent contractions produce an abnormal neck posture with muscle hypertrophy and, eventually, cervical spine degeneration.

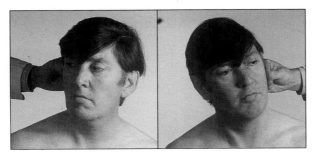

Fig. 4.29 *Left accessory nerve lesion.*

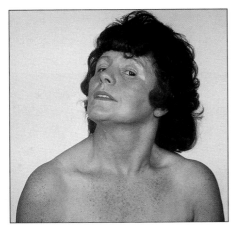

Fig. 4.30 *Spasmodic torticollis.*

THE TWELFTH CRANIAL NERVE (HYPOGLOSSAL)

Disturbances of twelfth nerve function result from interruption of the cortico-bulbar projections to the hypoglossal nucleus or from lesions of the nucleus itself or the peripheral course of the nerve.
- Unilateral upper motor neuron lesion. Usually has little effect, although the tongue may deviate slightly to the paralysed side

- Bilateral upper motor neuron lesions result in a pseudo-bulbar palsy. Features include dysphagia, dysarthria and emotional lability. The tongue is stiff and moves slowly. There is weakness of voluntary palatal movement, although with a brisk gag reflex exaggerated jaw jerk

The usual causes are:

- Cerebrovascular disease
- Motor neuron disease
- Unilateral lower motor neuron lesion. In a unilateral lesion of the hypoglossal nerve (**Fig. 4.31**), there is ipsilateral atrophy with fasciculation and protrusion to the paralysed side. Causes of a unilateral lower motor neuron lesion include malignant invasion of the skull base
- Bilateral lower motor neuron lesion. Usually part of a bulbar palsy, co-existing with involvement of other lower brainstem motor nuclei, leading to dysphagia and dysarthria. The tongue is wasted and immobile and fasciculates on both sides (**Fig. 4.32**). Causes of a bilateral lower motor neuron lesion include polio, motor neuron disease and Chiari malformation

> - Isolated lesions of the lower cranial nerves are uncommon
> - A bulbar palsy is the result of a lesion affecting cranial nerves IX–XII
> - A pseudo-bulbar palsy affects the same cranial nerves but through involvement, bilaterally, of their cortico-bulbar projections. It is associated with a brisk jaw jerk

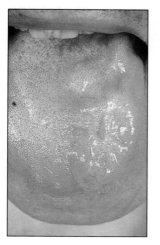

Fig. 4.31 Left hypoglossal nerve lesion.

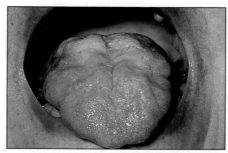

Fig. 4.32 Bilateral tongue wasting in motor neuron disease.

chapter 5

Vertigo, Dizziness and Ataxia

VERTIGO, DIZZINESS AND ATAXIA

Intensive investigation of patients with ill-defined dizziness or giddiness who have no physical signs on examination is seldom justified. Careful history taking is essential to define what is meant by the complaint and whether it includes a sense of rotation, either of the self or of the environment (vertigo). Patients with acute vertigo are likely to have a disturbance of the vestibular apparatus or its central connections, although vertigo can also figure in the aura arising from an epileptic discharge in one or other temporal lobe. Vertiginous patients are ataxic but many patients with ill-defined dizziness appear to have a normal gait despite their complaints. Patients who are ataxic in the absence of vertigo are likely, if their sensation is normal, to have a cerebellar system disorder.

The differential diagnosis of patients with vertigo, dizziness or giddiness is wide; as many as one-quarter will be left without a specific diagnosis (**Fig. 5.1**). Aspects of the history that are critical in reaching a diagnosis include:

- Is the symptom triggered by a particular environment, for example, a supermarket?
- Is the symptom triggered by a particular manoeuvre, for example, lying down in bed or by standing?
- Is the symptom accompanied by aural symptoms, for example, tinnitus or deafness?
- Is the symptom paroxysmal or constant?
- Are there accompanying symptoms that suggest the source of the problem?
- Are there objective accounts of gait ataxia?

Certain aspects of the examination are important when assessing the dizzy patient. With an acute, end-organ, vestibular disorder, certain clinical findings are characteristic:

- There is a jerk nystagmus on forward gaze with the fast phase to the side opposite the lesion
- The patient describes vertigo to the side opposite the lesion
- The patient past-points a stationary target on the side of the lesion
- The patient falls to the side of the lesion

Distribution of some of the diagnoses in 444 patients whose main complaint was vertigo, dizziness or giddiness	
Primary psychiatric disorder	109
Unknown	96
Acute vestibulopathy	69
Syncope	37
Epilepsy	36
Post-traumatic	31
Cerebrovascular disease	30
Benign positional vertigo	22
Other	14

Fig. 5.1 *Distribution of some of the diagnoses in 444 patients whose main complaint was vertigo, dizziness or giddiness.*

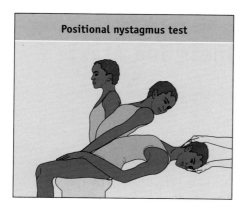

Positional nystagmus test

Fig. 5.2 *Testing for positional nystagmus (Barany's manoeuvre).*

In patients with vertigo caused by a central lesion, these findings become less clear cut. The nystagmus may change the direction of its fast phase according to the direction of gaze and may show vertical components (implying the presence of a brainstem lesion).

If the patient describes vertigo in a certain posture, the Barany manoeuvre is performed (**Fig. 5.2**). The patient is seated on the edge of the couch with the head rotated first 90° to the right and then 90° to the left. From each of those positions, the head and trunk are extended so that the head lies at approximately 30° below the horizontal plane. Any nystagmus is noted, whether it appears after a latent period, whether it fatigues or whether it returns as the patient resumes the upright posture.

PRIMARY PSYCHIATRIC DISORDERS

Dizziness, giddiness and even true vertigo are frequent components of an anxiety state and occur in over 50% of patients with hyperventilation syndrome. In this syndrome, the dizziness can be triggered by certain environments, for example, a supermarket, and a typical attack is reproduced by asking the patient to hyperventilate. Other symptoms in the attacks include faintness, paraesthesiae, chest pain and anxiety. Many older patients who have had an acute vestibular insult lose their confidence in walking, remaining house-bound long after the acute episode has resolved.

ACUTE VESTIBULOPATHY (VESTIBULAR NEURITIS)

Symptoms of acute vestibulopathy

- Acute vertigo
- Altered balance
- Nausea and often vomiting
- Normal hearing

The condition is probably the consequence of a virus affecting the vestibular nerve trunk. Typically, it follows evidence of an upper respiratory tract infection. It tends to resolve over 1–2 months.

The clinical findings are those of an acute peripheral vestibular disorder. The nystagmus is horizontal with rotatory components.

Caloric tests establish the presence of canal paresis ipsilateral to the lesion. Approximately two-thirds of patients recover canal function.

Vestibular sedatives, for example, dramamine, are used in the acute stages for symptomatic relief.

SYNCOPE AND EPILEPSY

Dizziness with or without vertigo is often prominent in patients with vaso-vagal attacks. The accompanying symptoms usually make the diagnosis straightforward. In some patients, attacks of dizziness are related to postural hypotension, typically drug-induced. The drugs most often responsible are those used for treatment of hypertension, the phenothiazines, diuretics and tricyclic antidepressants.

Vertigo is a recognized part of an epileptic aura arising usually from the temporal cortex. It can be accompanied by tinnitus and contralateral paraesthesiae. The attacks may be associated with rotation of the body or of the head and eyes.

BENIGN POSITIONAL VERTIGO

Symptoms of benign positional vertigo

- Brief attacks of rotational vertigo triggered by certain movements
- Often spontaneous but can follow head injury
- Any age group
- The attacks remit, usually within weeks but recur after intervals of up to several years in approximately one-quarter of patients

The patient complains of attacks of vertigo either on getting out of bed or on first lying down in bed. The diagnosis is established by a typical response to head positioning.

- Attacks are triggered by rapid change from the sitting to the head-dependent position
- A latent period of a few seconds occurs before the symptoms and signs emerge
- The nystagmus is rotatory, with the fast phase in the direction of the lowest ear
- The nystagmus and vertigo fatigue within 60 s
- A return of nystagmus in the opposite direction can occur when the patient becomes upright
- The phenomenon fatigues with repeated testing

The condition is thought to be related to displacement of otoconial debris on to the cupola of the posterior semi-circular canal.

Management of the condition is based on physical manoeuvres designed to dislodge the otolithic material from the posterior semi-circular canal. Patients are asked to trigger attacks by lying down sideways with their head supported on the bed. Having held the triggering position for 30 s they then take up the opposite position for a further 30 s. The process is repeated rapidly approximately five times and then every 3 h until there have been no attacks triggered for 48 h. Drug therapy is of very limited value. Rarely, transection of the posterior ampullary nerve is performed for patients with intractable symptoms.

MÉNIÈRE'S DISEASE

Ménière's disease is encountered infrequently in neurological practice.

Symptoms of Ménière's disease

- Typically, attacks last a few hours
- Rotational vertigo, preceded by slight deafness and tinnitus
- Patients may experience syncopal sensations and some briefly lose consciousness
- Between attacks the patient is symptom-free but later increasing tinnitus and progressive deafness appear

The condition usually begins in middle-life and tends to run in families. After some years, bilateral involvement appears in approximately 50% of patients. It is secondary to endolymphatic hydrops, usually caused by impaired endolymph resorption.

Acute attacks are managed symptomatically. Betahistine, on a long-term basis, reduces the frequency of attacks. For patients with intractable disease, selective vestibular nerve section relieves the attacks of vertigo but has no effect on the hearing loss.

CENTRAL VESTIBULAR DISORDERS

DISABLING POSITIONAL VERTIGO

It has been suggested that some patients with disabling attacks of positional vertigo have cross-compression of the vestibular branch of the auditory nerve by a vessel, usually the anterior or posterior inferior cerebellar artery. The exact status and specificity of the condition is questioned. As an alternative to microvascular decompression, carbamazepine can be tried in patients thought to have the disorder.

Various disorders of the brainstem or cerebellum can mimic vestibular neuritis, including cerebrovascular disease and multiple sclerosis. Paroxysmal attacks of dysarthria, vertigo and ataxia occur in multiple sclerosis and relate to the presence of a plaque in the region of the pons. The attacks resolve with carbamazepine. A positional nystagmus without vertigo is indicative of a lesion in the brainstem or vestibulocerebellum.

- Most patients with attacks of dizziness or vertigo do not require extensive investigation
- Common causes of dizziness include postural hypotension, hyperventilation, vestibular neuritis and benign positional vertigo
- Central vestibular disorders are characterized by a direction-changing nystagmus with vertical components

ATAXIA

Ataxia, in the absence of vertigo, is likely to be the result of a disorder of the cerebellum or its pathways, assuming that psychological factors or sensory deficits are not relevant to the problem. The cerebellum is concerned with the co-ordination and smooth operation of skilled motor activity. Consequences of cerebellar lesions include: abnormalities of eye movement, broken pursuit, hypometric or hypermetric saccades and nystagmus.

> **Symptoms of cerebellar lesions**
>
> - Abnormalities of speech: slurring dysarthria, sometimes with jerky, explosive phonation
> - Abnormalities of limb control
> - Gait ataxia

The cerebellum can be divided phylogenetically into three components: the archicerebellum, the palaeocerebellum and the neocerebellum.

ARCHICEREBELLUM
The oldest part of the cerebellum, its principal connections are with the vestibular nuclei. It consists of the flocculonodular lobe and adjacent uvula and nodulus. Deranged function produces gait ataxia, vertigo and nystagmus. The fast component of the nystagmus is to the side of the lesion.

PALAEOCEREBELLUM
The second oldest part of the cerebellum, its principal connections are with the spinocerebellar tracts. The palaeocerebellum consists of the anterior lobe of the cerebellum and part of the posterior lobe. Deranged function produces ataxia of gait and lower limb incoordination.

NEOCEREBELLUM
The newest part of the cerebellum, its principal connections are to the sensorimotor cortex. The neocerebellum consists of the lateral lobes of the cerebellum. Deranged function leads to incoordination, tremor, ataxia to the side of the lesion, hypotonia, dysarthria and nystagmus.

ATAXIC DISORDERS – FAMILIAL

ATAXIA TELANGIECTASIA
- Inherited as a recessive condition
- Clinical features include ataxia, dysarthria, choreo-athetoid movements and peripheral neuropathy
- Telangiectasiae are found on the skin and conjunctivae (**Fig. 5.3**) but are often not visible at presentation
- There are deficiencies of both humeral and cell-mediated immunity
- Serum levels of immunoglobulin A and immunoglobulin G are depressed
- There is an increased incidence of malignancy, principally of the lymphoid system and breast

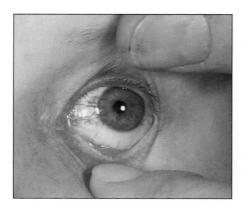

Fig. 5.3 *Ataxia telangiectasia.*

Abetalipoproteinaemia
- Inherited as a recessive condition
- Malabsorption of vitamins A, D, E and K is associated with depressed serum lipid levels, particularly cholesterol
- Clinical features include abnormal retinal pigmentation, ataxia, areflexia and proprioceptive loss
- Acanthocytes (spiky red blood cells) are found on examination of wet films
- The neurological deficit is partly responsive to vitamin E

Friedreich's ataxia
- Criteria for diagnosis include limb and gait ataxia, lower limb areflexia and electrophysiological evidence of a neuropathy
- Most patients present in the first part of the second decade of life
- Progression to a wheelchair existence is usual, with death in the early thirties
- Other clinical features include pyramidal signs (particularly extensor plantars), dysarthria, nystagmus and optic atrophy. Scoliosis is usual and pes cavus occurs in 50% of patients (**Fig. 5.4**)
- Cardiomyopathy is common and two-thirds of patients have an abnormal electrocardiogram
- There is a recognized association with diabetes mellitus
- The pathological changes centre on the spinocerebellar tracts, the posterior columns, the pyramidal tracts and the peripheral nerves
- There is no treatment. Localization of the gene to chromosome 9 allows prenatal diagnosis

Other early-onset ataxias
Other early-onset, familial ataxias are rare. They are inherited as recessive conditions. One resembles Friedreich's ataxia but the upper limb and knee reflexes are retained; optic nerve involvement does not occur and there is usually no scoliosis and no evidence of a cardiomyopathy. The prognosis is better than for patients with Friedreich's ataxia.

Late-onset familial ataxias
Principally, these are composed, pathologically, of olivopontocerebellar degeneration and cortical cerebellar degeneration. They are inherited as autosomal dominant conditions. Types I and II autosomal dominant cerebellar ataxias may have a supranuclear ophthalmoplegia and extrapyramidal features in addition to the ataxic syndrome. Type II

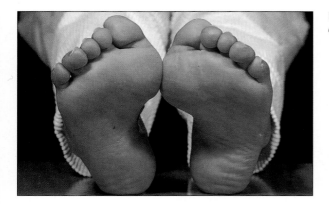

Fig. 5.4 *Friedreich's ataxia. Pes cavus.*

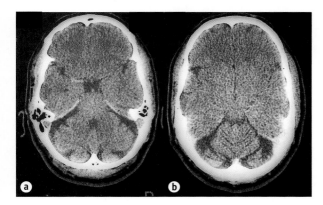

Fig. 5.5 *CT scan. Cerebellar and brainstem atrophy in a patient with sporadic late-onset ataxia.*

patients also have evidence of a pigmentary retinal degeneration. Type III is purely cerebellar.

Non-familial late-onset ataxia

The pathological basis for these patients' condition includes olivopontocerebellar atrophy, cerebello-olivary atrophy and cortical cerebellar atrophy. Some of the patients have a deficiency of glutamate dehydrogenase but this deficiency is found in other degenerative disorders. Imaging reveals cerebellar and brainstem atrophy (**Fig. 5.5**).

Neuroacanthocytosis

This condition can be inherited either as an autosomal dominant or recessive condition. It combines a movement disorder (typically chorea) with intellectual impairment, altered personality and an axonal neuropathy. Imaging reveals evidence of cerebral and caudate atrophy with, on magnetic resonance imaging, an abnormal signal from the caudate or lentiform nuclei. Light microscopy or scanning electron microscopy detects acanthocytes (red cells with spiny projections) and echinocytes (red cells with rounded projections [**Fig. 5.6**]).

Alcoholic cerebellar degeneration

Alcoholic cerebellar degeneration evolves gradually and affects gait more than limb function. Nystagmus is usually absent and the speech normal. Associated

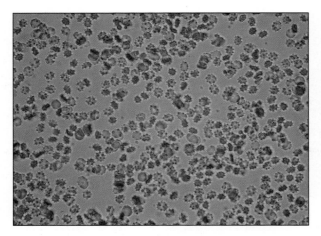

Fig. 5.6
*Neuroacanthocytosis.
Wright's-stained preparation
after 3 h incubation in
ethylenediaminetetraacetic
acid, illustrating increased
numbers of acanthocytes and
echinocytes.*

findings include an alcohol-related neuropathy. The condition seldom reverses, even
with abstinence.

Hypothyroid cerebellar degeneration
This disorder also principally affects gait. Other cerebellar signs are usually absent. The
diagnosis of hypothyroidism is generally evident and the condition tends to reverse with
replacement therapy.

Drug-induced cerebellar disorders
Acute cerebellar dysfunction occurs with alcohol intoxication and after an overdose with
many anticonvulsants. A persisting cerebellar syndrome is a recognized feature of chronic
phenytoin intoxication.

Ramsay–Hunt syndrome
Describes a syndrome of ataxia and myoclonus with generalized seizures in perhaps
one-half of the patients. It is inherited as an autosomal recessive condition. A
combination of cerebellar ataxia and myoclonus can also be inherited as a dominant
condition and some patients with a Ramsay–Hunt-like syndrome are found to have a
mitochondrial cytopathy.

Paroxysmal cerebellar ataxia
Can occur in recessive or dominant forms. Recessive forms include Hartnup's disease,
pyruvate dehydrogenase deficiency and pyruvate decarboxylase deficiency. There are at least
two autosomal dominant forms. In one, brief attacks of ataxia provoked by startle or
exercise are associated with myokymia and may respond to acetazolamide. In the other,
genetically distinct form, the attacks can last for several hours and are triggered by stress or
exercise. Attacks are normally very responsive to acetazolamide. Eventually, progressive
cerebellar ataxia may supervene.

Chiari malformations
Chiari malformations are divided into three types:
Type I – Herniation of cerebellar tonsils through the foramen magnum. Associated with
syringomyelia (**Fig. 5.7**). Type I malformation can present as syringomyelia, as a cluster of

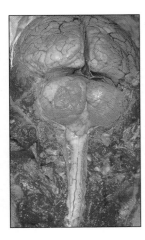

Fig. 5.7 *Chiari malformation*. *Tonsillar ectopia associated with an abnormal course of the upper cervical roots.*

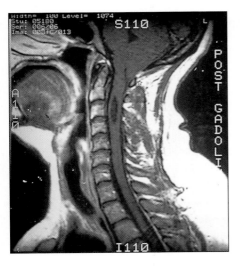

Fig. 5.8 *Chiari malformation*. *Magnetic resonance imaging showing ectopic cerebellar tonsils (star), associated with a syrinx in the cervical cord.*

lower cranial nerve symptoms and signs, usually with evidence of pyramidal and cerebellar deficit, or as cough headache (see p. 42). The displaced cerebellar tonsils are best identified using magnetic resonance imaging. Any associated syringomyelia is readily demonstrated (**Fig. 5.8**). The condition is treated by foramen magnum decompression.

Type II – Herniation of cerebellar tonsils and vermis. Associated with spinal or cranial dysraphism.

Type III – Rare. Herniation of entire cerebellum with a cervico-occipital encephalocoele.

Dandy–Walker syndrome

In this syndrome the cerebellar vermis is deficient, the cerebellum hypoplastic and the fourth ventricle enlarged. There is an associated hydrocephalus with partial absence of the corpus callosum. The skull is abnormally shaped with the confluence of the lateral sinuses directed upwards. The features are readily identified by magnetic resonance imaging. (**Fig. 5.9**). The cyst is shunted if its pressure is elevated.

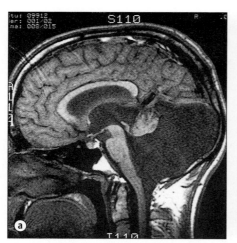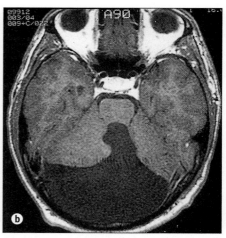

Fig. 5.9 Dandy–Walker syndrome. (a) *Sagittal T1-weighted magnetic resonance imaging. Enlarged posterior fossa, a large (cerebrospinal fluid containing) cyst in communication with the fourth ventricle and absence of the inferior vermis of the cerebellum.* **(b)** *Axial magnetic resonance imaging shows the cyst communicating with the fourth ventricle.*

Postanoxic myoclonus

This condition is frequently accompanied by cerebellar ataxia and dysarthria. It typically follows cardiac or respiratory arrest. The myoclonus occurs with action and can affect both limbs and trunk. Most patients have seizures. Drugs that enhance 5-hydroxytryptamine activity are valuable in treatment. Effective treatments include 5-hydroxytryptophan, in combination with carbidopa, clonazepam or sodium valproate.

- The cerebellum is frequently affected by cerebrovascular disease and multiple sclerosis
- Cerebellar degeneration is common in alcoholic patients, predominantly affects gait and is usually irreversible
- The Type I Chiari malformation can present with lower cranial nerve, pyramidal and cerebellar signs, with syringomyelia or with cough headache

chapter 6

Disorders of Higher Cortical Function

DEMENTIA

Various definitions of dementia exist. The definition used in the World Health Organization International Classification of Diseases, 10th Revision is:

Definition of dementia

A disorder characterized by both memory and thinking deterioration sufficient to impair personal activities of daily living. The memory impairment affects the registration, storage and retrieval of new information.

Other definitions have been used. All, to some extent, suffer from lack of quantification and all, at best, achieve a sensitivity of 90% when clinicopathological comparisons are made. The dementias are divided into early-onset (before 65 years old) and late-onset subtypes. Alzheimer's disease accounts for over one-half of the dementias. The most common other subtype is caused by vascular disease, either in isolation or in association with Alzheimer's disease (**Fig. 6.1**). The reversible dementias are those in which a specific trigger can be identified as responsible for the intellectual decline, the assumption being that if the trigger is treated, the process can be reversed (**Fig. 6.2**). Pseudo-dementia is a term applied to patients whose psychiatric disorder, usually depressive or schizo-affective, is considered responsible for the apparent intellectual decline.

Subcortical dementia is characterized by slowing of the thought process, altered behaviour, disturbances of speech other than aphasia and changes in gait and movement. It is a feature of many extrapyramidal disorders.

Pathological subtypes causing dementia (based on postmortem data)	
	%
Alzheimer-type	52.8
Arteriosclerotic	22.5
Alzheimer and arteriosclerotic	13.6
Other	8.3

Fig. 6.1 *Pathological subtypes causing dementia (based on postmortem data).*

Causes of reversible dementia	
Endocrinological	Hypothyroidism Hypoparathyroidism
Metabolic	Hepatic encephalopathy Vitamin B_{12} deficiency
Hydrocephalic	Normal pressure hydrocephalus
Tumour	Sub-frontal meningioma

Fig. 6.2 *Causes of reversible dementia.*

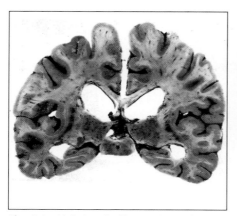

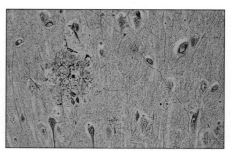

Fig. 6.4 *Alzheimer's disease.* Amyloid plaque in the hippocampus (mag X 280).

Fig. 6.3 *Alzheimer's disease. Coronal section showing widened cortical sulci and dilated lateral ventricles.*

ALZHEIMER'S DISEASE

PATHOLOGY

- Macroscopically, there is diminution of the cortex and subcortical white matter volume associated with dilation of the cortical spaces and enlargement of the lateral ventricles. The atrophy predominates in the frontal, temporal and occipital lobes (**Fig. 6.3**)
- Loss of cortical neurons
- Amyloid plaques, a central core containing amyloid surrounded by silver-staining elements derived from degenerated and enlarged neurites, are the critical pathological feature of Alzheimer's disease (**Fig. 6.4**). The major component of the amyloid is the amyloid peptide β-A4, derived from a larger transmembrane protein, amyloid precursor protein
- Neurofibrillary tangles are found in many conditions besides Alzheimer's disease and consist of silver-staining, dense, cytoplasmic, paired helical and straight filaments
- Congophilic angiopathy. The presence of amyloid in certain cerebral vessels which predisposes to their rupture. Found in approximately 40% of Alzheimer's disease patients

PATHOPHYSIOLOGY

- Substantial depletion of acetylcholine transferase and acetylcholine esterase is found, mainly in the temporal cortex
- Altered noradrenergic and 5-hydroxytryptamine activity
- β-A4 amyloid may be neurotoxic, possibly by altering neuronal calcium homeostasis and thereby altering neuronal susceptibility to the effects of excitotoxins such as glutamate

EPIDEMIOLOGY

The presenile and senile forms of Alzheimer's disease are now considered to be identical and the terms are no longer used.

- Age is the most important risk factor. Approximately 10% of the population over the age of 65 years have Alzheimer's disease and between 25 and 40% of those aged 85 years or over
- The female to male ratio is approximately 2:1
- Trauma appears to be an independent risk factor but perhaps only in people with a genetic predisposition

Genetic factors in Alzheimer's disease		
Type	**Gene**	**Chromosome**
Early onset	Amyloid precursor protein	21
Early onset	AD3	14
Late onset	Apolipoprotein E	19

Fig. 6.5 *Genetic factors in Alzheimer's disease.*

GENETIC FACTORS

A family history of Alzheimer's disease increases the risk of the disease four-fold. Familial forms are inherited as an autosomal dominant trait (**Fig. 6.5**). Mutations in the chromosome 14 locus are responsible for most early-onset, familial Alzheimer's disease. The apolipoprotein E gene on chromosome 19 has been implicated in late-onset Alzheimer's disease. Apolipoprotein E, a cholesterol transporting protein, has three common ($\epsilon2$, $\epsilon3$ and $\epsilon4$) and two uncommon alleles ($\epsilon1$, $\epsilon5$). $\epsilon3$–$\epsilon3$ is the most common genotype, present in approximately 65% of the population. The $\epsilon4$ allele elevates risk for Alzheimer's disease both in familial and non-familial, late-onset cases. The risk increase is at least partly due to an earlier age of onset in family members with $\epsilon4$–$\epsilon4$ compared with individuals without the allele.

- Alzheimer's disease accounts for over one-half of patients with dementia
- Amyloid plaques are the essential pathological feature of Alzheimer's disease
- At least one-quarter of the population over the age of 85 years have Alzheimer's disease
- The apolipoprotein E genotype $\epsilon4$–$\epsilon4$ confers a higher risk of both familial and non-familial, late-onset Alzheimer's disease

CLINICAL MANIFESTATIONS

Symptoms

Symptoms of Alzheimer's disease

- Memory loss (short term more affected than long term)
- Personality changes
- Depression
- Anxiety
- Other psychological features

Typically, the patient does not initiate the medical consultation. The vast majority of individuals who attend the neurology clinic complaining of memory loss, particularly in a younger age group, have depression, anxiety or other psychological factors triggering their complaint. Often friends or relatives have noticed a change in personality or an inability on the part of the patient to perform to their normal level in everyday decision making. Frequently, much of the history emanates from the relative. When the patient responds, there is often a tendency to deny or play down any problem and there may be a perceptible delay in word finding. It rapidly becomes apparent that short-term memory is more affected than long-term memory. The patient may have become less interested in their activities outside work and have problems remembering what they have just read. Note taking and list making are common and the patient may tend to lose direction in an unfamiliar environment. The mood may be altered. Some individuals will appear a little anxious, others become significantly depressed.

SIGNS

The examination of the patient in the early stages of the disease reveals little. There may be slight confusion about the date and the location of the interview. Speech can be a little hesitant but will not contain dysphasic errors. Short-term memory is clearly abnormal. Unless careful testing is performed, defects of praxis and gnosis are unlikely to be found. The routine neurological examination is likely to be normal. Initial screening with the Mini Mental State Examination is widely practised (**Fig. 6.6**). Early dementia is probable with a score of 24–27, although test results need to take account of the individual's education. A normal score does not exclude the diagnosis.

LATER STAGES

As the disease progresses, problems of language, praxis and gnosis become increasingly apparent. Personal care deteriorates. Extrapyramidal features often emerge with the appearance of primitive reflexes and, sometimes, myoclonus. Eventually, the patient is mute, bed-bound and doubly incontinent. The condition generally lasts between 7 and 15 years.

INVESTIGATION

Psychometry

The Mini Mental State Examination does not suffice. Formal psychometry is indicated, along with assessment of a possible depressive illness. Delayed recall is the best overall discriminator for early Alzheimer's disease.

Electrophysiology

Slowing of the dominant α rhythm occurs, along with the appearance of θ and δ activity. The P300 component of event-related potentials is either depressed or delayed in Alzheimer's disease, particularly if the test uses increasing memory loads.

Single photon emission computerized tomography

Measurement of cerebral blood flow using single photon emission computerized tomography shows a symmetrical reduction in grey matter perfusion, the degree of which correlates with the severity of the dementia. The earliest changes are found in the posterior temporoparietal cortex (**Fig. 6.7**).

Positron emission tomography

This shows bilateral reduction of oxygen use and glucose uptake, initially in the parietal and

Mini Mental State Examination

Orientation

1. What is the year, season, date, month, day? One point for each correct answer.
2. Where are we? Country, county, town, hospital, floor? One point for each correct answer.

Registration

3. Name three objects, taking one second to say each. Then ask the patient all three once you have said them. One point for each correct answer. Repeat the question until the patient learns all three.

Attention & calculation

4. Serial sevens. One point for each correct answer. Stop after five answers. Alternative: spell WORLD backwards.

Recall

5. Ask for names of objects asked in Question 3. One point for each correct answer.

Language

6. Point to a pencil and a watch. Have the patient name them for you. One point for each correct answer.
7. Have the patient repeat "No ifs, ands, or buts." One point.
8. Have the patient follow a 3-stage command. "Take the paper in your right hand; fold the paper in half; put the paper on the floor." Three points.
9. Have the patient read and obey the following: CLOSE YOUR EYES. (Write this in large letters.) One point.
10. Have the patient write a sentence of his or her own choice. (The sentence must contain a subject and an object and make some sense.) Ignore spelling errors when scoring. One point.
11. Have the patient draw two intersecting pentagons with equal sides. Give one point if all the sides and angles are preserved, and if the intersecting sides form a quadrangle.

Maximum score = 30 points

Fig. 6.6 *The Mini Mental State Examination.*

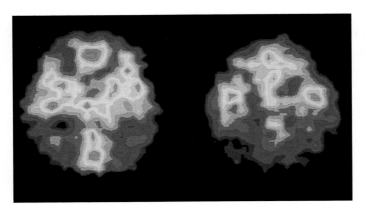

Fig. 6.7 Alzheimer's disease. *Single photon emission computerized tomography scan showing reduction of temporoparietal blood flow.*

temporal lobes but later involving the frontal lobes. The pattern can be shown to vary in different subgroups of Alzheimer's disease. The procedure can help to distinguish differing pathological types of dementia.

Computerized tomography

Brain imaging is carried out primarily to exclude other causes of dementia, for example, hydrocephalus or vascular disease. Simple measures of cortical sulcal width or ventricular volume correlate poorly with dementia. Specific measures of temporal lobe volume correlate better. Serial scanning can show progressive volume loss (**Fig. 6.8**).

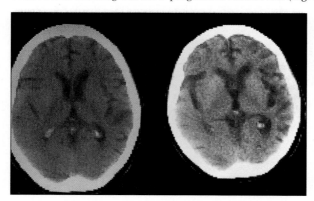

Fig. 6.8 *Alzheimer's disease.* *Serial computerized tomography scans showing progression of cortical atrophy and ventricular dilatation over a 2-year period.*

Magnetic resonance imaging

Quantitative measures of the temporal lobe, the hippocampus or amygdala have been used to study focal atrophy in Alzheimer's disease patients. The measures are complex and time consuming to apply and still fail inevitably to separate patients with early Alzheimer's disease from control individuals.

Blood tests

A full blood count, biochemical analysis and thyroid function tests are appropriate. A progressive dementia without focal signs is a very rare manifestation of pernicious anaemia or neurosyphilis but despite this, vitamin B_{12} levels and a serological test for syphilis are usually performed.

MANAGEMENT
Specific drug therapy

Tacrine, a cholinesterase inhibitor, has been shown to have a significant, although modest, effect on cognition in Alzheimer's disease patients. Perhaps 25–50% of the patients who tolerate the drug exhibit some benefit. The response is dose dependent. Hepatotoxicity occurs in at least 25% of patients.

Mood and behaviour management

Depressive symptoms occur in up to 50% of Alzheimer's disease patients. 5-hydroxytryptamine re-uptake inhibitors (e.g. sertraline) tend to be better tolerated than tricyclic antidepressants. Various behavioural disturbances (e.g. anxiety, agitation or aggression) may warrant drug therapy. Low doses of neuroleptics, for example, thioridazine, are recommended.

Other management issues

Competency – At a critical point, the individual will be unable to manage some or all of their affairs. A power of attorney allows that function to be taken over by a relative.

Institutional care – When the individual becomes so disabled that the family can no longer provide for their needs, institutional care becomes necessary. Carers tend to experience both depressive and physical symptoms when this transition becomes necessary and require on-going support.

Family support – The burden imposed on the family of a sufferer from Alzheimer's disease is difficult to overestimate. In addition to the support of the clinician and the paramedical staff, support from the Alzheimer's Disease Society is invaluable.

- Typically, a patient with Alzheimer's disease does not initiate the consultation
- There are seldom any focal neurological signs at the time of the first assessment
- Formal psychometry is usually essential to confirm the diagnosis of Alzheimer's disease, rather than relying on screening tests such as the Mini Mental State Examination
- The main role of brain imaging in the assessment of Alzheimer's is to exclude other pathologies

ARTERIOSCLEROTIC DEMENTIA (MULTI-INFARCT DEMENTIA)

Various types of vascular disease can underlie dementia, including multiple infarction, Binswanger's encephalopathy and the lacunar state. Various scales have been devised to allow a more confident clinical diagnosis of vascular dementia (**Fig. 6.9**).

The incidence of vascular dementia does not increase with age. Survival is shorter than for patients with Alzheimer's disease.

Fig. 6.9 *Vascular dementia indices.*

Vascular dementia indices	
Sudden onset	2
Stepwise course	1
Somatic complaints	1
Emotional incontinence	1
History or presence of hypertension	1
History of stroke	2
Focal neurological symptoms	2
Focal neurological signs	2
Patients with vascular dementia usually score more than 7	

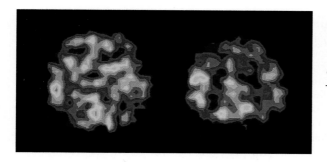

Criteria for diagnosing Lewy body dementia

- Fluctuating cognitive impairment with episodic confusion and lucid intervals

- At least one of:
  Visual or auditory hallucinations with or without delusions
  Mild spontaneous extrapyramidal features or neuroleptic sensitivity
  Repeated unexplained falls or transient clouding or loss of consciousness

- Clinical pattern persists over long periods

- No underlying physical illness to account for the fluctuating cognitive state

- Exclusion of stroke in history and by imaging

Fig. 6.11 *Criteria for diagnosing Lewy body dementia.*

In multi-infarct dementia, computerized tomography or magnetic resonance imaging reveals multiple infarction whereas single photon emission computerized tomography shows patchy blood flow reduction throughout the hemispheres (**Fig. 6.10**). Positron emission tomography, using 18F-fluorodeoxyglucose, reveals asymmetric cortical and subcortical changes.

Binswanger's disease (subcortical arteriosclerotic encephalopathy), a slowly progressive disorder albeit with fluctuations, leads to abnormalities of gait, sphincter control and pyramidal function similar to those seen in normal pressure hydrocephalus. Magnetic resonance imaging reveals striking periventricular signal change on T2-weighted images.

Patients identified as having a vascular cause for their dementia require meticulous control of relevant risk factors.

LEWY BODY DEMENTIA (DIFFUSE LEWY BODY DISEASE)

Diagnostic criteria have been suggested in an attempt to confidently separate this condition from Alzheimer's disease (**Fig. 6.11**). The disease is characterized by the presence of Lewy bodies in various parts of the cortex (**Fig. 6.12**), almost always accompanied by numerous Lewy bodies in the substantia nigra, as in Parkinson's disease. There are subtle

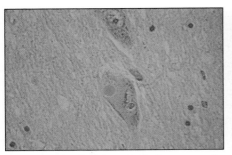

Fig. 6.12 *Cortical Lewy body in a case of Lewy body disease.*

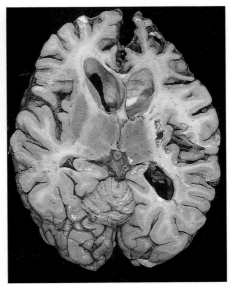

Fig. 6.13 *Pick's disease.* Axial plane section of brain. There is severe frontal lobe gyral atrophy.

morphological differences in the bodies found at these sites. Many patients with diffuse Lewy body disease have concomitant changes of Alzheimer's disease. The condition has an average duration of survival of 6 years. It responds poorly to antiparkinsonian therapy.

PICK'S DISEASE

Pick's disease is rare with a maximal prevalence among dementias of only 5%. It occurs in both sporadic and familial (autosomal dominant) forms. It generally presents at approximately the age of 60 years. Diagnostic criteria have been established: progressive dementia, predominance of frontal lobe features and behavioural changes that often precede overt memory impairment. The pathology concentrates on the frontal and temporal lobes (**Fig. 6.13**). Microscopic features include neuronal loss, spongiform gliosis and the presence of Pick bodies (intracytoplasmic inclusion structures).

OTHER DEMENTIAS

There is an almost endless list of conditions that can produce a dementia with a superficial resemblance to Alzheimer's disease. They include:
- Normal pressure hydrocephalus
- Prion disease
- Vitamin B_{12} deficiency
- Hypothyroidism
- Infections, for example, neurosyphilis
- Tumours, subdural haematomas, repetitive trauma

FOCAL DEMENTIAS

FRONTAL LOBE DEMENTIA

This condition occurs in men more than women and presents before the age of 65 years. Approximately one-half of the patients have a family history. Initial clinical features include altered language function and changes in behaviour and social conduct. Primitive reflexes emerge with extrapyramidal features. Later, the patient becomes mute. Histological features include frontotemporal atrophy with loss of large cortical neurons. Pick bodies are usually absent. Levels of choline acetyltransferase are comparable with those for control individuals. Imaging or blood flow studies confirm the predominant frontal lobe atrophy. Rarely, a frontal lobe dementia is accompanied by the features of motor neuron disease. The condition is usually inherited as an autosomal dominant form.

PRIMARY DYSPHASIC DEMENTIA (PRIMARY PROGRESSIVE APHASIA)

A degenerative process principally affecting the dominant frontotemporal lobe. It presents with a slowly progressive dysphasia without evidence of a more generalized disturbance of cognitive function. The condition is considered to be a subtype of Pick's disease.

PARIETO-OCCIPITAL ATROPHY

Characterized by asymmetrical atrophy of the parieto-occipital cortex. Clinical features include alexia, agraphia, anomia, disorders of visual fixation, visual agnosia and transcortical sensory aphasia. The pathological substrate varies. Imaging displays the characteristic distribution of the disease (**Fig. 6.14**).

- Arteriosclerotic dementia is the second most common cause of dementia
- Lewy body dementia combines characteristic cortical changes with brainstem pathology of the type seen in Parkinson's disease
- Certain focal dementias have been described, of which frontal lobe dementia is the most common

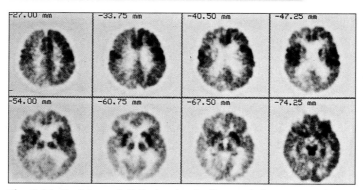

Fig. 6.14 *Parieto-occipital atrophy.* *Positron emission tomography scan. The impairment of cortical perfusion predominates posteriorly.*

APHASIA

Definition of aphasia

The loss or impairment of language caused by brain damage.

More than 99% of right-handed individuals have language function confined to the left cerebral hemisphere. The picture is more complex for left-handed individuals. Some 60% are left hemisphere dominant and 40% right hemisphere dominant but among both of these are individuals with bilateral language dominance.

An initial classification of aphasia can be made according to whether speech output is fluent or not. With fluent speech output, the lesion is posterior to the central sulcus and with non-fluent speech output, anterior to it; this classification may not be applicable in the acutely aphasic individual, in children with acquired aphasia and in many left-handed people with aphasia. Repetition is principally affected if the pathological process is in the perisylvian region. Comprehension defects in aphasic patients are of differing degree and may relate to the spoken word, the written word or both. Naming difficulty (anomia) is almost universal in aphasic patients but may display selective elements that allows some localization of the pathological process. Similarly, virtually all aphasic patients show disturbed writing ability.

CLASSIFICATION

Based on assessment of fluency, repetition, comprehension and naming, a classification of the major types of aphasia is possible (**Fig. 6.15**).

Classification of dyphasia				
	Fluency	**Repetition**	**Comprehension**	**Naming**
Broca's	Non-fluent	Abnormal	Relatively good	Abnormal
Transcortical motor	Non-fluent	Good	Relatively good	Abnormal
Wernicke's	Fluent	Abnormal	Abnormal	Abnormal
Conduction	Fluent	Abnormal	Good	Abnormal
Transcortical sensory	Fluent	Good	Abnormal	Abnormal

Fig. 6.15 *Classification of dyphasia.*

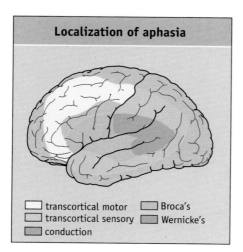

Localization of aphasia

transcortical motor ◻ Broca's
transcortical sensory ◻ Wernicke's
conduction

Fig. 6.16 *Anatomical sites associated with the various aphasic syndromes.*

Broca's aphasia

Non-fluent speech with relatively preserved comprehension. Repetition of speech is abnormal, as is naming. There is often a dysarthric element to the speech output. The lesion is in the region of the posterior inferior frontal lobe. The most common underlying pathology is cerebral infarction.

Transcortical motor aphasia

This has similar features to Broca's aphasia but the output is often repetitive as well as non-fluent and repetition is well preserved. The lesion is anterior to or superior to Broca's area and can follow infarction in the anterior cerebral territory.

Wernicke's aphasia

Output is fluent but with a loss of meaningful words and the use of paraphasias: substitution of a syllable (literal paraphasia), substitution of a word or phrase (verbal paraphasia) or the use of a nonsense word (neologism). Comprehension, repetition and naming are all substantially affected. The lesion is located in the posterior temporal region of the dominant hemisphere (**Fig. 6.16**).

Conduction aphasia

Conversational speech is fluent, with paraphasias. Articulation is intact. Comprehension is good but despite this, repetition is substantially affected. Naming and reading are impaired, although reading comprehension is relatively preserved. In some patients, the responsible lesion lies in the arcuate fasciculus, in others the lesion lies close to Wernicke's area.

Transcortical sensory aphasia

Speech is again fluent, comprehension severely defective but repetition strikingly preserved to the point where the patient inevitably incorporates the examiner's words into his or her own output (echolalia). The relevant lesion is probably in the border zone area around the posterior temporoparietal junction.

Other aphasic syndromes include anomic aphasia and global aphasia. The former has little localizing value and may be the end result in the recovery of a number of aphasic syndromes. In global aphasia, all language functions are substantially affected, typically, as the result of a substantial infarct in dominant middle cerebral artery territory.

PATHOLOGY

Many differing pathological processes lead to aphasia, of which the most common is undoubtedly cerebrovascular disease. Other processes sometimes responsible include tumour, trauma and infective processes.

MANAGEMENT

Most spontaneous recovery in aphasic individuals takes place within the first month. The role of speech therapy in stimulating further improvement beyond this time remains unsettled.

ALEXIA

This is an acquired disorder of reading function, distinct from dyslexia in which a developmental abnormality of reading exists.

ALEXIA WITH AGRAPHIA

In this condition the patient has reading difficulties, difficulty in comprehending written language and an inability to write, although copying of words may be relatively spared. Additional features that may or may not be present include visual field defects (on the right) and some degree of aphasia. The lesion is located in the region of the angular gyrus and is usually vascular in origin.

ALEXIA WITHOUT AGRAPHIA

Alexia without agraphia combines a severe reading inability with preservation of writing. Frequently, if the patient reads out the individual letters of a word, then the whole word follows. Most of the patients have a right homonymous hemianopia. There is frequently a severe colour-naming problem. Typically, there is a lesion in the left occipital cortex along with the splenium of the corpus callosum. The condition tends to resolve, although incompletely.

AGRAPHIA

Almost inevitably, patients with aphasia have some element of agraphia but agraphia is also found in other disorders. Disorders of writing can be classified into those of quality, of visuo-spatial organization, of spelling and of language content.

- Essential parts of the aphasia assessment include appraisal of fluency and measures of comprehension, repetition and naming
- Many left-handed individuals have mixed hemisphere dominance for speech
- The value of speech therapy in aphasic individuals remains unsettled

IDEOMOTOR APRAXIA

In order to diagnose this condition (or the other apraxias), it is necessary to show that the inability to carry out a motor command is not the result of a failure to understand the task and that the same task can be carried out in a different context.

Typically, the patient has difficulty in mimicking the use of an object when asked to do so. The performance improves if the patient is allowed to watch the examiner mimic the same task and, even more so, if the patient is allowed to handle the relevant object. An assessment of ideomotor apraxia should include appraisal of the orofacial musculature.

The anatomical pathway for the execution of a skilled motor task begins in Wernicke's area, and is transmitted through the arcuate fasciculus to the prefrontal area of the left hemisphere, then to the left motor cortex (for the right limbs) and across the corpus callosum to the right motor (cortex for the left limbs) (**Fig. 6.17**).

Ideomotor apraxia occurs, therefore, with lesions of the superior temporal region of the dominant hemisphere, of the arcuate fasciculus, of the premotor cortex or of the anterior corpus callosum.

IDEATIONAL APRAXIA

No single definition of this disorder has found acceptance, although the most widely used relates it to an inability to carry out a sequential motor task. The disorder has less localizing value than ideomotor apraxia and is often seen, for example, in demented patients. It is particularly liable to appear with frontal lobe damage.

LIMB-KINETIC APRAXIA

It is debatable whether this entity, referring to difficulty in fine movement typically of one hand, is truly apraxic or simply the manifestation of a subtle disorder of pyramidal function.

AGNOSIA

Definition of agnosia

Disorders of recognition in the absence of any impairment of elementary sensation.

Typically, the problem is confined to a single sensory modality, for example, vision. In some patients with visual agnosia, the problem is one of naming, the result of a disconnection of the appropriate cortical area from the speech centre. In the other form of visual agnosia, object recognition fails but the use of the object can be demonstrated when in the hand, allowing sensory data to bypass the defect of visual recognition. Such patients have damage to the visual association cortex in both hemispheres.

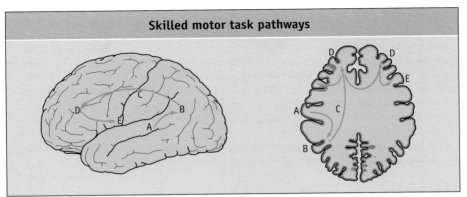

Fig. 6.17 *Pathways involved in the formulation and performance of a skilled motor task (a–e).*

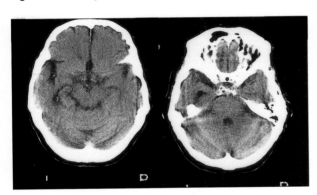

Fig. 6.18 *CT showing left temporal atrophy in a patient with primary dysphasic dementia.*

FOCAL SYNDROMES

THE FRONTAL LOBE

This leads to major effects on mood and behaviour with disinhibition and lack of concern. Spontaneous and inappropriate voiding of urine occurs with medial frontal lobe damage. There is an inability to perform complex mental tasks, with poor concentration. Abstract thinking is concrete. Various primitive reflexes are associated with frontal lobe lesions, including a grasp reflex, palmo-mental reflex and pout and suckling reflexes. Causative lesions include tumours, anterior cerebral artery occlusions, trauma, frontal lobe dementia and Pick's disease.

THE TEMPORAL LOBE

The temporal lobes are particularly concerned with memory function and its emotional content. Bilateral temporal lobe damage, for example, caused by herpes simplex encephalitis, produces a severe defect of memory function in which new memories are retained only fleetingly (Klüver–Bucy syndrome). In transient global amnesia, patients, for a period of a few hours, are unable to process or retain new information, although frequently they can still perform heavily learned, everyday tasks. The episodes seldom recur and recovery is complete. The aetiology remains uncertain. Unilateral temporal lobe atrophy is seen in primary dysphasic dementia (**Fig. 6.18**).

THE PARIETAL LOBE

Gerstmann's syndrome includes right–left disorientation, dyscalculia, dysgraphia and finger agnosia. Although originally considered to be caused by a lesion of the dominant parietal lobe, it can sometimes be seen with more diffuse pathologies. Furthermore, isolated elements of the syndrome can often be found with other parietal lobe features including constructional apraxia and aphasia. The non-dominant parietal lobe is concerned with the recognition of visual material. Certain tasks involving visuo-spatial function, for example, dressing, constructing diagrams and following a route, are dependent on non-dominant parietal function. Contralateral visual or sensory neglect is commonplace with parietal lobe lesions, particularly of the non-dominant hemisphere. Patients with right parietal pathology may ignore the affected left limbs or even deny their existence.

THE OCCIPITAL LOBE

Visual hallucinations caused by occipital lobe disturbances are usually unformed. In prosopagnosia, the individual has difficulty recognizing familiar faces, although not objects. The condition is often associated with a loss of colour perception (achromatopsia) and occurs with bilateral inferior occipital or occipitotemporal lesions. In visual disorientation, the patient is unable to localize an object in space even though fully aware of its presence. The condition is associated with bilateral parieto-occipital lesions but can sometimes, with a unilateral posterior parietal lesion, be confined to the contralateral half-field. Bilateral occipital infarction results in cortical blindness. The pupillary responses are normal. In some patients, there is denial of visual disability and confabulation of visual detail (Anton's syndrome).

- Ideomotor apraxia defines a disorder in which the ability to carry out skilled single motor tasks is lost
- Ideomotor apraxia occurs with lesions of the temporal lobe, the arcuate fasciculus, the prefrontal cortex and the corpus callosum
- A profound disorder of short-term memory function results from bilateral damage to medial temporal structures or their immediate connections

chapter 7

Cerebrovascular Disease

STROKE

Stroke is a useful term that allows discussion of the problem of cerebrovascular disease without assuming knowledge of the specific stroke mechanism. A more elaborate classification is based either on the temporal evolution of the event, its specific underlying pathology or its anatomical distribution.

Definition of transient ischaemic attack
A disorder of neurological function, thought to be ischaemic in origin, in which recovery takes place within 24 h.

Definition of reversible ischaemic neurological deficit
A disorder of neurological function, thought to be ischaemic in origin, in which recovery takes place over 3–5 days.

Definition of completed stroke
A disorder of neurological function, either ischaemic or haemorrhagic in origin, with deficit persisting beyond 5 days.

Definition of cerebral infarction
Death of brain tissue as a result of vascular occlusion. The occlusive process may affect either large or small vessels. The process is usually thrombotic or embolic.

Definition of cerebral haemorrhage
Haemorrhage within the brain substance.

Definition of subarachnoid haemorrhage
Haemorrhage into the subarachnoid space.

EPIDEMIOLOGY OF STROKE
- The third most common cause of death in the industrialized world
- Approximately 4.5 million stroke deaths each year, worldwide
- 20% of patients die within 30 days
- Subsequent mortality approximately 16–18% each year

- 90% of survivors have residual deficit and 30% are incapacitated
- Overall stroke incidence is declining
- Stroke mortality has substantially fallen in most industrialized countries in the past 20 years
- Stroke incidence is two and half times higher in Black than in White populations
- Intracranial atherosclerosis is more common in Black and Asian populations, whereas extracranial disease is more common in White populations
- For every 100 strokes (excluding subarachnoid haemorrhage), approximately 90 are caused by infarction and 10 caused by haemorrhage

RISK FACTORS FOR STROKE

- Arterial hypertension is the main risk factor for all stroke types
- Both systolic and diastolic blood pressure are independent risk factors
- Smoking increases the risk of stroke by 50%
- Polycythaemia and thrombocythaemia are both risk factors for ischaemic stroke
- Diabetes increases ischaemic stroke incidence by between two and a half and three and half times
- There is an increased concordance rate of stroke among monozygotic twins compared with dizygotic twins
- Presence of lipoprotein-a (LP[a]) is an independent risk factor for ischaemic stroke but lipid abnormalities are less relevant than they are for coronary artery or peripheral vascular disease
- Impaired cardiac function increases the risk of ischaemic stroke
- Non-rheumatic atrial fibrillation is associated with a five-fold increase in ischaemic stroke incidence

---

- The temporal definitions used for cerebrovascular events (transient ischaemic attack, reversible ischaemic neurological deficit, etc.) do not necessarily predict a particular pathological process
- Stroke incidence is declining, almost certainly the consequence of improved blood pressure control
- 90% of strokes, excluding subarachnoid haemorrhage, are ischaemic

---

CEREBRAL INFARCTION

PATHOLOGY

The outcome of cerebral ischaemia is determined by whether the process is global (e.g. after cardiac arrest) or focal (e.g. caused by a single vessel occlusion).

Global ischaemia affects the neurons most susceptible to ischaemia, particularly certain pyramidal and striatal neurons, and Purkinje cells and concentrates on the border zones between the territories of the major cerebral vessels.

Focal ischaemia produces a central zone of severe cell loss (although sparing glial cells if reperfusion occurs within an hour) surrounded by a penumbra in which ischaemic damage is less severe and potentially more reversible.

Infarction occurs with thrombus formation within the vessel, embolization to it from a proximal source or a global failure of perfusion pressure. Thrombus formation within the larger cerebral vessels is uncommon apart from in the basilar system. Within the smaller cerebral vessels, hypertension leads to thickening of the vessel wall with secondary fibrinoid degeneration (lipohyalinosis). The result is a lacunar infarct (**Fig. 7.1**). Occlusion of the larger cerebral vessels is usually embolic, the material derived from either the major extracranial vessels or the heart itself. Emboli originating from the neck arteries are composed of a fibrin–platelet mixture or cholesterol. The material is liable to form part of an atheromatous plaque, with fibrin–platelet deposition following damage to the endothelium of the vessel, typically triggered by a plaque haemorrhage (**Fig. 7.2**). Global perfusion failure occurs with cardiac arrest or severe hypotension. The areas of the brain most affected are at the margins of the territories of the major cerebral vessels (watershed infarction) (**Fig. 7.3**).

When cerebral infarction follows embolic occlusion, rapid break-up of the embolus can lead to reperfusion of the infarcted area, with subsequent extravasation of blood through damaged arterial walls (haemorrhagic infarction).

The cerebral oedema after infarction is both intracellular and extracellular. It reaches a maximum approximately 5 days after onset of the infarct. Obscuration of the cortical sulci occurs along with midline and transtentorial shift. With large infarcts, secondary compression of the brainstem results in ischaemic change and haemorrhage there and significantly contributes to mortality (**Fig. 7.4**). In the later stages, the infarcted area contracts leaving a focus of necrotic neurons associated with capillary proliferation and macroglia.

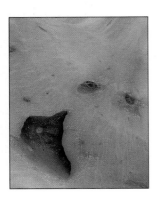

Fig. 7.1 Multiple lacunes in the right putamen.

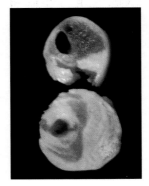

Fig. 7.2 Carotid endarterectomy specimen. *Severe stenosis with recent plaque haemorrhage.*

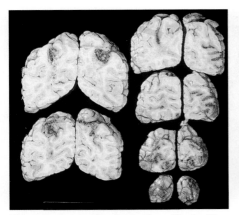

Fig. 7.3 Coronal brain sections illustrating watershed infarction consequent to cardiac surgery.

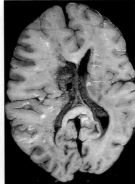

Fig. 7.4 Large acute infarct in left middle cerebral artery territory with focal haemorrhagic infarction and subfalcine herniation.

PATHOPHYSIOLOGY

As a result of ischaemia, the cell membrane is depolarized, leading to calcium ion influx and a variety of metabolic effects, including the failure of mitochondrial oxidative phosphorylation. At the same time, glutamate release alters cell membrane permeability to sodium, potassium and calcium ions. Water influx follows, leading to cerebral oedema. Other metabolic disorders include a fall in intracellular and extracellular pH caused, initially, by lactic acid production, with associated focal vasodilatation.

Areas of cerebral infarction are liable to lose their autoregulatory capacity, that is the capacity of vessels to alter their calibre in response to metabolic or neurogenic stimuli. A syndrome of luxury perfusion, in blood flow terms, is the occurrence of inappropriately high blood flow in an area adjacent to an infarct, relative to blood flow in the analogous area in the contralateral hemisphere.

Initially, after infarction, luxury perfusion is caused by loss of autoregulation. Later, it is the consequence of capillary sprouting (neovascularization). Luxury perfusion, defined metabolically, is an area in which there is a greater blood flow than is warranted by the metabolic rate (**Fig. 7.5**).

- Surrounding the zone of severe ischaemia in a cerebral infarct lies a penumbra of ischaemic tissue in which the damage is potentially reversible
- Infarction occurs with thrombosis, embolism, rare vasculopathies and a global reduction of perfusion pressure
- Cerebral oedema is an important cause of morbidity and mortality in cerebral infarction
- Major changes in ischaemic brain tissue include glutamate release, alteration of cell membrane permeability to calcium ions and lactic acidosis

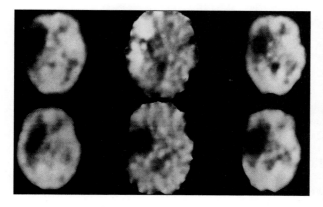

Fig. 7.5 *Positron emission tomography scans showing an infarct in the left temporoparietal region: at 8 h (upper) and 4 days (lower).* *The scans on the left indicate cerebral blood flow as expressed by emission from labelled CO_2. The scans on the right show metabolic activity as expressed by oxygen extraction. The middle scans indicate the oxygen extraction ratio. At 8 h there is an area of critical perfusion, replaced at 4 days by an area of luxury perfusion.*

CLINICAL MANIFESTATIONS

Large vessel disease

Antedating completed strokes in some patients are transient attacks of neurological dysfunction in the same arterial territory (transient ischaemic attacks [TIAs]). Most TIAs last only a few minutes. Some patients with longer TIAs have evidence of infarction on imaging. Over a follow-up period of 5 years, approximately one-third of TIA patients will progress to a completed stroke. The vast majority of TIAs are embolic in origin but a similar clinical picture can occur with non-vascular processes, for example, tumour and hypoglycaemia. Risk factors in carotid TIA patients with stenoses exceeding 70%, which add to the subsequent risk of stroke, include the severity of the carotid stenosis, the presence of ulceration or distal intraluminal thrombus on angiography and hemispheric as opposed to retinal TIA.

Symptoms of large vessel disease

- Most large cerebral infarcts present abruptly or evolve over a few hours. A more leisurely evolution is unusual, although it is seen with some basilar occlusions. Typically, infarcts from cardiogenic emboli evolve most rapidly of all
- Altered consciousness at onset is extremely unlikely with hemispheric infarction. Epilepsy may appear later (in approximately 5–10% of patients)
- Headache can equally well occur with cerebral infarction as with cerebral haemorrhage

Internal carotid territory

Atheroma commonly forms at the carotid bifurcation. Symptom formation or stroke resulting from the disease is caused by embolization from the site or complete occlusion of the internal carotid artery.

Symptoms of cerebral infarction in internal carotid territory

- Amaurosis fugax (transient monocular blindness)
- Dysphasia (if the dominant hemisphere is affected)
- Contralateral hemisensory or hemimotor disturbances

Evidence for an embolic basis for temporary vision loss is sometimes found in the form of cholesterol emboli within the fundus (**Fig. 7.6**). The degree of deficit with carotid occlusion (there may be none) is dependent on alternative avenues for sustaining flow distally, either through the circle of Willis or through branches of the external carotid. In such cases, the ipsilateral superficial temporal artery may be conspicuously distended (**Fig. 7.7**).

Anterior cerebral artery territory

This usually results from embolization but can occur as a consequence of vasospasm after subarachnoid haemorrhage (SAH), from an anterior communicating aneurysm or from subfalcine herniation (**Fig. 7.8**).

113

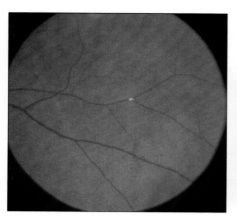

Fig. 7.6 *Multiple cholesterol emboli.*

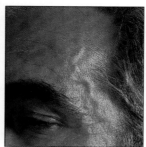

Fig. 7.7 *Distended superficial temporal artery in a patient with internal carotid occlusion.*

Anterior cerebral territory infarction

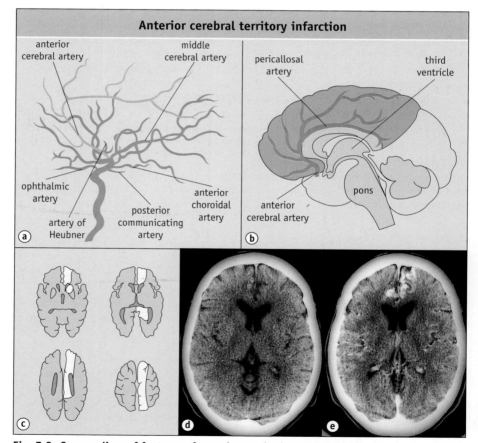

Fig. 7.8 *Compendium of features of anterior cerebral artery occlusion. (a) Angiographic localization of anterior cerebral artery. (b) Distribution of anterior cerebral artery (medial aspect of hemisphere). (c) Distribution of infarct in four brain sections. (d and e) Precontrast and postcontrast CT scans showing bilateral enhancing infarcts.*

The deficit is dependent on whether or not there is involvement of the artery of Heubner.

- Distal lesions produce weakness predominating in the lower limb, with sensory loss, and, in some cases, apraxia
- Proximal lesions produce a more complete hemiplegia. With both lesions there may be frontal lobe release signs and a transcortical motor aphasia if the dominant hemisphere is affected

Middle cerebral artery territory

Occlusions may occur in several areas with differing results (**Fig. 7.9**).

Main stem occlusion – Severe disability with a contralateral motor and sensory deficit, a homonymous hemianopia and a global aphasia if the dominant hemisphere is affected. Anosognosia, spatial disorientation and neglect may be prominent.

Occlusion of deep perforators – Usually caused by main vessel occlusion but with cortical sparing as a result of collateral circulation. It produces predominantly a contralateral hemimotor deficit.

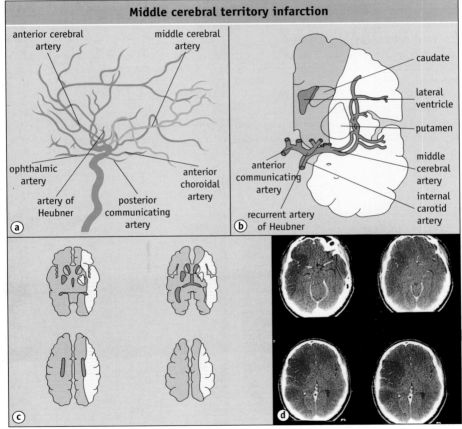

Fig. 7.9 *Compendium of features of middle cerebral artery occlusion.* (*a*) *Angiographic localization of middle cerebral artery.* (*b*) *Distribution of middle cerebral artery (coronal section).* (*c*) *Distribution of infarct in four brain sections.* (*d*) *CT appearance.*

115

Occlusion of superior trunk – Contralateral motor and sensory deficit with relative sparing of the leg. The temporal lobe is unaffected.

Occlusion of inferior trunk – Superior quadrantic hemianopia, visuo-spatial disorder (non-dominant hemisphere) or Wernicke-type aphasia (dominant hemisphere).

Occlusion of cortical branches – Deficit depends on area of cortex affected.

Posterior circulation territory

If the subclavian artery is occluded or severely stenosed proximal to the origin of the vertebral artery, reversed flow down the vertebral artery may occur when the limb is exercised (subclavian steal syndrome). Although the radiological finding is common, convincing cases of hindbrain ischaemia during exercise of the limb are rare.

Vertebral artery disease

Extracranial vertebral artery occlusion may be asymptomatic if the contralateral vertebral artery is of wide calibre. More distal vertebral stenosis or occlusion can lead to distal embolization, reduced flow in the distribution of the posterior inferior cerebellar artery (lateral medullary syndrome) (**Fig. 7.10**) and cerebellar infarction.

Lateral medullary infarction

Ipsilateral to the infarct are found a Horner's syndrome, facial spinothalamic loss, palatal paresis and cerebellar signs. Contralaterally, there is limb spinothalamic loss. The gait is unstable.

Cerebellar infarction

This is often the consequence of an intracranial vertebral artery occlusion. Clinical features include headache, dizziness and ipsilateral cerebellar signs with ipsilateral brainstem signs, for example, gaze paresis and facial paresis. Oedema can lead to obstruction of the fourth ventricle and hydrocephalus (**Fig. 7.11**).

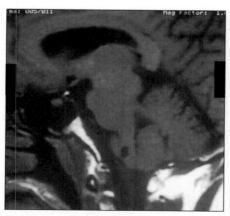

Fig. 7.10 Lateral medullary infarct.
Sagittal T1-weighted MRI.

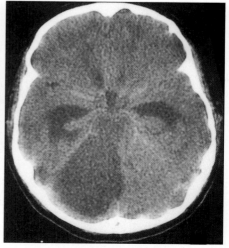

Fig. 7.11 Cerebellar infarction with secondary hydrocephalus. *CT appearance.*

Basilar artery disease

Proximal basilar occlusions tend to be thrombotic, distal ones embolic. With proximal occlusions, pontine damage tends to be conspicuous with tetraparesis, cranial nerve involvement and oculomotor signs, including gaze paresis, internuclear ophthalmoplegia or one-and-a-half syndrome (see p. 72). Distal basilar occlusions produce midbrain damage with pupillary abnormalities, abnormalities of vertical gaze and an altered state of consciousness.

POSTERIOR CEREBRAL ARTERY TERRITORY

Most posterior cerebral artery occlusions (**Fig. 7.12**) are embolic, although some occur during herniation of the brain through the tentorial notch.

Proximal occlusions produce infarction of the occipital lobe and the medial and inferior aspects of the temporal lobe, together with parts of the thalamus and midbrain. With distal occlusions, the deeper structures are spared. Clinical features include:

- Contralateral homonymous hemianopia that may be complete, quadrantic or paracentral

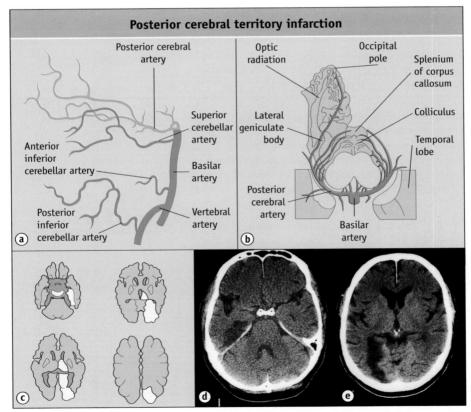

Fig. 7.12 Compendium of features of posterior cerebral artery occlusion. (*a*) Angiographic localization of posterior cerebral artery. (*b*) Distribution of posterior cerebral artery. (*c*) Distribution of infarct in four brain sections. (*d and e*) CT appearance.

- Thalamic infarction leads to contralateral sensory loss sometimes with spontaneous pain and hypersensitivity to contact (thalamic syndrome)
- Combined infarction of the left occipital lobe and the splenium of the corpus callosum results in alexia without agraphia
- Infarction of the angular gyrus can produce a combination of right–left disorientation, finger agnosia, dyscalculia and dysgraphia (Gerstmann's syndrome). Various combinations of these findings can occur with lesions in this area and the existence of a specific syndrome is debatable
- Visual agnosia can occur with left posterior cerebral territory infarction
- Prosopagnosia (difficulty in recognizing familiar faces) is seen with some right posterior cerebral territory infarcts
- Bilateral posterior cerebral occlusions (usually caused by a distal basilar embolus) produce bilateral occipital lobe infarction. Cortical blindness with a denial of disability may follow (Anton's syndrome)

- TIAs are followed by stroke in approximately one-third of patients over a 5-year follow-up
- Most carotid territory ischaemic strokes are caused by embolic material derived from the heart or the neck vessels
- Proximal basilar artery occlusions tend to be thrombotic, distal ones embolic

---

MULTIPLE TERRITORY INFARCTION

When multiple territory infarction has occurred, dementia may be added to the deficits imposed by the individual lesions. The presence of multiple territory infarction raises the possibility of embolization from a proximal source, particularly the heart (**Fig. 7.13**). Early identification of cardiogenic emboli is important as a recurrence rate of 20% is reported within 2 weeks of the first event. It has been estimated that cardiogenic embolism accounts for one in six ischaemic strokes (**Fig. 7.14**).

Sources of cardiogenic embolization	
Cardiac dysrhythmia	e.g. Atrial fibrillation
Left ventricular dysfunction	e.g. Myocardial infarction Ventricular aneurysm
Valvular diseases	e.g. Rheumatic heart disease Prosthetic valves Mitral valve prolapse Endocarditis
Paradoxical emboli	e.g. Patent foramen ovale
Rarer causes	e.g. Atrial myxoma

Fig. 7.13 *Sources of cardiogenic embolization.*

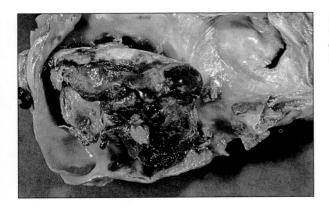

Fig. 7.14 *Mitral stenosis with a large thrombus almost completely filling the left atrium.*

Features of cardiogenic embolism

- Non-progressive onset
- Specific arterial territory involvement
- Isolated hemianopia
- Wernicke's aphasia
- Ideomotor apraxia

SMALL VESSEL DISEASE

LACUNAR INFARCTION

Arterial hypertension is the major risk factor for lacunar infarction. Most lacunes are less than 1 cm in diameter. They occur predominantly in the basal ganglia, thalamus and pons. Large lacunes are thought to be caused by atheromatous occlusion of small intracerebral arteries. Clinically, lacunar infarcts tend not to be preceded by TIAs. The deficit is liable to evolve more slowly than with large infarcts and is not associated with headache or seizures. Certain clinical patterns are suggestive of a lacunar aetiology:

- Pure motor hemiplegia
- Dysarthria: clumsy hand syndrome
- Ataxic hemiparesis
- Hemisensory stroke

BINSWANGER'S ENCEPHALOPATHY (SUBCORTICAL ARTERIOSCLEROTIC ENCEPHALOPATHY)

This is associated with diffuse loss of the subcortical white matter, probably caused by ischaemia secondary to degenerative changes in the relevant arterioles (**Fig. 7.15**). The

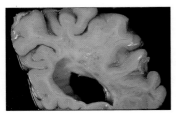

Fig. 7.15 *Binswanger's encephalopathy.* Coronal brain slice of right parieto-occipital region. The affected white matter is somewhat granular with preservation of subcortical 'U' fibres.

119

clinical picture includes progressive dementia, pyramidal signs, incontinence and gait disorder. There is a close relationship, pathologically, between the changes of Binswanger's disease and lacunar infarction.

- Cerebral emboli from the heart tend to produce a sudden, non-progressive deficit with a liability to early recurrence
- Lacunar infarction results from lipohyalinosis in small perforating arteries, the consequence of hypertension
- Binswanger's encephalopathy is one of the causes of vascular dementia and has a characteristic appearance on MRI

INVESTIGATION

Blood tests

Certain blood tests should be done in all patients with ischaemic stroke or TIA. Others will be confined to younger patients or when certain features in the history or examination suggest their necessity (**Fig. 7.16**). Some of the more esoteric test results can be influenced by the stroke event itself and may have to be repeated later.

Blood tests in stroke or transient ischaemic attack	
All patients	Full blood count
	Erythrocyte sedimentation rate
	U & E
	Glucose or glucose tolerance test
	Cholesterol
	Prothrombin time
	Partial thromboplastin time
Additional tests in younger patients	Serological test for syphilis
	Triglyceride
	Lipoproteins
Tests that may be suggested by particular clinical features	Anti-phospholipid antibodies
	Protein C
	Protein S
	Antithrombin III
	Factor V leiden

Fig. 7.16   *Blood tests in stroke or transient ischaemic attack.*

Cardiological tests

A standard 12-lead electrocardiogram should be performed in all stroke or TIA patients. The value of more prolonged electrocardiogram monitoring is questionable unless the history is particularly suggestive of cardiac dysrhythmia.

If patients with known or clinically evident cardiac disease and those with a history of arrhythmia are excluded, the value of routine echocardiography in stroke or TIA patients is debatable, although it is advisable in all young patients, say, under 45 years of age.

Transthoracic two-dimensional echocardiography is the initial test of choice but transoesophageal echocardiography is indicated if cardiac embolism is strongly suspected or if the left atrium and appendage require careful appraisal.

Non-invasive vascular screening

Oculoplethysmography and ophthalmodynamometry have been replaced by Doppler techniques in the evaluation of extracranial carotid disease. Colour-coded Doppler combines real-time haemodynamic Doppler measurements superimposed on a two-dimensional ultrasound image. The accuracy for identifying high-grade carotid stenoses approaches that of conventional intra-arterial angiography, although the technique sometimes wrongly identifies very severe stenoses as complete occlusions (**Fig. 7.17**). Abnormal or absent flow can be detected in the vertebral arteries. Transcranial Doppler techniques allow imaging of the origins of the major intracranial vessels. The technique can also identify circulating asymptomatic cerebral emboli in patients with relevant cardiac disease.

Magnetic resonance angiography

This is increasingly likely to replace conventional angiography for showing the state of the extracranial vessels.

Angiography

Angiography remains the investigation of choice in patients with carotid territory TIA or minor stroke for whom operative intervention is considered a possibility. Aortic flush angiograms have a very low morbidity in terms of cerebral complications but provide less information than images obtained after selective catheterization The addition of oblique views of the bifurcation substantially adds to the ease of diagnosing irregular or ulcerating plaques (**Fig. 7.18**).

Computerized tomography scanning

The computerized tomography (CT) scan is often normal in the first 24 h after an ischaemic stroke. Subsequently, a low-density area appears with contrast enhancement in approximately 70% of patients. The enhancement is most prominent approximately 2 weeks after onset and, rarely, can persist for several weeks. CT scanning is of limited value in detecting cerebellar and brainstem infarcts. Sometimes, thrombus formation within a cerebral vessel can be identified as a hyperdense area on precontrast views (**Fig. 7.19**).

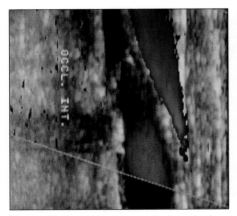

Fig. 7.17 *Carotid artery occlusion.* *Duplex scan. There is calcification beyond the occlusion.*

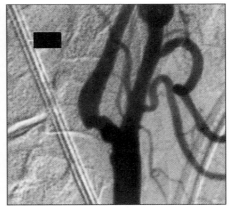

Fig. 7.18 *Plaque at the origin of the internal carotid artery.* *Carotid angiogram.*

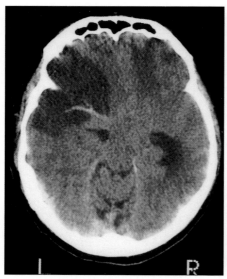

Fig. 7.19 *Thrombus within the left middle cerebral artery.* CT appearance.

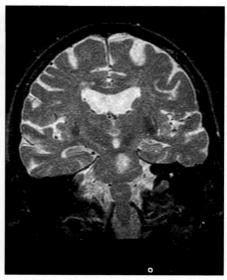

Fig. 7.20 *Infarct in the basis pontis.* Dual echo T2-weighted coronal MRI.

Magnetic resonance imaging

Magnetic resonance imaging (MRI) is more sensitive than CT for the detection of a recent ischaemic stroke. Abnormalities appear on MRI before being seen on CT and, initially, consist in an alteration of the signal gradient between the cortex and subcortex. MRI is far superior in the detection of brainstem and cerebellar strokes and is capable of detecting early haemorrhagic transformation. Areas of periventricular hyperintensity are found in patients with Binswanger's encephalopathy, which correlate with postmortem evidence of gliosis, demyelination and axonal loss. For most patients, however, MRI is unnecessary in the routine investigation of stroke (**Fig. 7.20**).

- A normal cardiological examination and electrocardiogram excludes the vast majority of cardiogenic causes of cerebral infarction
- Doppler studies of the neck arteries are a highly accurate screen for carotid stenosis, although they may have difficulty distinguishing a very severe stenosis from a complete occlusion
- CT scanning is a satisfactory imaging procedure for most stroke patients

MANAGEMENT

Primary prevention

A reduction in diastolic pressure of 5–6 mmHg produces a reduction of 41% in the stroke rate over 2–3 years, irrespective of initial diastolic level.

Patients under 60 years of age with lone atrial fibrillation but no other risk factors do not merit anticoagulation. Patients over 60 years old should be given either warfarin (to achieve an INR of 2–3) or aspirin, at a dose of 325 mg/day. Aspirin may not be effective in patients over 75 years of age, in whom warfarin, although effective, imposes an increasing risk of haemorrhage.

Stroke rate in patients with myocardial infarction admitted to hospital is approximately 1% and is most common in the first 24 h. If aspirin, in a dose of 162.5 mg/day is begun within 24 h of acute myocardial infarction, the 35-day non-fatal stroke rate is reduced by 46%.

Low-dose aspirin, supplementary to warfarin, in patients with prosthetic or tissue valve replacements and atrial fibrillation further reduces the risk of thrombo-embolism.

As yet there are no conclusive data as to whether patients with asymptomatic severe carotid disease should have surgery.

Secondary prevention

Patients who have had an embolic event in relationship to atrial fibrillation should be anticoagulated. A 22% reduction in non-fatal stroke occurs in patients with TIA or minor stroke treated with aspirin. Both men and women respond. The drug appears to be effective in preventing lacunar infarction. The optimal dose for aspirin is not yet fixed. Options range from 75 to 1200 mg/day. Alternative drugs for those intolerant of aspirin include sulphinpyrazone and dipyridamole.

Carotid surgery

For patients with carotid stenoses exceeding 70% who have experienced TIAs or minor strokes in the relevant carotid territory, surgery improves stroke-free survival. The surgical hazard (in terms of disabling stroke or death) is approximately 2%. Patients with less than 70% stenoses do not benefit.

- A reduction of diastolic pressure significantly reduces stroke incidence
- Patients with lone atrial fibrillation have a five times higher stroke risk than those in sinus rhythm
- Aspirin reduces stroke rate in TIA patients by approximately 20%
- Carotid surgery is indicated for symptomatic carotid stenosis of greater than 70%

Management of the completed stroke

Blood pressure control – Elevated blood pressure is seldom treated in the acute stages of stroke, unless there is concomitant cardiac failure. A transient rise in blood pressure after stroke is common. Overzealous correction of raised blood pressure is liable to further depress flow in areas lacking autoregulation.

Cerebral oedema – Cytotoxic oedema is probably more important than vasogenic oedema in ischaemic stroke. Steroids are without effect. Glycerol possibly reduces oedema with a beneficial effect on death rate. If there is coning, temporary reversal is achieved using 20% mannitol.

Haemodilution – No firm evidence for benefit exists.

Thrombolysis – The most effective agent is recombinant tissue plasminogen activator. No firm evidence exists for its role, how soon after stroke it needs to be given and by what route.

Calcium channel blockers – These are probably of no value.

Other measures

Fluid balance – Dehydration, with its effects on viscosity and blood flow, should be avoided.

Avoidance of pulmonary embolism – Preventative therapy lowers the risk of deep-vein thrombosis. Either low-dose heparin (500–1000 U/day) is given intravenously or low-molecular weight heparin subcutaneously.

Stroke units – Patients undergoing intensive rehabilitation after stroke probably benefit in terms of duration of hospital stay, likelihood of discharge, walking and transfer capacities and scores on activities of daily living. Benefit is less likely in older patients, individuals with severe disability and patients with cognitive impairment.

Depression is common after stroke and should be treated vigorously with antidepressants.

Programmes designed to improve motor outcome have not been adequately tested. Arm function after stroke reaches maximal recovery within 2 months of onset.

Speech and swallow therapy – The role of speech therapy in influencing speech outcome after stroke remains unclear. Similarly, it is not established that intensive swallow therapy supervised by a therapist in patients with dysphagia after stroke is any more successful than simple diet and swallow advice to patients and their carers.

Outcome

The principal factors predicting poor outcome after stroke are:
- Altered consciousness
- Complete paralysis
- Hemianopia
- Cognitive deficit
- Incontinence

- Blood pressure control is seldom necessary immediately after stroke onset
- Cerebral oedema associated with stroke is resistant to drug therapy
- Patients benefit from admission to a Stroke Unit provided they do not have severe disability

---

OTHER CAUSES OF CEREBRAL INFARCTION

DISSECTION

Perhaps 2% of first strokes are caused by arterial dissection. Intramural haematoma formation leads to constriction of the arterial lumen, with the hazard of thrombus formation and distal embolization. The dissection may be spontaneous, secondary to trauma or associated with anomalies of the arterial wall.

INTERNAL CAROTID DISSECTION

Tends to occur in middle-aged individuals and typically begins approximately 2 cm above the carotid bifurcation. Medial dissection is the rule extracranial; it predominates in middle-aged adults and is often associated with arterial wall disease. Subintimal dissection occurs intracranially in younger individuals.

CLINICAL MANIFESTATIONS

Presentations include:
- Unilateral headache, sometimes with neck pain. Horner's syndrome is found in 50% of patients
- Carotid territory ischaemia in the form of transient ischaemia or completed stroke
- Other cranial nerve dysfunction, particularly the hypoglossal nerve
- Ipsilateral pulsatile tinnitus, perhaps in one-third of patients
- Subarachnoid haemorrhage (for intracranial dissections)

INVESTIGATION

Doppler studies can strongly suggest the diagnosis but more specific information is obtained from MRI, magnetic resonance angiography or conventional angiography. Radiological appearances include a tapering occlusion of the internal carotid artery, double-lumen formation, a long stenotic channel (string-sign) and pouching or pseudo-aneurysm formation (**Fig. 7.21**).

OUTCOME AND MANAGEMENT

Dissected arteries re-open in the majority of survivors. Recurrence of the dissection is rare. There are no exact figures for prognosis, although a significant number of patients die in the acute stage or have residual deficit. The patient with extracranial carotid dissection is anticoagulated with heparin and then warfarin. Serial Doppler studies are used to determine the duration of treatment, which averages approximately 6 months.

Vertebrobasilar dissection

Less common than carotid dissection and may be either extracranial or intracranial. Extracranial vertebral dissections tend to affect the distal portion of the artery and are commonly bilateral. They predominate in women. Very characteristic is a pain ipsilateral to the dissection in the region of the neck and the mastoid process. Intracranial vertebral dissections predominate near to the origin of the posterior inferior cerebellar artery. Many of the patients with intracranial vertebral dissections present with SAH rather than with ischaemic events in vertebrobasilar territory. Basilar dissections are rare and usually fatal. Predisposing factors include trauma, neck manipulation and hypertension. In addition to typical angiographic findings, CT or MRI may show thrombus formation within the vertebral or basilar system (**Fig. 7.22**). Anticoagulation is used, certainly for the extracranial cases.

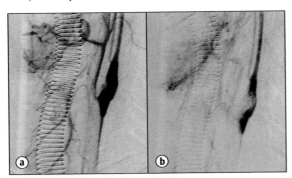

Fig. 7.21 *Carotid dissection.* *(a) Contrast remains in the proximal segment of the internal carotid artery (ICA). (b)The ICA then progressively tapers distally.*

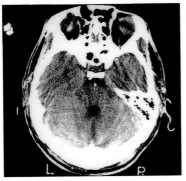

Fig. 7.22 *Vertebrobasilar dissection.* *CT showing high-density signal in the basilar artery (precontrast).*

Vasculitis

Many different conditions either have vasculitis as a major component or as part of a broader spectrum of pathologies. They include polyarteritis nodosa, systemic lupus erythematosus and various drug-induced conditions (see p 287–289).

Primary angiitis of the central nervous system, a vasculitic disorder with cellular infiltration, leads to headache, confusion, intellectual decline and focal neurological events. The erythrocyte sedimentation may be modestly raised. The cerebrospinal fluid often shows a lymphocytosis with a moderately raised protein concentration. Angiography may reveal focal areas of stenosis alternating with segments of dilation. The condition is usually treated with corticosteroids and cyclophosphamide.

Amphetamines can induce stroke, usually of a haemorrhagic type but sometimes ischaemic, possibly then caused by a vasculitis. A similar picture is seen with phenylpropanolamine. Cocaine abuse has been associated with both haemorrhagic and ischaemic stroke.

Pregnancy-associated stroke

Vasoconstriction of intracerebral vessels can occur in association with pre-eclampsia or eclampsia. Features include headache, seizures and focal neurological deficit. CT sometimes shows low-density areas that later resolve, as do the clinical deficits in most patients.

Antiphospholipid syndrome

Clinical signs that have been attributed to the presence of antiphospholipid antibodies include a migraine-like condition, retinal ischaemia and an encephalopathic condition with stroke-like events. Other features described include venous thrombosis, multiple spontaneous abortions and livedo reticularis. Some of these patients appear to have a variant of systemic lupus. The mechanism of the stroke is uncertain.

Radiation-associated carotid disease

An atherosclerotic process triggered by neck irradiation can develop some years after initial exposure, leading then to cerebral ischaemia (**Fig. 7.23**).

CADASIL

Cerebral autosomal dominant arteriopathy with subcortical infarcts and leukoencephalopathy (CADASIL) has been mapped to chromosome 19. Typically, it presents in the third decade of life with attacks of migraine with aura. Within 10 years, recurrent ischaemic events, often in the form

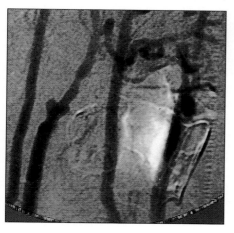

Fig. 7.23 Irradiation damage of the neck vessels after therapy for carcinoma of the thyroid. The right internal carotid artery is occluded at its origin, whereas the left has a distal stenosed segment.

of lacunar infarcts, have appeared, followed later by dementia. The vascular process principally affects leptomeningeal and perforating arteries and consists of an infiltration of the vessels' media by a material of unknown origin. MRI reveals multiple subcortical infarcts with a diffuse white matter disorder.

- Perhaps 2% of first strokes are caused by dissection
- Extracranial carotid and vertebral dissection are treated with anticoagulants
- 50% of carotid dissections are associated with a Horner's syndrome. Vertebral dissection is commonly associated with severe ipsilateral neck and occipital pain
- The possession of antiphospholipid antibodies probably increases stroke risk

CEREBRAL HAEMORRHAGE

Intraparenchymal haemorrhage is responsible for approximately 10% of all strokes. The major cause other than trauma is hypertension (**Fig. 7.24**).

RISK FACTORS
Hypertension, previous cerebral infarction, coronary artery disease and diabetes mellitus are all risk factors for cerebral haemorrhage.

HYPERTENSIVE CEREBRAL HAEMORRHAGE

PATHOLOGY
In hypertensive individuals, there is an increased incidence of small aneurysms (micro-aneurysms), predominating in the small penetrating arteries supplying the deep areas of the brain and the junction of grey and white matter in the subcortex (**Fig. 7.25**). The distribution of the aneurysms follows that of hypertensive-related intraparenchymal haemorrhage and includes the putamen, thalamus, cerebellum, pons and the subcortical white matter. Superficial, lobar haemorrhage is more likely to be related to vascular malformation, amyloid angiopathy or a bleeding diathesis.

Causes of intraparenchymal haemorrhage
- Trauma
- Hypertension
- Vascular malformation
- Aneurysm
- Amyloid angiopathy
- Bleeding diathesis
- Tumours
- Drugs

Fig. 7.24 *Causes of intraparenchymal haemorrhage.*

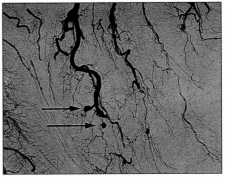

Fig. 7.25 *Aneurysms (arrowed) on the lateral branches of a main striate artery in a hypertensive patient.*

CLINICAL MANIFESTATIONS

Symptoms

Symptoms of hypertensive cerebral haemorrhage

Focal neurological deficit (in about 80% of patients)
Alteration of consciousness (in about 50% of patients)
Headache (in about 40% of patients)
Vomiting (in about 30% of patients)
Seizures (in about 10% of patients)

Symptoms generally evolve over minutes or hours but exceptionally can evolve over several weeks with headache, personality change, seizures and progressive hemiparesis. The distribution of the haematoma can be predicted, to some extent, from the presenting signs.

PUTAMENAL HAEMATOMA

Clinical features include contralateral motor and sensory deficits with conjugate ocular deviation to the side of the lesion.

THALAMIC HAEMATOMA

The predominant limb signs include contralateral sensory loss and involuntary movement, including dystonia or chorea. With medial thalamic involvement, the eyes may deviate away from the side of the lesion. Sometimes, there is a combination of ocular deviation, convergence and constricted pupils. Alteration of the state of consciousness is common.

PONTINE HAEMATOMA

Large pontine haematomas occupy the central pons, sometimes extending to the midbrain and fourth ventricle (**Fig. 7.26**). The patient is usually comatose with a tetraparesis, decerebrate rigidity, paresis of horizontal eye movements and small or very small but reactive pupils. Smaller, basal, lateralized haematomas produce a contralateral hemiparesis, sometimes with ataxia whereas lateral tegmental haematomas produce various oculomotor disturbances, including internuclear ophthalmoplegia, one-and-a-half syndrome and gaze paresis (**Fig. 7.27**).

CEREBELLAR HAEMATOMA

Most cerebellar haematomas occur in the region of the dentate nucleus. A minority of patients have severe headache or depressed consciousness. Presenting symptoms include vomiting (60%), headache (40%), vertigo (33%), ataxia, altered consciousness and dysarthria. With expansion, secondary brainstem compression occurs, leading to gaze paresis and pyramidal signs.

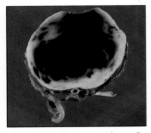

Fig. 7.26 *Cross-section of the pons showing a hypertensive haemorrhage.*

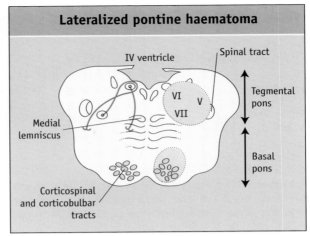

Fig. 7.27 *Basal and lateral tegmental pontine haematomas.*

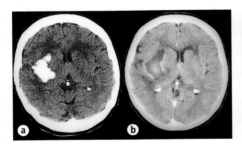

Fig. 7.28 *Cerebral haematoma.* (*a*) Acute stage. (*b*) Resolving to hypodense zone with marginal enhancement. CT scan.

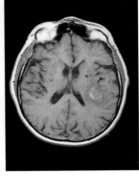

Fig. 7.29 *Haematoma scanned at 48 h.* A small area of hyperintensity caused by methaemoglobin is surrounded by hypointensity caused by a combination of blood and oedema. T1-weighted MRI.

INVESTIGATION

Computerized tomography

CT scanning identifies virtually all symptomatic haematomas but provides limited information about any associated vascular malformation. The procedure identifies any rupture of the haematoma into the ventricular system. At a later stage, the lesion may show enhancement, often with a ring pattern (**Fig. 7.28**).

Magnetic resonance imaging

The MRI appearance of an intraparenchymal haemorrhage depends on the age of the haemorrhage. Within 6–12 h of onset, deoxyhaemoglobin has formed within the red cells, leading to hypointensity on T2-weighted images. After 2–3 days, the deoxyhaemoglobin is converted to methaemoglobin in a centripetal fashion leading to increased signal on both T1- and T2-weighted images (**Fig. 7.29**). Eventually, haemosiderin accumulates in the margins of the haematoma, producing a rim of hypointensity on T2-weighted images.

Angiography

Is generally not considered in typical hypertensive haematomas.

PROGNOSIS AND MANAGEMENT

- 30-day mortality for intraparenchymal haemorrhage is approximately 30%
- Approximately 50% of patients with intraparenchymal haemorrhage make a complete or good recovery
- Poor outcome is predicted by large haematomas, depressed level of consciousness and increasing age. Intraventricular extension of the haematoma has also been identified as a poor risk factor
- Surgical intervention is seldom undertaken for supratentorial haematomas
- Surgical intervention for cerebellar haematomas is considered for patients with large haematomas who have a depressed level of consciousness or acute hydrocephalus
- Medical management includes hyperventilation and osmotic diuretics in patients with acutely elevated intracranial pressure. Steroids are worthless

---

- Hypertension is the most important risk factor for non-traumatic cerebral haemorrhage
- CT is the most valuable screening procedure
- Angiography is seldom indicated for hypertensive haematomas
- Surgical intervention is seldom indicated except for some cases of cerebellar haematoma

---

VASCULAR MALFORMATIONS

PATHOLOGY

Capillary telangiectasiae are common but usually clinically silent. Venous angiomas contain multiple low-pressure channels draining to a single central vein that usually then passes to the periphery of the structure. They are usually silent. Cavernous haemangiomas (cavernomas) predominate in the subcortex and contain thin-walled sinusoidal spaces. Arteriovenous malformations (AVMs) contain dilated arteries and veins joined by cavernous spaces in place of capillaries.

EPIDEMIOLOGY

Presentation is usually before the age of 30 years. Men are affected slightly more often than women. Approximately 10% of patients with AVMs have one or more berry aneurysms.

CLINICAL MANIFESTATIONS

Presentation is with headache, seizures or haemorrhage, which may be intraparenchymal or subarachnoid in distribution. The association between AVMs and recurrent unilateral headache remains uncertain.

INVESTIGATION

For AVMs, precontrast CT shows a mixed density lesion, sometimes with areas of calcification. Enhancement identifies the nucleus and the dilated draining veins (**Fig. 7.30**).

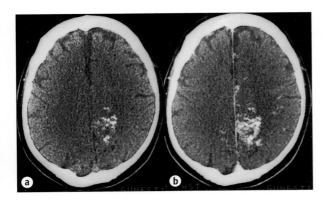

Fig. 7.30 *Partly calcified AVM. (a)* Precontrast and *(b)* postcontrast CT.

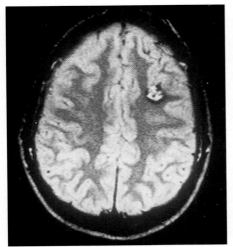

Fig. 7.31 *Cavernous angioma. There is a hyperintense core surrounded by a zone of hypointensity. T2-weighted MRI.*

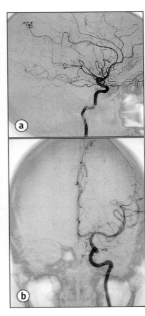

Fig. 7.32 *Right para-sagittal AVM. (a)* Lateral *and (b)* anteroposterior angiography.

MRI changes are influenced by whether the lesion has bled and its nature. For AVMs, in the absence of blood, the scan shows distended vascular spaces, with flow void secondary to rapid flow and turbulence. Cavernomas show a central nucleus that appears hyperintense on T1 and T2 images with a surrounding hypointensity on T2 images, reflecting the accumulation of haemosiderin in the surrounding brain tissue (**Fig. 7.31**).

Angiography

Angiography defines the feeding vessels and draining veins. Both external and internal carotid artery injection may be needed when defining feeders to hemispheric AVMs (**Fig. 7.32**). Some angiomas are not visualized because either they are too small, their vessels have thrombosed or an adjacent haematoma is compressing the relevant vessels. Cavernomas are not identified, probably because of the low rate of blood flow through them.

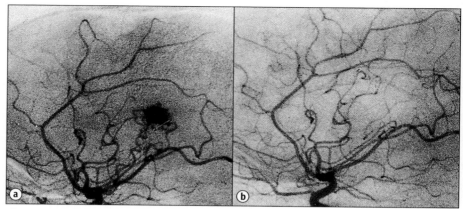

Fig. 7.33 *AVM treated by stereotactic radiotherapy.* *Lateral views (a) before and (b) after treatment.*

PROGNOSIS

- The risk of rebleeding after haemorrhage from a cerebral AVM is 6% in the first year and 2–4% each year thereafter (the same rate as in patients without a history of haemorrhage)
- Combined mortality and morbidity after haemorrhage from an AVM approaches 50%
- A proportion of patients with AVMs without evidence of haemorrhage show progressive intellectual impairment

MANAGEMENT

The three main techniques are direct surgical approach, embolization and radiation therapy. Larger AVMs are sometimes treated with partial embolization before surgical excision. The morbidity of surgery is influenced by the size and position of the AVM. Overall combined morbidity and mortality is approximately 10%. Postoperative neurological deficit tends to improve. Stereotactic radiosurgery is of value for small (less than 3 cm) surgically inaccessible lesions. Approximately three-quarters are obliterated 2 years after treatment, during which there is still a risk of rebleeding. A small proportion of patients develop radiation necrosis (**Fig. 7.33**). Cavernomas and angiographically occult AVMs are managed surgically.

AMYLOID ANGIOPATHY

In this condition, which presents in middle-aged and elderly people, deposition of amyloid occurs in leptomeningeal and cortical arteries, often associated with the presence of senile plaques in the cerebrum. Secondary degeneration of the arterial wall leads to fibrinoid necrosis and micro-aneurysm formation. Rupture of the affected vessels produces superficial, often multiple, haematomas in the parietal, temporal and occipital lobes.

COAGULATION DISORDERS

Intracerebral haemorrhage is a recognized hazard of anticoagulant therapy and can occur in thrombocytopaenia, whatever the cause. In anticoagulant-related cases, the risk correlates with the degree of prolongation of the prothrombin time. The clinical deficit often evolves over several days and has a high morbidity and mortality. Despite the underlying indication for warfarin, the patient should be treated with vitamin K and fresh frozen plasma. Bleeding into the brain is a recognized hazard in patients with either factor VIII or factor IX deficiency (**Fig. 7.34**).

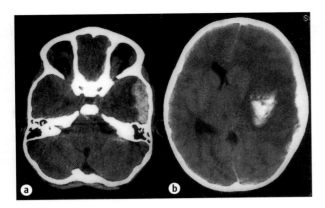

Fig. 7.34 Subdural (a) and intracerebral haematoma (b) in a patient with factor IX deficiency.

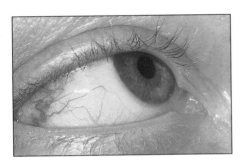

Fig. 7.35 Dilated conjunctival vessels in a patient with a dural fistula.

DRUGS

Various substances of abuse are known to cause intracerebral haemorrhage. They include amphetamines and cocaine.

TRAUMA

Traumatic haematomas are found most often in the frontal, temporal and occipital lobes. They may co-exist with subdural haematomas and evidence of cerebral contusion.

- AVMs present with bleeding much earlier than saccular aneurysms
- Angiography sometimes fails to show AVMs and usually fails to show cavernomas
- Larger AVMs are best managed by embolization and surgery, smaller AVMs by radiosurgery

DURAL ARTERIOVENOUS MALFORMATIONS

The arterial supply of these usually small lesions is normally derived from branches of the external carotid artery with drainage into one of the large sinuses. They can present with subdural haemorrhage, with evidence of raised intracranial pressure or with focal signs.

Malformations of the cavernous sinus either drain anteriorly via an ophthalmic vein or posteriorly via the petrosal sinus. Those draining anteriorly produce mild proptosis, dilated conjunctival vessels and, in some cases, a sixth nerve palsy (**Fig. 7.35**). The patient may complain of hearing a high-pitched noise. The preferred treatment is embolization.

133

SUBARACHNOID HAEMORRHAGE (SAH)

SAH is usually caused by rupture of a berry (saccular) aneurysm. Occasionally, an AVM is responsible. Less common causes include head injury, intracranial dissection, bleeding diathesis and cortical venous thrombosis.

PATHOLOGY AND PATHOPHYSIOLOGY

Saccular aneurysms are found at the bifurcations of the major cerebral vessels at the base of the brain. Approximately 85% occur in the anterior circulation (**Fig. 7.36**). Some 20% are multiple. Microscopy shows that the smooth muscle coat and the elastic lamina of the intracranial artery end at the neck of the aneurysm, the wall of which is composed of fibrous tissue. There is no evidence for a congenital defect of the vessel wall. The development of the aneurysm has been attributed to haemodynamic stress, exacerbated by hypertension and certain connective tissue disorders.

Vasospasm appears approximately 3–5 days after the onset of SAH and is present, angiographically, in 30–70% of patients, one-half of whom are symptomatic. Cerebral blood flow studies show a regional or global reduction in blood flow.

Perhaps 20% of patients develop hydrocephalus but at least one-half of these are asymptomatic.

EPIDEMIOLOGY

- Some 5% of the population over the age of 20 years have a saccular aneurysm
- The average annual incidence rate of rupture is approximately 11 per 100 000
- Annual mortality rate is approximately 4.3 per 100 000
- SAH from aneurysmal rupture reaches a peak incidence in the early fifties
- There is an association between saccular aneurysm and fibromuscular dysplasia in the carotid artery
- Familial aneurysms are recognized
- The risk of SAH is increased in first-degree relatives of patients with SAH

CLINICAL MANIFESTATIONS

Symptoms

Presentation of saccular aneurysm includes the effect of compression on adjacent structures, the consequences of a substantial SAH and manifestations caused by a minor leak from the aneurysm.

Symptoms of subarachnoid haemorrhage

- Sudden onset, violently painful headache
- Vomiting
- Neck stiffness
- Alteration of consciousness
- A lesser bleed occurring in the days or weeks before presentation

Compression of adjacent structures can, for example, produce a third nerve palsy caused by compression by a posterior communicating or terminal carotid aneurysm (**Fig. 7.37**).

A substantial bleed results in headache, vomiting, neck stiffness and alteration of consciousness. Retrospective analysis indicates that in some patients with SAH, a lesser bleed has occurred in the days or weeks before presentation. The minor bleed is

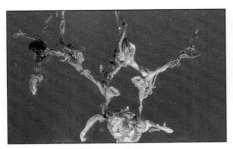

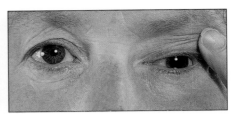

Fig. 7.37 *Third nerve paresis caused by a posterior communicating aneurysm.*

Fig. 7.36 *Aneurysms. There are aneurysms at the top of the basilar artery, two along the right middle cerebral artery and one on the anterior communicating artery.*

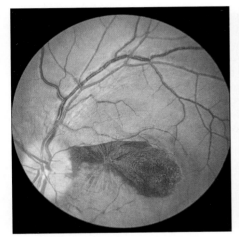

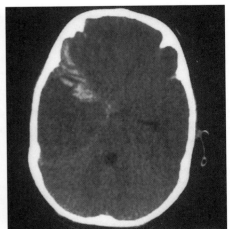

Fig. 7.38 *Subhyaloid haemorrhage.*

Fig. 7.39 *Subarachnoid blood in the left Sylvian fissure. CT.*

characterized by a sudden, fairly severe, usually occipital headache resolving spontaneously within a few days.

Signs

- Meningeal irritation. The patient has neck stiffness and a positive Kernig's sign. The signs may be absent in the comatose patient
- Subhyaloid haemorrhage secondary to a sudden rise in intracranial and, consequently, retinal venous pressure (**Fig. 7.38**)
- Focal signs determined by the site of the aneurysm; for example, in an anterior communicating aneurysm there may be bilateral lower limb pyramidal signs

INVESTIGATION

Computerized tomography

CT is the initial investigation of choice. It detects subarachnoid blood in 90% of patients when the scan is performed within 24 h of onset. The distribution of the blood may allow prediction of the likely site of the aneurysm (**Fig. 7.39**). The presence of diffuse blood or local thick clots correlates with a worse prognosis. In a small proportion of patients, the aneurysm itself is identified.

Magnetic resonance imaging

MRI as yet has not replaced CT in the early assessment of suspected SAH, although with appropriate techniques it may be more useful in detecting subarachnoid blood. Aneurysms less than 4 mm in size are not visualized.

Cerebrospinal fluid examination

Cerebrospinal fluid examination remains necessary if CT (or MRI) is negative. The mean duration of persisting red cells in the cerebrospinal fluid after SAH is 9 days, with a range of 4–19 days. Haemolysis of red cells starts after approximately 12 h. The mean duration of xanthochromia, in one study, was 20 days. Spectrophotometry can identify haem breakdown products in the supernatant even when visual inspection has been normal. If cerebrospinal fluid examination is delayed, a moderate depression of glucose concentration may be found and later, a mild mononuclear pleocytosis.

Angiography

Retrospective analysis of angiography in patients confirmed to have one or more aneurysms at postmortem has indicated an 89% yield from the procedure (bilateral carotid angiography succeeded by vertebral angiography). If repeat angiography is performed, the figure rises to approximately 96%. Negative studies are more likely if vasospasm is present. The distribution of the vasospasm gives some indication of the site of aneurysmal rupture (**Fig. 7.40**). Negative angiograms also appear more likely when the blood is primarily localized, on CT, in the perimesencephalic cisterns.

PROGNOSIS

- Approximately 45% of patients die within the first 3 months
- The risk of rebleeding within the first month is approximately 33% and is maximal in the first 2 weeks
- For long-term survivors, the rebleeding rate is approximately 3% per annum
- Prognosis correlates closely with the clinical grade of the patient and the amount of subarachnoid blood

MANAGEMENT

- Early surgery (within 3 days) is now advocated, certainly for the better risk patients
- Immediate use of nimodipine reduces the incidence of cerebral infarction and improves outcome through an effect on vasospasm
- Postoperative angiograms are normally performed, although uncertainty exists over the eventual significance of the finding of a small residual portion of the aneurysm proximal to the clip
- Unruptured aneurysms, found incidentally, are usually operated on
- Electrothrombosis via an endovascular approach may increasingly displace conventional surgery in the management of saccular aneurysms (**Fig. 7.41**)

- Perhaps 5% of the population have saccular aneurysms
- Mortality from SAH is in the region of 40–50%
- CT scanning is the initial investigation of choice in suspected SAH
- Early surgery is recommended

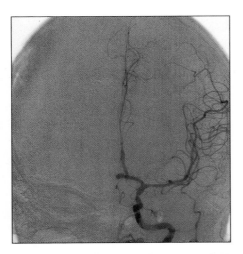

Fig. 7.40 *SAH. Angiogram showing an anterior communicating aneurysm with spasm in the anterior cerebral artery distally.*

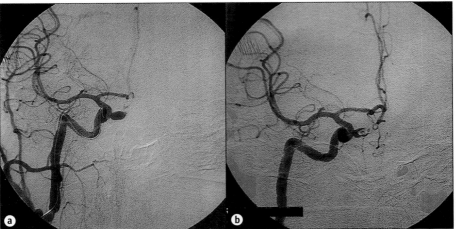

Fig. 7.41 *Ophthalmic artery aneurysm (a) with endovascular coil (b) in situ.*

THUNDERCLAP HEADACHE

In this condition, a sudden severe headache mimicking SAH prompts admission and investigation. By definition, CT and cerebrospinal fluid examination are negative. Follow-up suggests the condition is benign. Perhaps 20% of patients have further, similar attacks, whereas many later have features of tension headache or migraine.

GIANT ANEURYSMS

Giant aneurysms, defined as those exceeding 25 mm in diameter, represent approximately 5% of all intracranial aneurysms. The presentation is more often a reflection of mass effect than SAH. Some of the aneurysms are saccular, others are fusiform, arising in degenerate basilar or carotid arteries. Within the cavernous sinuses, compression can lead to involvement of the third, fourth and sixth cranial nerves, the first and second divisions of the trigeminal nerve and the ocular sympathetic fibres. These aneurysms can be shown by CT, MRI or angiography. They are seldom approachable by direct surgery but balloon occlusion is sometime feasible.

CEREBRAL VENOUS THROMBOSIS

In most patients with venous thrombosis, occlusion of one or more of the major sinuses is associated with variable involvement of the cortical veins. Isolated cortical vein thrombosis is rare. The condition may be idiopathic but recognized associations include disease processes affecting the vessel wall (e.g. Behçet's disease), a hypercoagulable state (e.g. the use of the oral contraceptive, pregnancy and the puerperium, antithrombin III deficiency) and alteration of blood flow.

Pathological changes include cerebral oedema and either haemorrhage or haemorrhagic infarction. The clinical features are dependent on the site of the pathological process.

With cavernous sinus thrombosis, there is unilateral proptosis and chemosis, associated with an ophthalmoplegia. The condition is often triggered by sepsis in the paranasal sinuses, consequently, the patient appears acutely ill with fever and severe headache. With superior sagittal sinus thrombosis there is headache, raised intracranial pressure and seizures, features that may also be encountered in thrombosis of the deeper veins.

INVESTIGATION

CT scanning is usually abnormal but specific changes (either the cord sign, the visualization of a thrombosed vein on precontrast views, or the δ sign – an empty triangular shape in the posterior aspect of the superior sagittal sinus on postcontrast views) are relatively uncommon (**Fig. 7.42**).

MRI is the imaging technique of choice and shows changes reflecting the age of the lesion. When combined with magnetic resonance angiography, virtually all patients can be identified, with only those with predominant cortical vein involvement requiring conventional venous-phase angiography.

In apparently idiopathic cases, a clotting screen should be performed, including a platelet count, measurement of antithrombin III, protein C and protein S and factor V leiden.

MANAGEMENT

Intravenous heparin is given to patients with cerebral venous thrombosis even if initial scanning has shown haemorrhagic elements to the brain lesion. After a period that has not been defined the patient is switched to warfarin therapy. Direct thrombolytic therapy (e.g. instillation of urokinase into the region of the affected vessel) is also capable of achieving recanalization. Seizures are managed symptomatically. Steroids are probably without benefit.

EXTRADURAL HAEMATOMA

Extradural haematoma is usually caused by bleeding from the middle meningeal artery. A skull fracture is identified in 90% of patients. Typically, the patient recovers after a head injury, then develops headache, focal symptoms and a deteriorating level of consciousness. The sequence is more protracted if the bleeding is venous rather than arterial. CT or MRI reveals a lens-shaped mass over the surface of the cortex. Treatment is surgical.

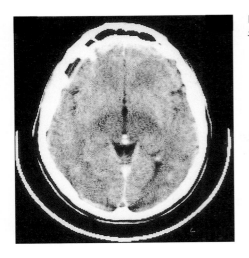

Fig. 7.42 *Cerebral venous thrombosis.* *CT showing the δ sign.*

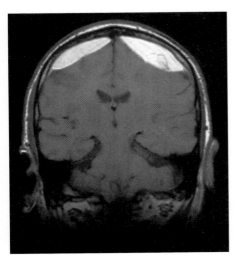

Fig. 7.43 *Subacute subdural haematomas.* *MRI reveals a bilateral, high-intensity signal on a T1-weighted image.*

SUBDURAL HAEMATOMA

Patients with acute subdural haematoma can present in a similar fashion to those with extradural haematoma or may present in coma without a history of a lucid interval after the head injury. There is often associated cerebral contusion. The lesion appears on CT as a high-density mass with displacement of underlying brain tissue. In subacute patients, the lesion is of mixed density on CT, whereas on MRI there is a high-intensity signal on T1-weighted images (**Fig. 7.43**).

Chronic subdural haematomas are often difficult to diagnose. Presenting symptoms include headache, seizures and dulling of intellectual function. At times the state of consciousness varies between alertness and drowsiness. CT or MRI are definitive in establishing the diagnosis. Some patients can be managed conservatively.

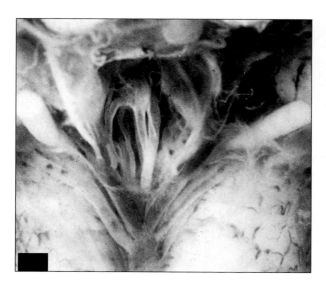

Fig. 7.44 Moya moya. *Anterior view of the termination of the basilar artery with multiple hypertrophic arterial branches extending towards the midbrain and thalamus.*

MOYA MOYA

Moya moya mainly occurs in women. Stenosis, congenital hypoplasia or occlusion is found in the terminal parts of both internal carotid arteries and in their main branches. In addition, multiple small anastomotic channels occur in the region of the circle of Willis and the pia mater (**Fig. 7.44**). The younger patient presents with ischaemic events, the adult with intracerebral or subarachnoid haemorrhage. Angiography identifies both the occluded and anastomotic vessels. Extracranial or intracranial by-pass procedures reduce the frequency of ischaemic events.

HYPERTENSIVE ENCEPHALOPATHY

Hypertensive encephalopathy is triggered by a sudden elevation of blood pressure, often in a previously normotensive individual. The brain is swollen with evidence of fibrinoid necrosis in medium- and small-sized cerebral vessels. Clinical features include headache, vomiting, alteration of the level of consciousness and seizures. CT or MRI shows areas of altered signal that resolve when the blood pressure is satisfactorily controlled.

- Giant aneurysms usually present with mass effect
- MRI, with magnetic resonance angiography, is the screening procedure of choice in cerebral venous thrombosis
- Cerebral venous thrombosis is treated with anticoagulation
- Some subdural haematomas can be managed conservatively

chapter 8

Parkinson's Disease and Other Extrapyramidal Disorders

PARKINSON'S DISEASE AND OTHER EXTRAPYRAMIDAL DISORDERS

Clinical classification of parkinsonian syndromes

1. Idiopathic Parkinson's disease
2. Symptomatic parkinsonism
   Postencephalitic
   Drug-induced
   Toxic
   Traumatic
   Arteriosclerotic
   Normal pressure hydrocephalus
3. As part of a neuronal degenerative disorder
   Multisystem atrophy
   Progressive supranuclear palsy
   Corticobasal degeneration
   Diffuse Lewy body disease

Parkinson's disease is defined clinically as the combination of bradykinesia, rest tremor, cogwheel rigidity and the impairment of postural reflexes.

Using these criteria, some 20% of patients at postmortem examination will prove have a pathology other than idiopathic Parkinson's disease (IPD). If to these are added asymmetrical onset and the absence of atypical features and possible other aetiologies, the predictive accuracy rises above 90% but approximately one-third of genuine patients are then excluded.

IDIOPATHIC PARKINSON'S DISEASE

AETIOLOGY

The aetiology remains unknown. A very similar (but not identical) clinical and pathological entity follows exposure to 1-methyl-4-phenyl-1,2,3,6-tetrahydropyridine.

Complex 1 of the mitochondrial respiratory chain is deficient in the substantia nigra. Decreased glutathione and glutathione peroxide activity is found in the substantia nigra, which could lead to a reduced ability to clear hydrogen peroxide generated from increased dopamine metabolism.

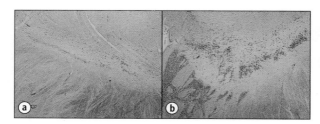

Fig. 8.1 *Atrophic substantia nigra (a) compared with normal control (b).*

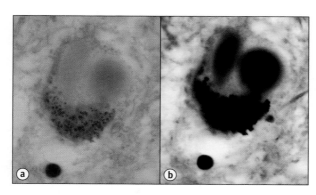

Fig. 8.2 *Parkinson's disease. Lewy body in the substantia nigra pars compacta. (a) H&E, (b) modified Bielschowsky silver technique.*

PATHOLOGY

The changes concentrate on the substantia nigra and locus coeruleus. The substantia nigra shows a loss of at least 50% of its melanin-containing cells, maximally in the central part of the zona compacta. Alongside these changes is found a characteristic cytoplasmic inclusion: the Lewy body (**Figs 8.1 and 8.2**).

PATHOPHYSIOLOGY

Bradykinesia

The pathophysiology is unclear. Fast, ballistic movements are most affected.

Rigidity

Rigidity is probably secondary to enhancement of long-latency stretch reflexes.

Tremor

Tremor is possibly related to rhythmic neuronal discharges within the thalamus and is associated with alpha-gamma co-activation.

Epidemiology

Varying prevalence reported: 30–300 per 100 000; perhaps 60–80 000 patients in the UK.
- Increases with age
- More common in men
- Higher risk for those in rural residence and with herbicide or pesticide exposure
- Reduced risk in cigarette smokers
- Approximately 10–15% of parkinsonian patients have a relative with the disease
- Autosomal dominant forms of Parkinson's disease are described but have atypical features
- Survival, on treatment, comparable with age-matched controls

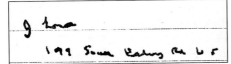

Fig. 8.3 *Parkinson's disease.* Micrographia.

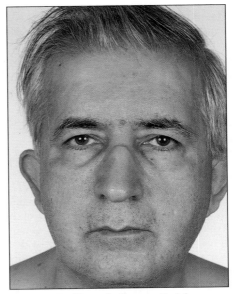

Fig. 8.4 *Parkinson's disease.* Facial appearance.

CLINICAL MANIFESTATIONS

Symptoms

Symptoms of Parkinson's disease

- Bradykinesia
- Tremor
- Rigidity
- Autonomic symptoms

Bradykinesia

Typically, asymmetrical at onset and during the initial course of the disease. Upper limb involvement leads to slowing of fine movement. Patients comment on change in dressing and eating speed. Writing becomes smaller (**Fig. 8.3**). The patient and relatives notice a change in walking speed. Typically, one arm swings less than the other. There are difficulties in turning in bed and rising from a chair. The posture becomes stooped. Relatives often comment on the patient's impassivity (**Fig. 8.4**). Speech volume becomes reduced.

Tremor

A rest tremor is estimated to be present at onset in 70% of patients and during the course of the disease in 75%. Patients have usually noticed the resting element to the tremor and that it is asymmetrical. Typically, the tremor begins in one upper limb with involvement of the corresponding lower limb approximately 2 years later. Occasionally, the disease produces tremor of the jaw, lips or tongue. Rarely, it affects the head or voice.

143

Rigidity

Patients sometimes complain of muscle stiffness or pain. The condition can present with a 'frozen shoulder' picture.

Autonomic symptoms

Urinary urgency and constipation occurs.

SIGNS

Bradykinesia

The diagnosis can often be suspected by simple observation of the patient as they walk into the consulting room and during the course of history taking. Despite the stress of speaking to a strange doctor, parkinsonian patients tend to remain still and impassive. Bradykinesia of the upper limb can be assessed by asking the patient to 'polish' the back of one hand with the other or repetitively to tap the back of the hand with the fingers of the other hand. Typically, there is a delay in initiation of movement, followed by a decline in its range and speed. The noise of the tapping fingers fades. Writing a standard passage allows objective assessment of bradykinesia and its response to treatment. Facial impassivity produces a fixed expression, with infrequent blinking.

Tremor

Classically, a resting tremor occurs at approximately 3–4 Hz. A combination of flexion and extension of the fingers with a pronator–supinator movement of the forearm is common, as is 'pill-rolling' of the fingers. The tremor is inhibited briefly by a purposive movement, for example, the finger–nose test. A postural tremor at a faster rate can also occur.

Rigidity

Produces an increase in muscle tone throughout the range of movement of the joint. It can be confined to one limb or even part of it. If subtle, it can be brought out by activating muscles in another part of the body. Rigidity is best assessed in the neck and the wrists. Cogwheeling is a fluctuant increase in tone, whose rate corresponds to the postural rather than the resting tremor frequency.

Postural reflexes

The posture becomes stooped and patients have increasing difficulty in maintaining posture when pushed suddenly either backwards or forwards (**Fig. 8.5**).

Gait

Stride length diminishes. More steps are needed when changing direction. The more affected arm swings less. In more advanced cases, the patient freezes when trying to initiate walking.

OTHER FEATURES

Dementia

A true, cortical, dementia has been reported with varying frequency in parkinsonian patients. Perhaps 15–20% show manifestations eventually. Dementia is more likely in older patients, those with a longer duration of disease, in men and in those with more parkinsonian disability. Disturbance of frontal lobe function, in the absence of dementia, is common, with thought slowing, apathy and inanition.

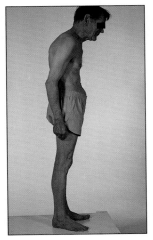

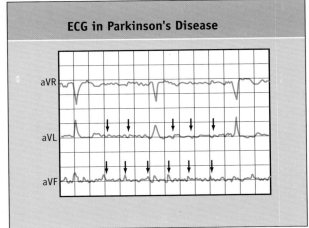

Fig. 8.5 *Parkinson's disease.* Stooped posture.

Fig. 8.6 *Parkinson's disease.* Electrocardiogram showing a tremor artefact (arrows).

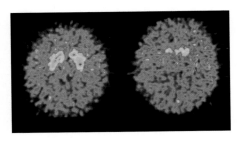

Fig. 8.7 *Parkinson's disease.* Positron emission tomography scan showing reduced fluorodopa uptake in the basal ganglia (right) compared with a normal control (left).

Eye signs

A variety of eye signs occur. There is a reduced frequency of blinking, with impaired convergence and up-gaze, although these latter signs are common in an elderly population. Particularly characteristic is the tendency for the patient to blink as they alternate gaze from one side to the other.

- The clinical diagnosis of IPD is apt to be incorrect in some 20% of patients
- The condition is typically asymmetrical at onset
- A postural tremor occurs as well as the classic resting tremor
- Dementia occurs in a significant proportion of the patients

INVESTIGATION

Evidence for a parkinsonian tremor may be found inadvertently as an artefact on the electrocardiogram (**Fig. 8.6**). Imaging reveals some degree of ventricular dilatation and cortical atrophy, particularly in atypical patients. Positron emission tomography scanning, using 6-[18F]-fluoro-dopa shows reduced uptake of the isotope, particularly in the putamen and, maximally, contralateral to the more affected side (**Fig. 8.7**). Subcutaneous apomorphine has been used diagnostically, with a positive response in terms of symptom relief being interpreted as evidence in favour of IPD. A significant proportion of patients with IPD fail to respond, whereas some parkinsonian patients without IPD respond.

MANAGEMENT

The management of IPD is detailed in **Figure 8.8**.

Management of idiopathic Parkinson's disease
• Neuroprotection
• Drugs   Anticholinergics
Amantadine
Dopa
Dopamine agonists
Apomorphine
• Surgery
• Physiotherapy
• Speech therapy
• General support

Fig. 8.8 *Management of Parkinson's disease.*

Neuroprotection

Selegiline (a monoamine oxidase B inhibitor) prevents Parkinson's disease developing in primates receiving 1-methyl-4-phenyl-1,2,3,6-tetrahydropyridine. Its use has been advocated on the grounds that monoamine oxidase B inhibition could prevent some of the oxidative stress believed to be a factor in causing neuronal damage in IPD. The dosage is 10 mg in the morning. The most recent data suggest that the drug delays the need for dopa by exerting a symptomatic effect, rather than by neuroprotection. It use is possibly associated with an increased mortality.

Anticholinergics

These are of limited value, have considerable side effects (dry mouth, constipation) and commonly cause confusion in the elderly. No effect on bradykinesia is seen and only seldom do they influence tremor. Benzhexol is most commonly prescribed, in doses of 2–10 mg daily.

Amantadine

This exerts a very mild effect through stimulating dopamine release; it is seldom used.

Dopa

Failure to respond is unusual in IPD. Treatment is initiated when the patient's symptoms and disability demand it. Many patients are initially followed without active drug intervention.

Initial treatment is with either Sinemet® (Du Pont) or Madopar® (Roche), probably preferably in the slow-release form. Benefit is seen in all aspects of the condition, although the tremor often proves stubbornly resistant. By 5 years from initiation of therapy, only approximately one-quarter of the patients continue to have a good, stable response. An average dose is approximately 800 mg dopa each day.

Dopamine agonists

Most experience has been obtained with bromocriptine. Perhaps only one-third of patients respond and many experience side effects, including nausea, headache, dizziness and confusion. Patients on agonist treatment alone are much less likely to develop long-term complications such as dyskinesias and fluctuations. The dosage of bromocriptine averages approximately 35 mg/day. Pergolide and lysuride are other agonists that can be used, the former being preferred. Dosage starts at 50 µg/day, increasing to a maximum of 3 mg/day. Some authorities favour initial treatment with low-dose dopa and pergolide.

Apomorphine

Used when sudden off-periods appear (see *Fluctuations*). Given by subcutaneous injection. Often causes nausea, controlled by domperidone.

Late problems with drug therapy

Lessening effect – The majority of patients show a lessening response after approximately 5 years of treatment.

Movement disorders – Various movement disorders, including dyskinesias and dystonic postures emerge. Some coincide with the period of maximum benefit from the treatment (peak dose), others are biphasic or appear during off-periods. Treatment is difficult (**Fig. 8.9**). Reduction of dopa dosage is beneficial for some but at the expense of exacerbating the parkinsonian features.

Fluctuations – After some 5 years of treatment, fluctuation of response is commonplace. Initially, it takes the form of a wearing-off effect before the next dose. Eventually, unpredictable oscillations in response occur (on–off), together with disabling episodes of immobility ('freezing'). Fluctuations are postponed by delaying treatment with dopa initially and by the use of small doses. Strategies to lessen these problems include combinations of standard and slow-release preparations, the addition of pergolide, the avoidance of high-protein meals and the use of apomorphine.

Surgery

Unilateral thalamotomy lessens or eliminates contralateral tremor and rigidity but has no effect on bradykinesia. Stroke occurs in approximately 5–10% of patients. Pallidotomy lessens tremor and rigidity and can reduce dopa-induced dyskinesias. Thalamic stimulation can suppress tremor and dopa-induced dyskinesias. Foetal substantia nigra transplants into the striatum are viable and are capable of producing clinical benefit. Their role has not yet been established.

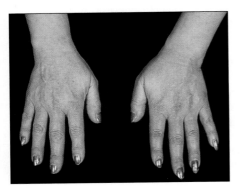

Fig. 8.9 *Parkinson's disease. Abducted left little finger as a dystonic response to dopa.*

- Failure to respond to dopa should raise doubts about the diagnosis
- Lessening of the initial response is almost universal after 5 years of therapy
- Slow-release dopa preparations probably offer advantages over conventional forms
- Surgery can play a role, particularly in the management of tremor and dyskinesias

Physiotherapy

Valuable in retraining walking patterns and in teaching transfer techniques.

Speech therapy

Can help in improving speech and swallow techniques and, later, in providing communication aids.

General support

The urinary urgency and frequency may respond to dopa or to low-dose oxybutynin. Depression is commonplace and can be treated by a tricyclic antidepressant, although at the risk of exacerbating constipation. Confusional states can emerge and may require neuroleptic therapy. Involvement of the social services and the support of the Parkinson's Disease Society is invaluable.

SYMPTOMATIC PARKINSONISM

POSTENCEPHALITIC PARKINSON'S DISEASE

This form originally followed the pandemic of encephalitis lethargica in the early part of the twentieth century. It still occurs sporadically and represents a different pathological entity from IPD. In addition to parkinsonian features, there are prominent autonomic symptoms, behavioural changes and oculogyric crises, in which sustained ocular deviation, usually upwards, can last for minutes or hours (**Fig. 8.10**).

DRUG-INDUCED PARKINSON'S DISEASE

Typically due to a phenothiazine, tetrabenazine or reserpine. Tremor is usually an insignificant part. It can be reversed by drug withdrawal. A parkinsonian picture can follow toxic exposure (e.g. carbon monoxide), and trauma (e.g. boxing), and occur with arterial disease (usually multiple lacunar infarcts) and in normal pressure hydrocephalus.

PARKINSONISM IN OTHER CONDITIONS

MULTISYSTEM ATROPHY

Typically, this constitutes a combination of autonomic symptoms (caused by intermediolateral degeneration of the spinal cord), cerebellar signs (caused by olivopontocerebellar atrophy [**Fig. 8.11**]) and parkinsonism (caused by striatonigral degeneration). Autonomic symptoms include impotence, incontinence and postural hypotension. Classic, pill-rolling tremor is uncommon. The parkinsonian features may respond initially to dopa. Pyramidal signs appear in the majority of patients. An anal or urethral sphincter electromyogram indicates degeneration of Onuf's

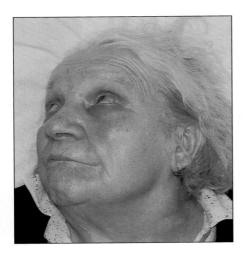

Fig. 8.10 *Oculogyric crisis in postencephalitic parkinsonism.*

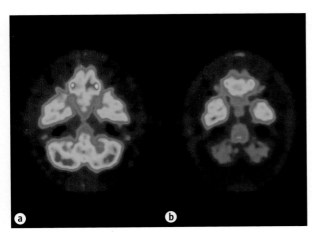

Fig. 8.11 *Olivo-ponto cerebellar atrophy.* Positron emission tomography scan showing a normal control (*a*) and a patient with OPCA (*b*); the latter shows brainstem and cerebellar hypometabolism.

nucleus in the spinal cord in 90% of patients. Inspiratory stridor occurs in one-third of patients. Severe disability within a few years is common.

PROGRESSIVE SUPRANUCLEAR PALSY – STEELE–RICHARDSON–OLSZEWSKI SYNDROME

Progressive supranuclear palsy occurs later in life and is associated with pathological changes in the substantia nigra, locus coeruleus, pons, midbrain, dentate and subthalamic nuclei, globus pallidus and nucleus basalis. The oculomotor palsy initially affects downward saccadic movements with preservation of pursuit and reflex movements. Later, up-gaze is affected, then horizontal saccades. Subsequently, pursuit movements and reflex movements are lost (**Fig. 8.12**). Other features include parkinsonism, altered gait, dysarthria and declining memory. Axial rigidity is profound, leading to hyperextension of the neck. Only occasionally is the condition responsive to dopa. Some patients, with typical pathological features, fail to develop an ophthalmoplegia.

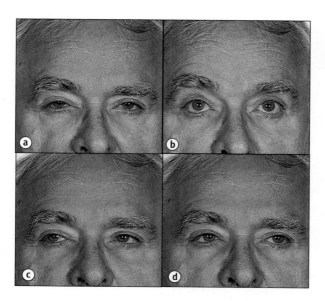

Fig. 8.12 *Failure of down-gaze (a) with partial sparing of up-gaze (b) and horizontal gaze (c and d).*

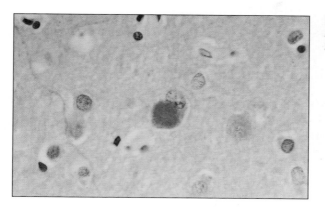

Fig. 8.13 *Cortical Lewy body in a case of cortical Lewy body disease.*

CORTICOBASAL DEGENERATION

This condition shares some features with progressive supranuclear palsy. It usually presents with a clumsy or stiff arm with rigidity, akinesia and apraxia on examination. The arm may be held in a dystonic posture or show myoclonic jerks. Involvement of the lower limbs leads to gait disorders and loss of motor control. Eventually, all four limbs are affected. Supranuclear eye movement disorders appear, more in the vertical than horizontal plane. Cognition is relatively spared. There is no specific treatment.

DIFFUSE LEWY BODY DISEASE

This consists of a parkinsonian syndrome along with a severe dementia. The brainstem pathology is that of Parkinson's disease. The cortex contains numerous Lewy bodies and in addition may show Alzheimer-type pathology. Progression of disability is more rapid than in IPD (**Fig. 8.13**).

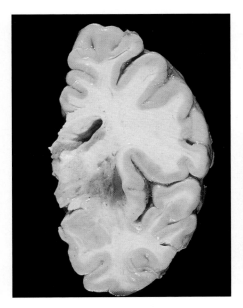

Fig. 8.14 *Wilson's disease. Cavitation and discoloration of the putamen with lesser changes in the caudate nucleus and globus pallidus.*

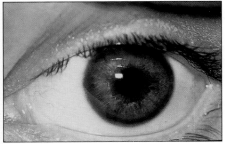

Fig. 8.15 *Wilson's disease. The Kayser–Fleischer ring.*

- A parkinsonian picture is seen in many pathological processes
- The diagnosis of Parkinson's disease is rendered unlikely by the presence of early dementia, falls early in the course of the disease and the presence of pyramidal signs
- Most of the parkinsonian syndromes have limited dopa responsiveness

WILSON'S DISEASE

Inherited as an autosomal recessive condition, this leads to copper deposition in various organs, particularly the liver and the brain. Onset is usually in childhood, with liver disease or, less commonly, renal disease or haemolytic anaemia. Individuals with adult-onset (seldom beyond 40 years old) present with neurological or psychiatric features. Pathological changes include cirrhosis and putamenal atrophy with cavitation (**Fig. 8.14**). Serum caeruloplasmin levels are depressed and urinary excretion of copper is increased. Imaging reveals ventricular dilatation, cortical atrophy and an abnormal putamenal signal. Various movement disorders occur, including tremor, dystonia and choreo-athetoid movements. Dysphagia and dysarthria are prominent. Alteration of mood and behaviour is seen. In patients with neuropsychiatric involvement, a Kayser–Fleischer ring is visible, the result of copper deposition in Descemet's membrane of the cornea. Slit-lamp microscopy may be required to identify the pigment (**Fig. 8.15**).

Treatment is with chelating agents (D-penicillamine or trientine) or with zinc, which blocks uptake of copper from the intestine. Most of the recovery is seen in the first 2 years of treatment.

MOVEMENT DISORDERS

CLASSIFICATION
- Tremor
- Dystonia
- Chorea
- Athetosis
- Ballismus
- Tics
- Myoclonus
- Drug-induced disorders

TREMOR

Definition of tremor

Rest	Present when limb fully supported against gravity.
Action	During any voluntary muscle contraction.
Postural	During maintenance of a particular posture.
Kinetic	During any type of movement.
Intention	Exacerbation of kinetic tremor as the planned movement nears completion.
Task-specific	During a particular skilled action, for example, writing.

Physiological tremor
Physiological tremor is a normal phenomenon, exacerbated by agitation or fatigue.

Essential tremor
Essential tremor is a postural tremor predominating in the upper limbs. It occurs as an autosomal dominant condition but also in a sporadic form. Later, involvement includes the legs, head, face, voice and tongue. One-half of the patients respond to alcohol but the tremor returns in an exaggerated form approximately 4 h later. Some response occurs to either primidone or propranolol in most patients.

Tremor is also seen with certain drugs (e.g. salbutamol and sodium valproate), in cerebellar disease, with midbrain lesions (rubral tremor), with certain neuropathies (e.g. with Ig M paraproteinaemia) and in association with dystonia.

Primary orthostatic tremor
Tremor of the legs appears on standing, leading to unsteadiness. The condition may respond to clonazepam or phenobarbitone.

DYSTONIA
A syndrome of sustained muscle contractions, frequently causing twisting and repetitive movements or abnormal postures.

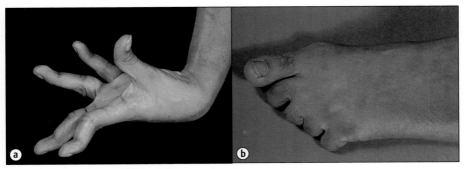

Fig. 8.16 *Dystonic posturing of the hand and foot.*

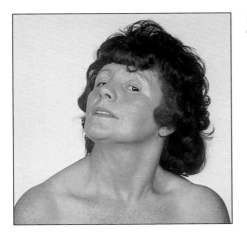

Fig. 8.17 *Spasmodic torticollis.* A characteristic head posture.

Classification

- Focal dystonia affects a single body part, for example, the eyelids
- Segmental dystonia is either cranial, axial, brachial or crural
- Generalized dystonia
- Hemidystonia. Ipsilateral arm and leg

Dystonia can be classified as idiopathic (either sporadic or familial) or symptomatic. Familial forms often show autosomal dominant inheritance. In such families, the dystonia may be focal, segmental or generalized and even the generalized forms tend to begin focally before spreading to other areas (**Fig. 8.16**). Symptomatic dystonia occurs in a wide variety of neurological disorders, both metabolic and structural. The diagnosis of symptomatic dystonia is usually suggested by the presence of additional neurological signs, for example, an extensor–plantar response or an oculomotor disorder.

FOCAL DYSTONIAS

Spasmodic torticollis

Leads to sustained or episodic contraction of neck muscles, with abnormal head posture (**Fig. 8.17**). Secondary degeneration of the cervical spine is likely in patients with long-standing disease.

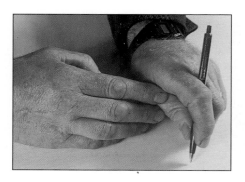

Fig. 8.18 *Writer's cramp. Abnormal hand posture.*

Blepharospasm

Intermittent eyelid contraction can eventually become so persistent that the patient is effectively blind. In some patients, the spasms can be relieved by touching the eyelid.

Oromandibular dystonia

Leads to involuntary movements of the tongue and mouth, typically triggered by eating or speaking. Dysphagia and dysarthria occur.

Spasmodic dysphonia

Affects the laryngeal muscles, leading either to a strangulated quality to the voice or to a breathy quality according to whether the cords are respectively adducted or abducted.

Writer's cramp

Patients describe a discomfort in the hand, associated with the use of excessive force and the adoption of an abnormal writing posture (**Fig. 8.18**).

DOPA-RESPONSIVE DYSTONIA

Typically presents in the first decade with abnormal foot posturing or a gait disorder. There is often a marked diurnal variation, worsening as the day progresses. It is likely to be accompanied by bradykinesia and rigidity. A dominantly inherited condition, it shows a dramatic response to low-dose dopa.

Investigation of dystonia

Imaging is unhelpful for idiopathic torsion dystonia and for the focal dystonias.

Extensive investigation may be needed to exclude secondary causes of dystonia, including imaging; screening for lysosomal enzymes, urinary amino acids and long-chain fatty acids; copper studies; haematological investigation including bone marrow; and a search for acanthocytes.

Treatment of dystonia

Anticholinergic therapy is sometimes helpful but large doses are needed and side effects are common. Dopa is probably worth giving as a therapeutic trial in case the problem is an atypical dopa-responsive dystonia. Botulinum toxin is of considerable value for the treatment of focal dystonia. It acts by reducing release of acetylcholine from the presynaptic motor terminal. It is the treatment of choice for spasmodic torticollis, spasmodic dysphonia associated with adduction of the cords, blepharospasm and some types of oromandibular dystonia. Its effect lasts 3–4 months, after which the injections have to be repeated. Thalamotomy is of potential value in patients with disabling widespread dystonia.

- Probably all patients with neurological manifestations of Wilson's disease have a Kayser–Fleischer ring
- All younger patients developing dystonia should be given a trial of dopa
- Some of the focal dystonias are most effectively treated with botulinum toxin

CHOREA, BALLISMUS AND ATHETOSIS

Definition of chorea, ballismus and athetosis

Chorea.   Erratic, unpredictable, non-repetitive muscle contractions.
Athetosis. Similar movements but more distally distributed and writhing in quality.
Ballismus. Violent, flinging movements, predominantly proximal and often unilateral (hemiballismus).

Chorea, athetosis and ballismus are best regarded as a continuum of movement disorders with similar underlying pathophysiology.

Chorea

Patients often convert their involuntary movements into an apparently purposive action in order to disguise them better. The condition is associated with an inability to maintain muscle contraction and a tendency for the reflexes to be 'hung-up' (pendular).

Sydenham's (rheumatic) chorea

Arises some months after the acute illness and is largely confined to children between 5 and 15 years old. It is thought to be related to auto-antibodies reacting with the caudate nucleus. It sometimes relapses or becomes more chronic in adult life.

Huntington's disease

Inherited as an autosomal dominant disorder, the relevant gene lies on chromosome 4. The caudate nuclei become severely atrophic, with microscopic change predominating in the small and medium spiny neurons of the basal ganglia (**Fig. 8.19**). Mild to moderate cortical atrophy is also present. No single excitatory amino acid receptor is selectively decreased. Onset is usually in the third and fourth decades but 10% present before the age of 20 and 10% beyond the age of 60. Juvenile patients are more likely to show paternal transmission, a fulminant course and predominant rigidity. Clinical features include chorea, ataxia, dementia, personality change and abnormal saccadic eye movements. Measurement of caudate atrophy on computerized tomography incompletely differentiates the condition from Alzheimer's disease. Magnetic resonance imaging abnormalities depend on whether the condition has presented in a rigid or choreic form. Positron emission tomography scanning shows a reduced striatal metabolism and single photon emission computerized tomography shows altered caudate and putaminal blood flow (**Fig. 8.20**). There is no specific treatment. Tetrabenazine or reserpine will help suppress abnormal movements but both are capable of

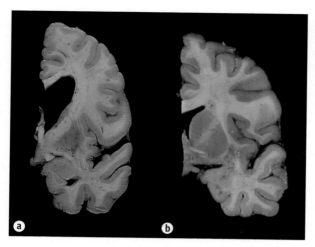

Fig. 8.19 *Huntington's disease.* *Coronal section (a) showing a dilated lateral ventricle with caudate and lentiform atrophy compared with a normal coronal section (b).*

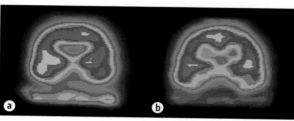

Fig. 8.20 *Huntington's disease.* *Single photon emission computerized tomography scan showing reduced caudate blood flow (a) compared with normal (b).*

causing a depressive illness. Screening of at-risk relatives can identify those likely to develop the disease. The technique should be used with extreme caution because of the potential emotional reaction to a confirmation of an individual's at-risk status.

Neuroacanthocytosis

A rare condition that usually presents in the third or fourth decade. Typical features include movement disorders (chorea, tics, dystonia), extrapyramidal features, seizures, psychiatric symptoms, dementia and an axonal neuropathy. Various forms of inheritance have been proposed. Light microscopy or scanning electron microscopy shows acanthocytes (red cells with spiny projections) usually with echinocytes (red cells with rounded projections) (**Fig. 8.21**). There is no specific treatment.

Other forms of chorea

Chorea is also seen in pregnancy, with the oral contraceptive, in systemic lupus erythematosus, in polycythaemia rubra vera and in thyrotoxicosis. Ballismus can similarly be triggered by many different pathological processes. Hemiballismus is particularly associated with lesions of the contralateral subthalamic nucleus. Drugs used for its treatment include reserpine, tetrabenazine and haloperidol.

- Chorea, athetosis and ballismus should be regarded as a continuum
- The carriers of the Huntington's disease gene can be identified

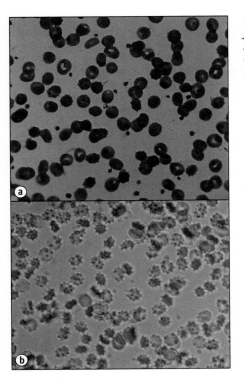

Fig. 8.21 Neuroacanthocytosis. (a) Wet film with saline dilution and (b) Wright-stained preparation after 3 h incubation in ethylenediaminetetraacetic acid, illustrating both acanthocytes and echinocytes.

TICS

Tics result either in movement (motor tics) or vocalization (vocal tics). Simple tics are sudden, brief, repetitive, isolated movements, whereas complex tics result in repeated, more sophisticated motor acts, for example, scratching, and touching the nose. Vocal tics may produce nothing more than a grunt or actual verbalization.

Gilles de La Tourette's syndrome

A familial disorder inherited as a dominant condition with incomplete penetrance. It is more common in men. The tics may persist during sleep. Associated behavioural disturbances occur, including obsessive–compulsive disorders. Coprolalia, the uncontrollable desire to utter obscenities, occurs in less than one-half of the patients. The tics predominate in the face, head and neck. They can be voluntarily suppressed for brief periods. There are no specific investigations. Haloperidol, pimozide and fluphenazine are used to suppress the tics.

Myoclonus

Sudden, short-lived, shock-like movements. The movements may be rhythmic or arrhythmic. Additional classification is made according to whether the myoclonus is cortical, brainstem or spinal in origin. Arrhythmic myoclonus is seen in various structural, toxic or degenerative disorders of the central nervous system. Rhythmic myoclonus is usually caused by a brainstem or spinal lesion. Palatal myoclonus produces a repetitive contraction of the soft palate and adjacent structures. It may result from a lesion of the Guillain–Malleret triangle (usually vascular or traumatic) or be idiopathic. Some forms of myoclonus respond to sodium valproate or clonazepam. Postanoxic myoclonus is helped by 5-hydroxytryptophan.

DRUG-INDUCED DISORDERS

Acute dystonic reactions can occur within hours or days of commencing neuroleptic medication. Reactions include opisthotonos, torticollis, retrocollis and oculogyric crises. Metoclopramide is particularly liable to produce such a reaction. Treatment consists in administration of intravenous benztropine or diazepam.

Acute akathisia produces both an inner sense of restlessness and external evidence of inappropriate muscle activity. It is triggered by dopaminergic blocking agents and usually improves when they are withdrawn.

Tardive dyskinesia typically leads to repetitive tongue and lip movement. Choreic and dystonic features may be seen. The movements are triggered by long-term neuroleptic therapy (**Fig. 8.22**). If possible, the causative agent should be withdrawn, although this can cause a temporary exacerbation of the condition.

Neuroleptic malignant syndrome is a potentially fatal disorder triggered by neuroleptic therapy but also seen with metoclopramide, tetrabenazine, lithium or tricyclic antidepressants. Extrapyramidal features include tremor, rigidity, salivation, retrocollis, oculogyric crises and chorea. Autonomic features include hyperthermia, sweating, tachycardia, hypertension or hypotension, and urinary retention. The level of consciousness is often altered. Creatine kinase levels are typically elevated. The condition usually starts within a few days of starting the relevant drug therapy and is more likely to develop with high-dose or intramuscular therapy. The condition is thought to be caused by a functional dopamine blockade at the postsynaptic receptor site. The causative agent is withdrawn and bromocriptine, along with dantrolene used, to control the manifestations of the condition.

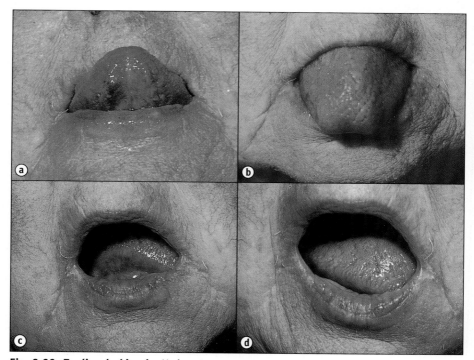

Fig. 8.22 *Tardive dyskinesia. Various tongue postures.*

chapter 9

Cerebral Tumour and Hydrocephalus

CEREBRAL TUMOUR

The prevalence of intracranial tumour lies between 3 and 8.4 per 100 000 of the population. The figure rises with age. The incidence of cerebral tumour is probably stable. The prognosis for patients with glioblastoma has not altered significantly in the past 15 years. Some of the tumours encountered in the brain are listed in **Figure 9.1**. Primary brain lymphoma, at one time rare, accounts for 5% of the total and predominates in the immunocompromised individual.

CLASSIFICATION OF CEREBRAL TUMOURS

Diffuse astrocytomas (the most common type) are classified into three grades according to the degree of malignancy:
- Astrocytoma (I)
- Anaplastic astrocytoma (II)
- Glioblastoma multiforme (III)

PATHOLOGY

Glioblastoma accounts for approximately 50% of the total. Typically, it contains both necrotic and haemorrhagic areas and occurs as a single focus around the junction of grey and white matter in the cerebral hemisphere (**Fig. 9.2**). Spread occurs along white matter pathways within the hemisphere, across the corpus callosum or along the ependyma. Seedling deposits are sometimes conveyed via the ventricular system but extracranial metastases are rare.

Primitive neuro-ectodermal tumours include medulloblastomas, pineoblastomas and neuroblastomas and consist of largely undifferentiated neoplasms occurring in childhood

Intracranial tumours

- Glioma
- Metastasis
- Meningioma
- Pituitary adenoma
- Sarcoma
- Haemangioblastoma
- Craniopharyngioma
- Neurinoma

Fig. 9.1 Intracranial tumours.

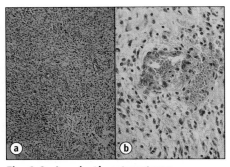

Fig. 9.2 Anaplastic astrocytoma.
(**a**) Cellular tumour with dark nuclei and solid fibrillary eosinophilic background.
(**b**) Evidence of vascular hyperplasia with proliferated endothelial and perithelial cells.

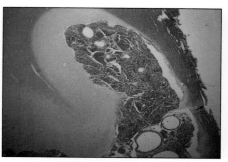

Fig. 9.3 *Primitive neuro-ectodermal tumour.* Dense cellular mass of dark-staining tumour cells lying in the subarachnoid space above the corpus callosum (blue) and cingulate gyrus cortex (pink).

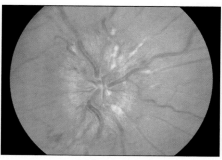

Fig. 9.4 *Acute papilloedema in a patient with cerebral tumour.*

and containing glial, neuronal and rhabdomyoblastic components. The tumours are liable to disseminate along cerebrospinal fluid (CSF) pathways and can infiltrate the cortical sulci, the basal cisterns or the spinal nerve roots (**Fig. 9.3**).

CLINICAL MANIFESTATIONS OF CEREBRAL TUMOURS

The clinical manifestations represent the combination, in varying degree, of non-specific features, focal symptoms and signs and false localizing signs.

Non-specific features

General symptoms of cerebral tumours

- Headache
- Nausea and vomiting
- Seizures
- Altered mentation

Headache – Occurs in the majority of patients with intracerebral tumour. An early morning predominance is relatively uncommon. The pain is not necessarily severe. For supra-tentorial tumours, in the absence of papilloedema, the headache is ipsilateral to the tumour in approximately 80% of patients.

Nausea and vomiting – The former is more common. One or other occurs in approximately 50% of patients with cerebral tumour and is more likely if the tumour lies below the tentorium.

Seizures – Over 50% of patients with frontal lobe tumours have seizures, sometimes as a presenting complaint, sometimes in the form of status epilepticus. Seizures are less common with tumours in the posterior hemisphere.

Papilloedema – Occurs more often with infra-tentorial than supra-tentorial tumours. It is often asymptomatic but may result in transient visual obscurations, typically induced by changes of posture (**Fig. 9.4**).

Altered mentation – Apathy and inertia are symptoms common to tumours at any site but more so for those in the frontal lobe or corpus callosum.

Focal symptoms and signs

Frontal lobe – Produces altered mood and behaviour, with contralateral pyramidal signs. Incontinence is common. Primitive reflexes emerge, for example, a contralateral grasp reflex in the hand or foot.

Parietal lobe – Sensory symptoms and signs predominate. Contralateral sensory or visual suppression is likely when the non-dominant hemisphere is affected. The visual defect may predominate in the inferior half-field but is more often complete. Dressing apraxia is found with lesions of the non-dominant lobe.

Temporal lobe – Speech disturbance is likely with tumours of the dominant hemisphere. A superior quadrantic homonymous hemianopia may be found, along with a contralateral motor deficit. Complex partial seizures are characteristic of temporal lobe pathology but are also found with posterior frontal lesions.

Occipital lobe – Visual field abnormalities are the most prominent feature of occipital neoplasms.

False localizing signs

False localizing signs are defined as signs that cannot be explained on the basis of the immediate, local, effects of the tumour. The most common false localizing sign found in association with a cerebral tumour is a unilateral or bilateral sixth nerve palsy (**Fig. 9.5**). Other cranial nerve palsies are less common but include those of the third, fourth and fifth nerves. Uncal herniation can either compress the contralateral cerebral peduncle against the tentorium, producing a hemiparesis ipsilateral to the tumour, or against the posterior cerebral artery, producing a contralateral homonymous hemianopia caused by occipital lobe infarction.

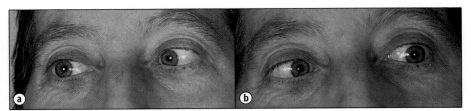

Fig. 9.5 *Bilateral sixth nerve palsies in a patient with glioblastoma multiforme.*

INVESTIGATION OF MALIGNANT BRAIN TUMOURS

- Plain radiographs are not justified. Calcification may be detected in up to 50% of oligodendrogliomas
- The electroencephalogram is almost always abnormal with tumours involving the cerebral cortex but the changes are non-specific
- Formal angiography is seldom performed for assessing the vasculature of cerebral tumours as magnetic resonance angiography is usually adequate for that purpose
- Computerized tomography (CT) scan appearances are influenced by the degree of malignancy. Approximately one-half the hypodense lesions shown on CT, interpreted as low grade astrocytomas, are found to be higher grade, more aggressive tumours. Glioblastoma multiforme produce a mixed density pattern with oedema and enhancement after contrast injection (**Fig. 9.6**)
- Magnetic resonance imaging (MRI) is the most sensitive imaging technique. With gadolinium, the tumour is found either to be more extensive or even multifocal when compared with its CT appearance (**Fig. 9.7**)

161

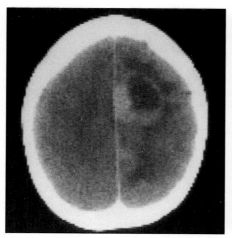

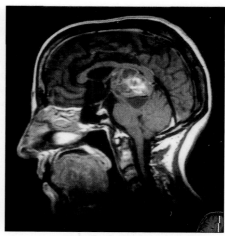

Fig. 9.6 *CT showing ring enhancement in a glioma.*

Fig. 9.7 *MRI with gadolinium showing a high brainstem glioma.*

- Stereotactic biopsy is generally undertaken to confirm the diagnosis of glioma, although seldom in the older (greater than 60 years) patient who has substantial disability by the time of presentation. The morbidity is usually less than 5% and the mortality less than 1%. The procedure remains necessary partly because, at best, only 95% of malignant brain tumours can be confidently diagnosed on CT and partly because the histological appearance can influence choice of therapy

MANAGEMENT OF MALIGNANT BRAIN TUMOUR

Cytoreductive surgery (tumour debulking)

Generally, tumour invasion occurs for at least 2 cm beyond either its macroscopic boundary or that defined by enhanced CT. Extensive tumour and peritumour excision would inevitably severely jeopardize brain function. Immediately, surgery can reduce focal neurological deficit and lessen seizure frequency. Its effect on survival is uncertain.

External beam brain irradiation

Usually approximately 60 Gy are given in 30 fractions, resulting in a survival time of 9–11 months for anaplastic astrocytoma and glioblastoma. Higher doses fail to improve survival and are associated with a significant risk of radionecrosis. The additional use of nitrosourea with the radiotherapy slightly prolongs survival time.

Corticosteroid therapy

A dramatic reduction of tumour oedema occurs with corticosteroid therapy. The effect is relatively short lived. The steroids (usually given as dexamethasone up to 16 mg/day) are continued until radiotherapy has been completed. Sometimes they are continued thereafter as alternate-dose prednisolone, although with little evidence for longer-term benefit.

Interstitial radiotherapy

Sometimes used for patients with recurrent disease. Radioactive seeds are implanted stereotactically in the tumour. The procedure is associated with a substantial risk of adjacent radionecrosis and its role is uncertain.

Other approaches

On theoretical grounds, more focal treatment could be achieved by introducing gene material directly into the tumour cells, which then renders them sensitive to a particular cytotoxic agent. For example, herpes simplex thymidine kinase can be introduced into tumour cells using a retroviral vector that then renders the cells sensitive to gancyclovir. As yet the approach has not produced benefit in humans.

The whole patient

The condition is distressing to deal with and often handled ineptly. Although many specialities are involved in the patient's care, it is important to identify one individual to whom the patient can relate and from whom information can be obtained.

- Brain tumour manifestations include non-specific features such as headache, specific symptoms and signs related to the site of the lesion, and false-localizing signs produced by distortion of the intracranial contents
- Stereotactic biopsy is generally required to confirm the diagnosis but is avoided in the elderly patient with severe disability and typical scan appearances
- Radiotherapy prolongs survival. The overview of a caring physician is critical

OTHER TUMOURS

METASTASES

Up to 20% of patients with systemic cancer have evidence of brain metastases at postmortem examination (**Fig. 9.8**). Up to 40% of intracerebral tumours are metastatic (the figure varies widely from series to series) and, of these, approximately two-thirds are multiple. The most common sources for these tumours are lung, breast, kidney and skin (melanoma).

The lesions are well demarcated and typically found at the junction of grey and white matter in the middle cerebral territory of the hemisphere. Other sites for spread include the brainstem, cerebellum and orbit. Typically, CT shows a mixed density lesion with substantial oedema and enhancement. MRI is more sensitive for the detection of these tumours. Treatment has little influence on survival, although occasionally excision of isolated renal metastases is followed by a considerable period of remission.

OLIGODENDROGLIOMA

Oligodendrogliomas occur in adults and predominate in the frontal lobes. They frequently contain calcium (**Fig. 9.9**). Although most are slow growing, anaplastic forms occur that have proved to be chemosensitive. A combination of procarbazine, lomustine and vincristine delays progression of disease by up to 36 months. The role of additional irradiation for these tumours is unsettled.

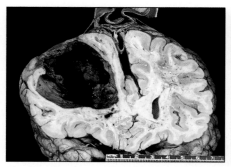

Fig. 9.8 *Cystic metastasis from a small-cell carcinoma of the lung.*

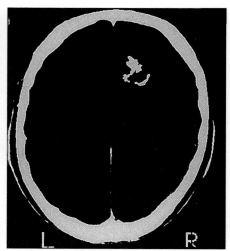

Fig. 9.9 *Oligodendroglioma.* CT with bony windows showing tumour calcification.

TUMOURS IN THE REGION OF THE VENTRICULAR SYSTEM

EPENDYMOMA

Occurs predominantly in children and arises principally from the region of the fourth ventricle. Spread can occur along the CSF pathways and extension into the subarachnoid space is possible. Radical excision is usually feasible.

CHOROID PLEXUS PAPILLOMA

This rare tumour originates within the lateral or fourth ventricle. CT shows striking contrast enhancement. Hydrocephalus is common. The tumour is excisable.

MALIGNANT LYMPHOMA

Spread of systemic lymphoma (usually of the non-Hodgkin's type) to the brain typically affects the meninges. Primary central nervous system lymphoma occurs close to the lateral ventricles or third ventricle and tends to remain confined to the parenchyma, although approximately 20% of patients have tumour cells in the CSF.

The majority of the tumours are large cell in type with more than 95% derived from B cells. They are liable to occur in both congenital and acquired immune deficiency states. Their incidence is markedly increased (350 times) in patients who have had renal transplants and they occur in up to 13% of AIDS patients. In AIDS patients, destruction of T cells by HIV-1 allows uncontrolled proliferation of B cells that have been latently infected with the Epstein Barr virus. Monoclonal Epstein Barr virus is found in virtually all the primary central nervous system lymphomas occurring in AIDS patients.

Some patients present with focal seizures or deficit but many display non-specific problems including lethargy, personality change and confusion. Imaging changes overlap with those produced by toxoplasmosis, with single or multiple lesions, typically showing oedema and ring enhancement (**Fig. 9.10**). In addition to showing tumour cells, in some patients, CSF examination can reveal Epstein Barr viral DNA.

Although corticosteroids produce tumour lysis and dramatic shrinkage of the mass, their

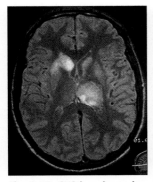

Fig. 9.10 *CNS lymphoma in an AIDS patient. There are enhancing lesions in the L thalamus and the R frontal regions. T1-weighted MRI.*

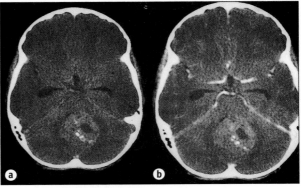

Fig. 9.11 *Medulloblastoma. (a) The CT scan shows a mixed-density growth with obliteration of the fourth ventricle. (b) After contrast, there is slight enhancement.*

use can hinder diagnosis when stereotactic biopsy is employed. For AIDS patients, radiotherapy prolongs survival by a few months. For patients who do not have AIDS, a combination of radiotherapy and chemotherapy is used.

MEDULLOBLASTOMA (CEREBRAL PRIMITIVE NEURO-ECTODERMAL TUMOUR)

Posterior fossa medulloblastomas account for approximately 20% of paediatric brain tumours. They usually arise from the superior vermis of the cerebellum and are liable to disseminate along the CSF pathways. Distant metastases occur infrequently. CT shows a mixed-density tumour with enhancement (**Fig. 9.11**). Hydrocephalus is almost inevitable. The tumours are highly radiosensitive and overall survival, for childhood patients, is approximately 60%.

COLLOID CYSTS

These tumours mainly present in early adult life. They arise in the anterior aspect of the third ventricle. Clinical features include headache, dementia, acute hydrocephalus and episodes resembling drop attacks. CT or MRI shows an intraventricular mass sometimes with slight enhancement. The tumours are benign and can be completely excised.

TUMOURS OF THE MENINGES, CRANIAL NERVES AND SKULL BASE

MENINGIOMA

Meningiomas arise from arachnoidal cap cells and represent 15–20% of all intracranial tumours. Differing pathological types are described; of significance alone is the presence of mitotic figures with brain invasion signifying a malignant form with a high likelihood of recurrence after surgery. The tumours display progestogen and Type II oestrogen binding sites. Cytogenetic analysis indicates that chromosome 22 loss or deletion is common, particularly in fibroblastic meningiomas. Some sporadic meningiomas have mutations of the

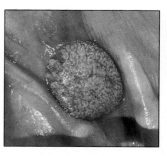

Fig. 9.12 *Incidental meningioma found at postmortem examination.* *The patient had been jaundiced.*

NF-2 gene. Sites where meningiomas arise include the dura over the cerebral convexity, the falx, the sphenoidal wing, the parasellar or suprasellar region and the tentorium (**Fig. 9.12**). Clinical features relate to the site of origin:

Sphenoidal wing	Ophthalmoplegia, mild proptosis and involvement of the ophthalmic division of the trigeminal nerve
Olfactory groove	Anosmia, personality change and visual failure
Parasagittal	Focal epilepsy or a focal motor or sensory deficit, predominantly in the leg
Parasellar	Evidence of chiasmatic compression

The typical CT appearance is a slightly hyperdense tumour close to the falx, tentorium or bone. Enhancement is often conspicuous but oedema relatively slight. Signal characteristics on MRI are similar to those of brain but again there is conspicuous enhancement.

The tumours are resectable but a recurrence rate of up to 20% has been reported even when total macroscopic removal has been achieved.

SCHWANNOMA

Neurofibromatosis is inherited as an autosomal dominant condition. The gene for Type 1 is located on chromosome 17 and for Type 2 on chromosome 22. Criteria have been recommended

Criteria for diagnosis of neurofibromatosis Types 1 and 2	
Criteria for the diagnosis of NF-1	**Criteria for the diagnosis of NF-2**
Two of the following eight criteria	**Any one of the three criteria below**

• Six café-au-lait spots over 15 mm in diameter (adults)
 	
• Multiple axillary or inguinal freckles
 	
• One plexiform neurofibroma or two or more neurofibromas of other types
 	
• Optic nerve or chiasmatic glioma
 	
• Lisch iris nodules (two or more)
 	
• Thinning of the cortex of long bones
 	
• Sphenoid dysplasia
 	
• A first degree relative with NF-1
	• Bilateral VIIIth nerve tumours (as determined by CT or MRI)
	• Unilateral VIIIth nerve tumour and first-degree relative with NF-2
	• Any two of the following plus first-degree relative with NF-2
	  a. plexiform neurofibroma
	  b. neurofibroma of another type
	  c. meningioma
	  d. glioma
	  e. schwannoma
	  f. presenile posterior cataract

Fig. 9.13 *Criteria for diagnosis of neurofibromatosis Types 1 and 2.*

for the diagnosis of each type (**Fig. 9.13**). Markers for Type 1 include café-au-lait spots, neurofibromas or plexiform neurofibromas and iris nodules. Type 2 is principally characterized by the presence of bilateral eighth nerve tumours (acoustic neurinoma or schwannoma).

ACOUSTIC NEURINOMA

Arises close to the mouth of the internal auditory meatus at the junction of the peripheral and central components of the nerve. With expansion, the tumour obtrudes into the cerebellopontine angle. Typically, the tumour presents with unilateral deafness. Other clinical features include vertigo, tinnitus and symptoms and signs of seventh and fifth nerve compression. Cerebellar signs and hydrocephalus are now rarely encountered.

Audiometry is abnormal in the vast majority of patients but the most sensitive electrophysiological investigation is brainstem auditory-evoked responses. A delay between the first and second components (N1–N2) is particularly suggestive. Bilateral abnormalities are common even with unilateral lesions. CT scanning is a relatively sensitive technique for detection of these tumours but the investigation of choice, particularly for intracanalicular tumours, is MRI (**Fig. 9.14**). The tumours can be resected but deafness is virtually inevitable and some degree of facial weakness common.

- Primary central nervous system lymphomas are associated with the immunocompromised patient
- Primary central nervous system lymphomas are radiosensitive
- Meningiomas occur at particular sites in the cranium. Although most are benign, the recurrence rate is relatively high
- Bilateral acoustic neurinomas are associated with the NF-2 gene

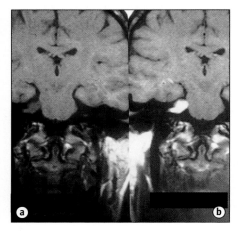

Fig. 9.14 *Acoustic neurinoma.* (*a*) *Before and (**b**) after gadolinium MRI.*

PINEAL TUMOURS

Pineal tumours include:

- **Pinealomas**   Pineocytoma
                          Pineoblastoma

- **Germinal tumours**   Germinoma
                          Embryonal carcinoma
                          Teratoma
                          Choriocarcinoma

Clinical features include the consequence of aqueduct compression, with hydrocephalus, various endocrinological disturbances (e.g. precocious puberty, hypogonadism and diabetes insipidus) and the effects of upper midbrain compression (Parinaud's syndrome). Ocular signs include impairment of up-gaze, convergence–retractory nystagmus on attempted up-gaze and light-near dissociated pupils.

Radiological findings include hydrocephalus, distortion of the posterior aspect of the third ventricle and compression of the quadrigeminal cistern. Calcification is found in both pineocytomas and teratomas. Some of the tumours are enhanced with contrast medium.

EPIDERMOID AND DERMOID CYSTS

Epidermoid and dermoid cysts present as a gradually expanding mass lesion. Rupture of cyst contents into the subarachnoid space can cause a chemical meningitis. CT shows a low-density lesion sometimes with calcification. The tumours are resectable.

Epidermoids are cystic growths that emanate from displaced epithelial cells whereas dermoids are similar but represent mature cystic teratomas.

CHORDOMAS

These arise principally from the sacrum and clivus, from primitive notochordal tissue. Clinical features of the latter result from compression of the brainstem, the lower cranial nerves, the hypothalamus or the region of the optic chiasm. Extensive bone destruction is common and can be best shown by CT. The tumours are managed by surgery combined with high-dose focal irradiation with cyclotron-derived protons.

HAEMANGIOBLASTOMA

Haemangioblastoma principally arises in the cerebellar vermis or hemisphere. Multiple lesions in the central nervous system and retina, associated with cystic changes in the kidney, pancreas and epididymis, occur in Von Hippel–Lindau disease. Typically, the haemangioblastoma consists of a small nodule in the wall of a cyst. Clinical features include hydrocephalus, a cerebellar syndrome or, rarely, a polycythaemic picture secondary to production of erythropoetin by the tumour. CT or MRI reveals a solid or cystic lesion. In the case of the latter, the scan shows a mural nodule undergoing enhancement (**Fig. 9.15**). The tumours are resectable.

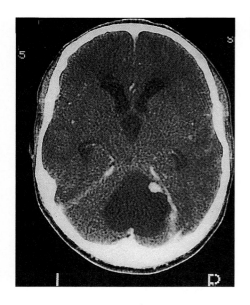

Fig. 9.15 *Haemangioblastoma.*
Postcontrast CT appearance.

PITUITARY TUMOUR

This accounts for 10–20% of intracranial tumours. More common in women.

Definitions of pituitary tumour types

Microadenomas	Less than 1 cm in diameter. Detectable clinically, only if endocrinologically active
Macroadenoma	Greater than 1 cm in diameter. May be detected because of endocrinological changes or mass effect

---

PATHOLOGY
Subtypes include:
Prolactinomas   Account for 20–30% of tumours removed at operation
Adrenocorticotropic hormone producing tumours   10–15%
Follicle stimulating hormone and luteinizing hormone producing tumours   10–15%
Growth hormone producing tumours   5%
Endocrinologically inactive tumours   20–30%

CLINICAL MANIFESTATIONS
Endocrinological effects include Cushing's syndrome, acromegaly, galactorrhoea and hypopituitarism with amenorrhoea, loss of secondary sexual characteristics, impotence and skin pallor.

Compression of the optic chiasm produces a bitemporal hemianopia (typically asymmetrical) or optic nerve or tract compression if the chiasm is postfixed or prefixed (**Fig. 9.16**).

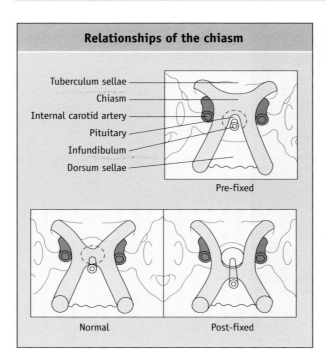

Relationships of the chiasm

Tuberculum sellae
Chiasm
Internal carotid artery
Pituitary
Infundibulum
Dorsum sellae

Pre-fixed

Normal

Post-fixed

Fig. 9.16 *The relationship of the chiasm to the pituitary fossa.*

Sudden expansion of the tumour, either because of infarction or haemorrhage leads to severe headache and ophthalmoplegia, and to signs of subarachnoid haemorrhage if the process is haemorrhagic (pituitary apoplexy).

INVESTIGATION

Plain radiographs are usually abnormal with a pituitary adenoma but are now seldom recorded. Angiography can show mass effect and, in some patients, tumour circulation, but is seldom indicated.

CT reveals an isodense or slightly hyperdense tumour, with calcification in approximately 20% of patients and enhancement in approximately 75%. Microadenomas are difficult to detect on CT.

MRI is the investigation of choice. Microadenomas appear as hypointense on T1-weighted images. Macroadenomas are readily detected and may contain areas of haemorrhagic or cystic necrosis (**Fig. 9.17**).

A random prolactin level will detect patients who have a prolactinoma. A comprehensive testing of anterior pituitary function is achieved by injecting, in turn, insulin, in a dose of 0.1 IU/kg, thyrotropin releasing hormone in a dose of 200 µg and gonadotropin releasing hormone in a dose of 100 µg. Blood samples for follicle stimulating hormone, luteinizing hormone, thyroid stimulating hormone, prolactin, glucose and cortisol are taken at 30-min intervals for 2 h. Specific precautions are needed when intravenous insulin is used.

MANAGEMENT

Large tumours with suprasellar extension are treated surgically via the transfrontal approach. Postoperative radiotherapy is used.

To lessen the risk of recurrence, smaller tumours can be approached trans-sphenoidally

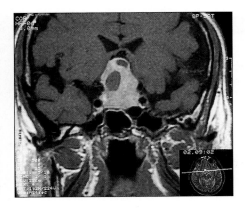

Fig. 9.17 *Pituitary adenoma.* T1-weighted MRI after gadolinium.

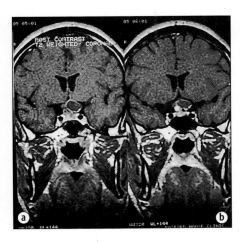

Fig. 9.18 *Craniopharyngioma.* (*a*) Before and (*b*) after gadolinium T1-weighted MRI.

via the nose. Prolactinomas are treated with a dopaminergic agonist, which reduces tumour size substantially without, however, producing cell death. The tumour therefore regrows when the drug is discontinued. Agonists used include bromocriptine, cabergoline and quinagolide. Serial visual fields are used, along with prolactin levels, for documenting response. Surgery is reserved for patients with rapidly deteriorating vision or those contemplating pregnancy.

CRANIOPHARYNGIOMA

Craniopharyngiomas represent approximately 3% of intracranial tumours and usually present before the age of 20 years. Virtually all arise in close relationship to the sella turcica. In children, they produce raised intracranial pressure or hypothalamic dysfunction. In adults, visual failure is the most common presentation.

Calcification is found in most of the tumours arising in childhood but less so for adult-onset patients. CT or MRI show a mass lesion that may be solid or partly cystic and shows uniform or rim enhancement (**Fig. 9.18**). The tumours are dealt with surgically.

GLOMUS JUGULARE TUMOURS

These tumours arise from paraganglionic tissue adjacent to the jugular vein but can also appear in the middle ear, on the tympanic branch of the glossopharyngeal nerve and on the postauricular branch of the vagus. In the middle ear, the tumours produce deafness, often with vertigo and tinnitus and facial weakness. Tumours around the region of the jugular foramen produce a combined palsy of the ninth, tenth and eleventh cranial nerves (**Fig. 9.19**).

The prominent vascular channels of the tumour can be shown by angiography. CT shows the tumour and any associated bone erosion. MRI reveals, on T2-weighted images, a mixed hypointense and hyperintense signal.

Management often combines direct surgery with tumour embolization.

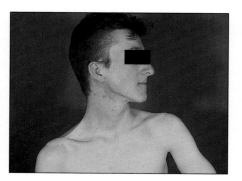

Fig. 9.19 *Glomus jugulare tumour.* Wasting of the right sternomastoid muscle.

- Approximately 60% of pituitary tumours are either prolactin producing or are endocrinologically inactive
- The visual defect produced by pituitary tumours depends on the relationship of the optic chiasm to the gland
- Prolactinomas can often be managed medically, using bromocriptine or an analogous drug
- MRI is the imaging technique of choice for pituitary tumour, craniopharyngioma and glomus tumour

NEOPLASTIC MENINGITIS

Leptomeningeal metastases occur in approximately 5% of all cancer patients. Outside the lymphomas and leukaemias, the tumours most often encountered come from the breast, bronchus, skin (melanoma) and gastrointestinal tract. AIDS-related lymphomatous meningitis is becoming increasingly common. Parenchymal brain metastases are found in approximately 40% of patients with leptomeningeal metastases.

CLINICAL MANIFESTATIONS

Clinical manifestations are a reflection of involvement of the cerebral hemispheres, cranial nerves and the spinal cord and roots.

Cerebral hemispheres
Features include headache, vomiting, seizures, focal weakness and alteration of the mental state.

The cranial nerves
Most commonly affected are the oculomotor nerves, the auditory nerve, the facial nerve, the optic nerve and the trigeminal nerve.

The spinal cord and roots
Features include weakness, numbness, spinal or radicular pain and sphincter disturbances.

INVESTIGATION
Cerebrospinal fluid
Approximately three-quarters of patients have a raised cell count, 90% a raised protein concentration and approximately two-thirds a depressed glucose concentration, based on multiple examinations. Malignant cells are found in the majority of patients, although multiple punctures may be needed and sometimes the positive findings are confined to fluid obtained from the cisterna magna or the ventricles. Various biochemical markers have been studied in the CSF, including β-microglobulin, lactate dehydrogenase, β-glucuronidase and β-human chorionic gonadotrophin. Various protein changes may occur, including abnormal immunoglobulin ratios and the presence of oligoclonal bands.

Imaging
CT abnormalities, using enhanced examinations, are found in approximately one-half of the patients and include sulcal obliteration, hydrocephalus, sulcal or cisternal enhancement and ependymal or subependymal enhancement. In addition, there may be evidence of parenchymal metastases.

MRI with gadolinium is a better technique with a higher yield of abnormal findings. Both MRI and CT myelography have been used for detecting spinal changes. Abnormalities include nerve root thickening, cord enlargement, subarachnoid nodules and pial enhancement of the cord (the last abnormality is seen with gadolinium-enhanced MRI) (**Fig. 9.20**).

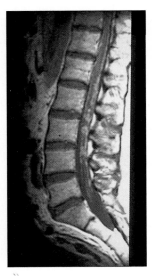

Fig. 9.20 *Multiple nodules of leptomeningeal cancer of lung origin undergoing enhancement.* *T1-weighted MRI.*

Treatment

Systemic chemotherapy is generally unsuccessful because of poor CSF penetration. Direct administration of drugs into the CSF is needed, although benefit here may be limited if there is obstruction to CSF flow. The agents used (single therapy suffices) are methotrexate, cytosine arabinoside or thiotepa. Results are disappointing. Existing neurological deficit seldom improves, although pain syndromes triggered by the disease process may settle. Median survival is of the order of 6 months. Craniospinal irradiation is used for leukaemic meningitis.

BENIGN INTRACRANIAL HYPERTENSION

Benign intracranial hypertension (pseudo-tumour cerebri) predominates in obese women of child-bearing age. A recent population survey of the UK produced an annual incidence for the whole population of 1 per 100 000. The condition is usually idiopathic but a similar picture can occur with certain drugs (e.g. nalidixic acid and the tetracyclines), during withdrawal of corticosteroid therapy and as the sole manifestation of venous sinus thrombosis.

CLINICAL MANIFESTATIONS

Symptoms of benign intracranial hypertension

- Headache. Typically of recent onset, generalized, often severe and exacerbated by straining
- Nausea is common, vomiting less so
- Visual symptoms include blurred vision, transient obscurations (typically triggered by posture change) and diplopia (secondary to a sixth nerve palsy)

SIGNS

- Fundus examination reveals papilloedema, sometimes with peripapillary haemorrhages (Fig. 9.21)
- Various field defects occur, including enlarged blind spots, inferonasal defects and (in the later stages) peripheral constriction or central scotoma
- A unilateral or bilateral sixth nerve palsy is the only other physical sign allowable

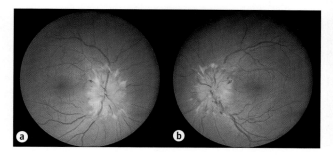

Fig. 9.21 Benign intracranial hypertension. Bilateral papilloedema.

INVESTIGATIONS

CT or MRI fails to show a mass lesion. The ventricles may be slightly narrowed or slightly dilated. CSF pressure is elevated but the constituents are entirely normal. Fluorescein angiography shows an increased vascularity of the optic disc with later leakage of dye from the disc margins.

MANAGEMENT

Acetazolamide is used, on the basis of its potential for reducing production of CSF by the choroid plexuses. Corticosteroids are of no definite value.

Although repeat lumbar puncture is often practised, there is no substantial evidence of a beneficial effect.

For intractable cases (most remit within a few weeks), either lumboperitoneal shunting can be performed or, when there is incipient visual failure, decompression of one or both optic nerves by creating a fistula, allowing the optic nerve subarachnoid space to communicate with the orbital contents.

- Leptomeningeal carcinoma usually arises from the breast, bronchus, skin (melanoma) or gastrointestinal tract
- CSF remains of value in diagnosing leptomeningeal carcinoma
- The only physical signs compatible with a diagnosis of benign intracranial hypertension are papilloedema, various visual field defects and sixth nerve palsies
- Most cases of benign intracranial hypertension resolve spontaneously
- Occasionally, creating a fistula in the subarachnoid space of the optic nerve is needed to prevent visual failure

HYDROCEPHALUS

In hydrocephalus there is a dilatation of the ventricular system, usually in association with an increase in intraventricular pressure. Obstructive hydrocephalus is intraventricular or extraventricular according to the site of the obstruction. Ex-vacuo hydrocephalus results from expansion of the ventricular system secondary to shrinkage of the adjacent brain tissue, caused, for example, by atrophy (**Fig. 9.22**).

AETIOLOGY

- Overproduction of CSF. Rare. Secondary to a choroid plexus papilloma
- Failure of resorption or obstruction of flow. The cause varies according to the age of presentation

AQUEDUCT STENOSIS

Presents either in childhood or adult life. The aetiology of the condition is unclear. Clinical features include:

- In infants, abnormal skull enlargement

175

Causes of hydrocephalus	
Lateral ventricular obstruction	Intraventricular tumour or haemorrhage
Obstruction of foramen of Monro	Suprasellar mass Tuberous sclerosis
Obstruction of third ventricle	Colloid cyst Suprasellar mass Chiasmatic glioma
Obstruction of aqueduct	Aqueduct stenosis Pineal tumour Arteriovenous malformation
Obstruction of fourth ventricle or outflow foramina	Cerebellar tumour Dandy–Walker syndrome Meningitis
Obstruction of subarachnoid space	Meningitis Subarachnoid haemorrhage Chiari malformation

Fig. 9.22 *Causes of obstructive hydrocephalus.*

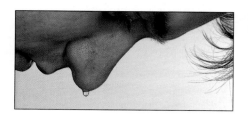

Fig. 9.23 *CSF rhinorrhoea in a patient with aqueduct stenosis.*

- In adults, epilepsy, dementia or CSF rhinorrhoea (**Fig. 9.23**)

Less commonly, an acute elevation of intraventricular pressure leads to headache and clouding of the state of consciousness.

INVESTIGATION OF HYDROCEPHALUS

In infants, cranial ultrasound provides an accurate assessment of ventricular size. Both CT and MRI define the degree of hydrocephalus. The size of the fourth ventricle indicates whether any obstruction is proximal or distal to that site. In addition, MRI provides information on flow within the aqueduct. Periventricular oedema around the frontal and occipital horns is conspicuous if the hydrocephalus has accumulated rapidly and is then an indication for shunting.

NORMAL PRESSURE HYDROCEPHALUS

Intracranial pressure monitoring indicates that in patients with normal pressure hydrocephalus who respond to shunting, abnormal pressure waves occupy at least 5% of the time and recur at intervals of up to two each minute, despite the fact that random CSF pressure measurements are normal. Some cases of normal pressure hydrocephalus follow head injury, meningitis or subarachnoid haemorrhage; others are of unknown cause.

CLINICAL MANIFESTATIONS

A typical triad of symptoms is described, with abnormal gait, dementia and altered micturition.

Features of normal pressure hydrocephalus

- Gait disturbance. Some patients are unable to initiate walking; others tend to take small, stuttering steps with an overall flexed posture
- Dementia. Initially, there is simply a dulling of thought with withdrawal and a lack of motivation. Later, a frankly dementing picture emerges
- Incontinence. Initially, the patient has urgency and frequency. Later, incontinence supervenes

---

INVESTIGATION

Removal of 50 ml of CSF can lead to a temporary improvement in cognition (assessed by the Mini Mental State Examination) and gait. There is a significant association between response to CSF removal and subsequent shunt responsiveness.

Lumbar or cisternal injection of a radioisotope sometimes leads to striking pooling of tracer within the lateral ventricles but the finding correlates poorly with shunt responsiveness.

CT or MRI shows dilatation of the ventricular system and relatively normal sulci. Periventricular lucencies are found, particularly with MRI.

MANAGEMENT

If the triad of symptoms is complete and an aetiological factor is involved, response to shunting occurs in approximately two-thirds of patients and is complete in one-half. If the triad is complete but no aetiological factor is present, only one-third of patients respond. Patients presenting with gait disturbance fare better. Outcome correlates poorly with any change in ventricular size. Shunt complications include infection, epilepsy and subdural haematoma (**Fig. 9.24**).

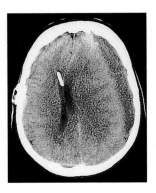

Fig. 9.24 *Normal pressure hydrocephalus.* *Subdural haematoma complicating previous shunting.*

MANAGEMENT OF RAISED INTRACRANIAL PRESSURE

In adults, the normal intracranial pressure lies between 0 and 10 mmHg. Initially, the presence of a mass lesion is partly compensated by a reduction in CSF volume and cerebral blood volume. When that compensatory mechanism fails, intracranial pressure rises, with the appearance of spontaneous waves of pressure (plateau and B waves).

Intraventricular pressure monitoring is the most accurate guide to the presence of intracranial hypertension. Active treatment is normally instituted if intracranial pressure exceeds 25 mmHg for more than 5 min.

Intravenous mannitol is of value as initial treatment in a patient with raised intracranial pressure and impending brain herniation. It is given as an intermittent bolus whenever the pressure rises above 25 mmHg.

Hyperventilation, by producing hypocapnoea, results in cerebral vasoconstriction. The effect does not persist for more than 24 h and may trigger cerebral ischaemia in its own right.

Continuous CSF drainage is sometimes used to control intracranial hypertension, particularly in patients with subarachnoid haemorrhage.

Corticosteroids (e.g. dexamethasone 16 mg/day) are very effective for the treatment of cerebral oedema associated with tumour or abscess. There is no evidence for their effectiveness in patients with head injury but some benefit is seen when high doses of methylprednisolone (30 mg/kg/day) are used in patients with spinal cord injury.

Barbiturates have not been shown to improve outcome in patients with intracranial hypertension secondary to trauma.

- Periodic abnormal pressure waves are found in the CSF in so-called normal pressure hydrocephalus
- Patients with an aetiology for their normal pressure hydrocephalus respond better to shunting than those without one
- There is a significant morbidity associated with shunting for normal pressure hydrocephalus, particularly the development of subdural haematoma
- Intracranial pressure monitoring identifies post-traumatic brain injury patients who are at risk
- Therapeutic intervention is still limited for the management of post-traumatic intracranial hypertension

chapter 10

Multiple Sclerosis and Other Demyelinating Disorders

MULTIPLE SCLEROSIS

DEFINITION OF MULTIPLE SCLEROSIS

A disease of the central nervous system, although, rarely, the condition is accompanied by peripheral nerve abnormalities. It is characterized, in the majority, by remissions and relapses and produces scattered areas of demyelination in the brain and spinal cord.

PATHOLOGY

The hallmark of the condition is central nervous system (CNS) demyelination (**Fig. 10.1**) with relative axonal preservation, although in the late stages, axonal degeneration appears.

Macroscopy

Some degree of cerebral and spinal cord atrophy is usually seen at postmortem. The characteristic lesion consists of a demarcated periventricular plaque of demyelination. Although the plaques predominantly occupy the white matter, cortical lesions are encountered. The plaques tend to be perivenular. The optic nerve, brainstem and spinal cord are all usually affected by the time of death.

Microscopy

The microscopic appearances are determined by the age of the lesion. Early, established lesions are hypercellular with partial myelin destruction and accumulation of myelin debris. The cells, which have a perivascular distribution, include macrophages (**Fig. 10.2**), plasma cells and lymphocytes. Later, cellularity diminishes, gliosis appears and severe oligodendrocyte loss is apparent. Some degree of remyelination is possible but usually ineffective in terms of functional improvement. Evidence for an abnormal immunological response has been found, suggested by the cerebrospinal fluid (CSF) changes encountered and supported by analysis of T cell function.

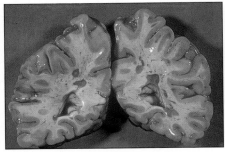

Fig. 10.1 *Multiple sclerosis. Numerous plaques of demyelination particularly in the periventricular areas.*

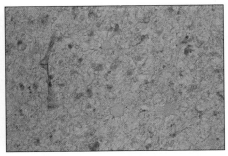

Fig. 10.2 *Lipid-containing macrophages in relation to a multiple sclerosis plaque (mag X 280).*

PATHOPHYSIOLOGY

Partial demyelination of CNS nerve fibres permits saltatory conduction to continue but at a considerably reduced velocity. At a critical level of myelin loss, conduction fails and does so more rapidly if the environmental temperature is elevated. Remyelination can restore conduction, although uncertainty exists over whether this is saltatory or continuous.

Conduction block is likely to cause symptoms. An inability to conduct a rapid train of impulses can be less readily correlated with clinical phenomena. The paroxysmal symptoms of multiple sclerosis (MS) probably reflect the lateral spread of excitatory impulses to contiguous fibre pathways. The exacerbation of symptoms by a rise in body temperature is readily explained by the blocking of partly demyelinated nerve fibres by rising temperature (**Fig. 10.3**).

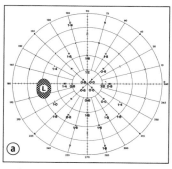
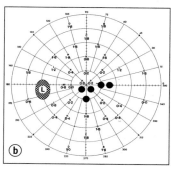

Fig. 10.3
Friedmann visual fields before (**a**) and after (**b**) a hot bath.

- The predominant pathology in MS is demyelination
- Later, axonal degeneration occurs
- Pathophysiological effects include conduction slowing and, eventually, conduction block

---

Epidemiology

- In the UK, Northern USA and Canada, the prevalence of MS is approximately 100 per 100 000 of the population
- The condition is more common in women than men with a ratio of approximately 2:1
- Peak incidence is reached at about the age of 30 years. Onset of the condition is rare in children and in adults over the age of 60 years
- The condition has been attributed to a previous viral insult to the nervous system of a genetically susceptible individual, with a subsequent abnormal immune response in the CNS
- There is no reliable evidence for recovery of viral material from MS brain.

Environmental factors in multiple sclerosis

North–South frequency gradient in the Northern Hemisphere (higher in the North) but the following exceptions apply:
- More prevalent in Italy than comparable latitudes
- North–West to South–East gradient in the USA

In the Southern Hemisphere, prevalence increases in more southerly latitudes

Fig. 10.4 *Environmental factors in multiple sclerosis.*

Natural history

A remitting–relapsing course of disease occurs in approximately 75% of patients with MS leaving the other 25% with a progressive course from onset. The median survival time is over 30 years. The parameters predicting shorter survival are as follows:

- Older age at onset
- Being male
- Cerebellar symptoms at onset
- Progressive course from onset

The frequency of relapse increases with time. The length of the first remission is inversely correlated with the likelihood of conversion to a more malignant course of the disease. A benign course is experienced by 30% of patients. Less than 20% of patients are markedly restricted within 20 years of onset.

Genetic factors in multiple sclerosis

- HLA association
  Class 1 antigens A3, B7
  Class 2 antigens (in whites: haplotype DRW15, DQW6, DW2)
- Racial variation in risk
- Family clustering
- An eight times excess of multiple sclerosis concordance in monozygotic twins

Fig. 10.5 *Genetic factors in multiple sclerosis.*

- MS is more common in women
- MS peaks at about the age of 30 years
- Most patients have remissions and relapses
- Both genetic and environmental factors operate

SYMPTOMATOLOGY

The initial symptoms of the condition are often so subtle that they excite little comment and perhaps are only recognized retrospectively. Inhibiting the ease of early diagnosis is the fact that comparable, vague symptoms can occur in individuals without disease of the CNS.

Early symptoms of multiple sclerosis

- Weakness
- Short-lived episodes of paraesthesiae
- Brief impairment of balance with vertigo and dizziness
- Sensory disturbances
- Clumsiness
- Diplopia
- Visual loss

Motor symptoms

The patient may complain of a short episode of weakness affecting one or more limbs or have noticed a tendency for the legs to feel heavy, perhaps when walking. Occasionally, the weakness is hemiparetic in distribution. Many patients with bilateral signs complain of only the more affected limb.

Sensory symptoms

The initial episode may consist of a sensory disturbance ascending from the legs to the trunk or symptoms occupying the periphery of all four limbs. In all such cases, enquiry should be made about a Lhermitte phenomenon, in which neck flexion produces brief fatiguable electric shock sensations in the spine, legs or, rarely, arms. The Lhermitte phenomenon is virtually pathognomonic of MS in a young individual, although it also occurs in cervical spondylosis, after neck trauma, in subacute combined degeneration of the spinal cord and after spinal irradiation.

Cerebellar symptoms

Most patients will have difficulty distinguishing a cerebellar from a motor deficit. The problem can result in hand clumsiness, a slightly unstable gait or, more rarely in the early stages, dysarthria.

Diplopia

The condition sometimes presents with an isolated sixth nerve palsy. Third nerve palsies are rare in MS (**Fig. 10.6**). Patients with an internuclear ophthalmoplegia seldom complain of diplopia. More often they describe ill-defined blurring of vision or dizziness. A few will have noticed a problem in horizontal tracking.

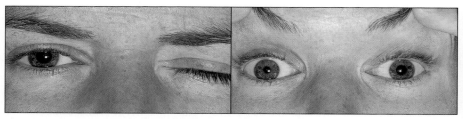

Fig. 10.6 *A third nerve palsy in multiple sclerosis.*

Visual symptoms

In optic neuritis, unilateral visual blurring or loss occurs, typically preceded by ocular pain and pain on eye movement. Occasionally, the condition is bilateral. Physical findings include an afferent pupillary defect and a central scotoma (**Fig. 10.7**). The optic disc initially may be normal or swollen. Recovery is usual.

Typically, early symptoms last for a few days or weeks before resolving. In some patients, an acute episode of this nature (e.g. of optic neuritis) is not followed by dissemination, despite many years of follow-up.

Many patients with remitting–relapsing disease eventually enter a progressive stage.

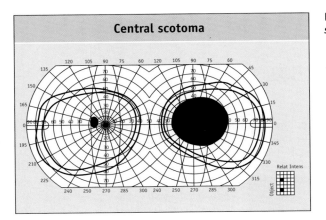

Fig. 10.7 *Right central scotoma.*

- Sensory, motor or visual symptoms predominate initially
- Patients should be asked to recall any brief neurological complaints that they have had in the past

Physical findings

In the early stages of the disease, certainly outside the time of a recent relapse, the physical examination shows little. Abnormalities may be confined to an afferent pupillary defect, depressed abdominal responses or a unilateral extensor–plantar response. Later, a characteristic, fixed pattern of deficit is seen. There is often temporal pallor of the optic discs (although that finding is often overdiagnosed in patients with MS). An internuclear ophthalmoplegia (**Fig. 10.8**) produces slowing of adduction compared with abduction, with nystagmus in the abducting eye; this may be bilateral or unilateral. The speech can become slurred. Pyramidal signs include weakness, hyper-reflexia and extensor plantar responses. The abdominal responses are lost. Some patients will complain of extensor or flexor spasms. The limbs become clumsy. Typically, there is altered or loss of lower limb vibration sense, with some depression of proprioception but relatively normal cutaneous sensation.

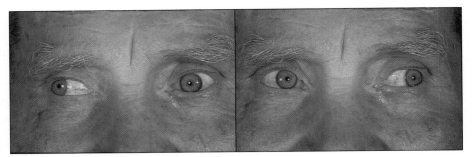

Fig. 10.8 *Bilateral internuclear ophthalmoplegia.*

183

OTHER FEATURES

Pain
Pain is sometimes conspicuous in patients with MS. In addition to painful limb spasms, some patients experience distressing dysaesthesiae in the limbs.

Facial myokymia
Facial myokymia (**Fig. 10.9**) results in a fine rippling motion occurring in part or the whole of the facial nerve distribution. The condition is distinct from benign eyelid myokymia. In young adults it is highly suggestive of the diagnosis but is also seen with pontine tumours.

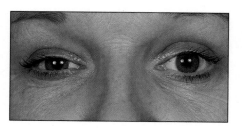

Fig. 10.9 *Facial myokymia causing narrowing of the right palpebral fissure.*

Epilepsy
Epilepsy occurs more commonly in people with MS than in the normal population. Both generalized and focal seizures are described.

Sphincter disturbances
Although bladder symptoms seldom appear at the onset of the disease, they are present in the majority of patients with established, disabling disease. Common problems include detrusor hyper-reflexia and detrusor sphincter dyssynergia, resulting in a mismatch of detrusor contraction and sphincter relaxation. Patients with detrusor sphincter dyssynergia typically complain of urgency and frequency of micturition but may then have problems in voiding. Incontinence is relatively common. Faecal urgency and incontinence, mercifully, are infrequent but constipation is commonplace in the later stages of the disease.

Sexual function
Erectile impotence has been reported in up to 40% of men with MS. It correlates with the presence of sphincter disturbances and the duration of the disease.

Uhthoff's syndrome
Up to 25% of patients with MS report that their symptoms are temporarily exacerbated by increasing temperature or exercise. It is worth asking individuals suspected of having MS whether their symptoms are worsened by a hot bath. Typically, symptoms appear with the appropriate trigger then settle after 20–30 min. Occasionally, similar symptom exacerbation can occur with other neurological disorders.

Bell's palsy
At times, a facial palsy of a Bell's type (**Fig. 10.10**) can be triggered by an MS plaque within the pons (**Fig. 10.11**). In many cases, the presence of other brainstem signs should suggest the possible diagnosis.

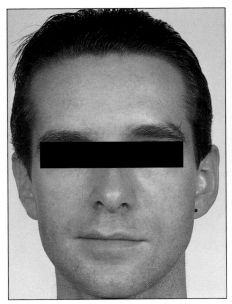

Fig. 10.10 *A lower motor neuron facial weakness in multiple sclerosis.*

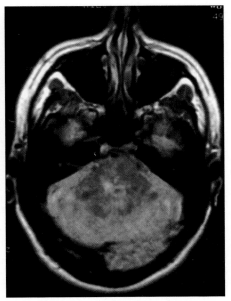

Fig. 10.11 *Magnetic resonance imaging showing a plaque* in the region of the seventh nerve nucleus in a patient with facial palsy.

- Depressed abdominal responses are said to be an early development in MS
- Enquiry should always be made about exacerbation of symptoms by exercise or by a hot bath

Paroxysmal symptoms

The most common of these is trigeminal neuralgia. It occurs in about 3% of patients with MS. The condition is usually indistinguishable from that occurring as a consequence of vascular cross-compression.

Paroxysmal symptoms in multiple sclerosis

- Trigeminal neuralgia
- Tonic seizures
- Dysarthria and ataxia
- Pain
- Itching
- Paraesthesiae
- Diplopia
- Akinesia

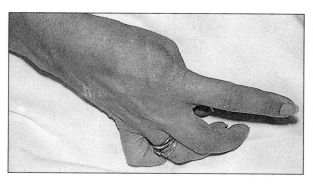

Fig. 10.12 *Tonic seizures.*

Tonic seizures

Frequent paroxysms of muscle contraction affect the upper limb, sometimes with involvement of the face or leg (**Fig. 10.12**). The fingers and wrists tend to flex whereas the lower limb extends. The attacks are brief but often rapidly recurrent and may be painful. Most of these attacks are rapidly controlled by carbamazepine.

Dementia and mood change

Dementia undoubtedly appears in some patients with MS but there is no agreement about its prevalence. It correlates with duration and severity of disease. A euphoric mood has been exaggerated as an MS feature. Depressive illness is more common.

INVESTIGATION

CSF Examination

See **Figure 10.13**.

Cell count – An elevated cell count, consisting mainly of lymphocytes, occurs in up to two-thirds of patients with MS and is more likely during an acute exacerbation. The cell count is less often elevated in older patients and in those with greater disability. It seldom, if ever, exceeds 50/mm^3. The presence of polymorphonuclear leukocytes suggests an alternative diagnosis.

Protein concentration – Elevated overall in perhaps one-quarter of patients but is unaffected by recent exacerbations. It seldom exceeds 1.5 g/l.

Immunoglobulin G (IgG) ratios – Elevated IgG ratios are found in up to 70% of patients with MS and increase according to the diagnostic certainty. There is some correlation between the number of clinical lesions and degree of disability with IgG levels.

Electrophoresis – Electrophoresis is used to detect oligoclonal bands in the IgG fraction of the CSF (**Fig. 10.14**). The abnormality reflects the synthesis within the CNS of multiple IgG fractions with distinct electrophoretic mobilities. The same pattern should be absent in a simultaneously run serum sample. Abnormal bands are found in up to 90% of patients with definite MS. Oligoclonal IgM can also be found, as can elevated levels of free kappa and lambda light chains. Oligoclonal bands are found in other conditions, including sarcoid, AIDS and subacute sclerosing panencephalitis.

Electrophysiology

Electrophysiological techniques, applied to the visual, auditory, somatosensory and motor pathways, have been used to detect subclinical pathology, allowing a more confident

Typical cerebrospinal fluid findings in a multiple sclerosis patient	
Protein	0.80 g/l
Cell count (all lymphocytes)	15/mm³
Immunoglobulin G/albumin	0.30
Immunoglobulin G index	1.05
Oligoclonal bands	positive

Fig. 10.13 *Typical cerebrospinal fluid findings in a patient with multiple sclerosis.*

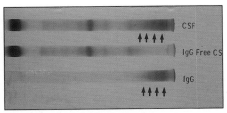

Fig. 10.14 *Oligoclonal bands in the cerebrospinal fluid.*

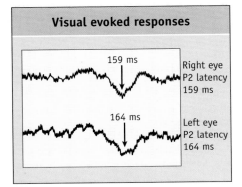

Fig. 10.15 *Visual-evoked responses showing bilateral delay.*

Magnetic resonance imaging criteria for multiple sclerosis

Any two of the following:
- A lesion adjacent to the body of a lateral ventricle
- A lesion below the tentorium
- A lesion ≥6mm in diameter

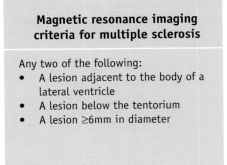

Fig. 10.16 *Magnetic resonance imaging criteria for multiple sclerosis.*

statement of dissemination of the disease process than could be made on the basis of clinical features alone.

Visual-evoked potentials

These are abnormal in up to 90% of patients with definite disease (**Fig. 10.15**). The degree of delay, often approximately 30 or 40 ms, is seldom seen with other neurological disorders.

Other electrophysiological techniques are less sensitive in detecting subclinical disease in the relevant pathway and are less frequently used for diagnostic purposes.

Imaging

Magnetic resonance imaging (MRI) provides not only a highly accurate diagnostic test for MS but also an insight into the natural history of the condition. It has replaced other imaging techniques. The MRI criteria for MS are listed in **Figure 10.16**.

Abnormalities are found in over 95% of patients with definite MS. Typically, periventricular white matter lesions are shown on T2 or proton density images (**Fig. 10.17**), along with abnormalities in the brainstem and cerebellum. Criteria have been established providing a high level of diagnostic specificity and sensitivity. Lesions within the corpus callosum, seen on a T2-weighted parasagittal scan, are particularly suggestive.

Enhancement with gadolinium is characteristic of new lesions, the enhancement resolving after approximately 4 weeks. Far more new lesions occur on sequential scans than can be

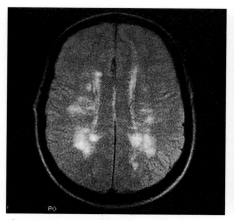

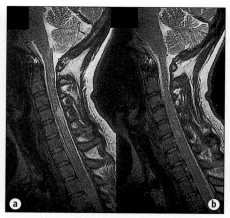

Fig. 10.17 *Typical white matter changes on magnetic resonance imaging in multiple sclerosis.*

Fig. 10.18 *Signal change in the spinal cord in multiple sclerosis. (a) = 1993. (b) = 1994.*

accounted for by clinical events. In patients with an isolated clinical syndrome (e.g. acute optic neuritis), the presence of signal change in other areas of the nervous system substantially increases the risk of subsequent clinical progression. Other conditions can result in periventricular or deep white matter signal change, whereas scattered small white matter lesions are increasingly common with age, probably reflecting small vessel disease. Neurosarcoidosis and various vasculitic syndromes can be particularly confused with MS in terms of their imaging characteristics. Spinal cord imaging has advanced rapidly and can allow identification of typical lesions or exclude other pathologies (**Fig. 10.18**).

- The most important CSF abnormality in MS is the presence of oligoclonal bands
- Visual-evoked responses are the most commonly abnormal electrophysiological investigation
- MRI is the investigation of choice in MS and almost always shows abnormalities in patients with established disease

MANAGEMENT

Acute exacerbations

Reasonably good evidence supports the use of corticosteroids in disabling acute attacks of the condition. Symptom duration is reduced, although without effect on the final outcome. The most common regime used is a 3–5 day course of intravenous methyl prednisolone 0.5–1 g/day, given as an intravenous bolus over 30 min, sometimes followed by a tapering oral dose. It has been suggested that such a regime, in patients with acute optic neuritis, lessens the relapse rate over the next 24 months, whereas conventional doses of oral prednisolone used for the same condition are liable to increase the risk of repeated attacks of optic neuritis over the next 24 months.

Alteration of disease course

Corticosteroids – are ineffective.

Azathioprine – has a slight advantage if the drug is given over a 2–3-year period in terms of disease progression.

Cyclophosphamide – (with or without other regimes.) No consistent evidence for any long-term benefit.

Methotrexate – has possible benefit in patients with chronic progressive MS using a low-dose, long-term regime (7.5 mg/week).

Copolymer 1 – when administered intramuscularly, this appears to reduce the relapse rate in patients with remitting–relapsing disease. No evidence of benefit exists for progressing disease. The substance, a synthetic polypeptide, alters the course of experimental allergic encephalomyelitis.

Cladribine – is a lymphocyte-specific nucleoside. Preliminary reports suggest it may alter the course of chronic progressive disease.

Interferon – Interferon γ increases the relapse rate in MS. Interferon β1b appears to reduce the relapse rate and severity of exacerbations in remitting–relapsing MS when given by subcutaneous injection every other day in a dose of 8 MIU over a 3-year period. The drug is now licensed in the USA and the UK. Serial MRI shows a reduction in the rate of new lesion formation. Overall disability appears unaffected. Side effects include flu-like symptoms and local reactions to the injections. Interferon β1a has also been shown to reduce the relapse rate and severity of relapses when used in a weekly intramuscular regime (6 MIU/week). In addition, the drug appears to have a significant effect on disease progression.

- Acute exacerbations are shortened by the use of corticosteroids
- Interferon β appears to alter some aspects of the natural history
- Methotrexate is possibly of value in chronic progressive MS

Symptom measures

Symptoms managed

- Fatigue
- Pain
- Weakness
- Spasticity
- Bladder function
- Impotence

Fatigue – Many patients with MS complain of chronic fatigue. Sometimes useful benefit is obtained from amantadine or pemoline (a CNS stimulant).

Pain – Disabling dysaesthesiae sometimes respond to amitriptyline.

Weakness – 4-aminopyridine, on theoretical grounds, is able to improve nerve conduction by blocking potassium channels in CNS synaptic excitatory nerve membrane. Measurable improvement in various motor functions has been recorded with the drug in patients with MS but the effects are small.

Spasticity – The three drugs used for spasticity are baclofen (up to 100 mg/day), dantrolene (up to 400 mg/day) and diazepam (up to 60 mg/day). Side effects are common and the results are often disappointing. Rarely, affected limbs become so flaccid that walking capacity is actually reduced. For intractable spasticity, intrathecal baclofen can be valuable. The drug is administered through an implanted pump.

Botulinum toxin is capable of reducing spasticity in muscles into which it has been injected. Considerable doses are needed for the proximal lower limb muscles and the possible role for this treatment is not yet established.

Bladder function – The first step in management of altered bladder function is to determine the predominant pathophysiology. Problems include detrusor hyper-reflexia and detrusor sphincter dyssynergia. Symptoms alone are not sufficient to enable a distinction to be made and it is probably wise to measure the residual urine after micturition before deciding management policy. The measurement can be accurately performed by ultrasound.

For patients with a low residual volume, oxybutynin, initially 2.5 mg bd, is given for symptom control. The dose can be increased to 5 mg tds. Alternatives are a tricyclic antidepressant or propantheline. For patients with a high residual volume, intermittent catheterization should be considered, along with oxybutynin if appropriate.

For troublesome nocturia, intranasal desmopressin (a vasopressin analogue) is useful. At bedtime, 10–20 mg is given and is effective for up to 8 h. Only one dose every 24 h should be given.

Urinary tract infection – Generally, short courses of high-dose antibiotics are preferable to prophylactic low-dose therapy.

Urinary diversion – The creation of an artificial bladder is seldom undertaken now but some patients benefit from a suprapubic catheter. Long-term indwelling catheters are best avoided.

Sexual dysfunction – For some men, intravenous papaverine helps overcome erectile incompetence.

> - Drugs exist for influencing spasticity, altered bladder function, impotence and abnormal fatigue in MS

Other measures

Physiotherapy – This can be of considerable value for improvement of spasticity, help with transfers in chair-bound patients and advice about walking aids.

Occupational therapy – If rational alteration of the home environment is to be attempted in order to maintain independence, occupational therapy appraisal is essential.

Speech therapy – This may be offered to patients with dysarthria and communication difficulties.

MS Society – This organization provides invaluable support to patients, their families and carers.

The role of diet – Marginal evidence exists for advising patients with MS to consume a diet low in animal fats, along with supplements of linoleic acid.

Hyperbaric oxygen – This is of no proven value, other than sometimes lessening bladder symptoms.

Particular situations

Pregnancy – There is no increased risk of relapse in pregnancy itself but there is in the first three months of the puerperium. Despite such relapses, pregnancy does not appear to confer a long-term effect on disease progression.

Vaccination, trauma – Although accounts are available of apparent immediate exacerbations triggered by vaccination or by various forms of trauma, case–control studies do not support such an association.

Childhood – Occasional cases appear before the age of 10 years. Investigators recently suggested that there are no major differences in the way the condition behaves in this age group compared with adults. It is particularly important to distinguish acute disseminated encephalomyelitis (**Fig. 10.19**) from MS, although this may be difficult at the onset of symptoms.

VARIANTS OF MULTIPLE SCLEROSIS

Marburg type

An acute, monophasic, demyelinating condition that leads to early death (**Figs 10.20 and 10.21**).

Schilder's disease

Some patients, described in the past under this umbrella, had leukodystrophy as opposed to demyelinating disease. Others patients, often children, have a rapidly advancing form of MS with predominant involvement of the posterior hemispheric white matter.

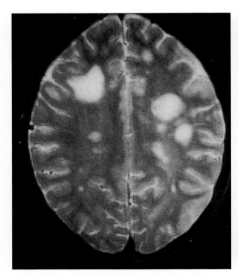

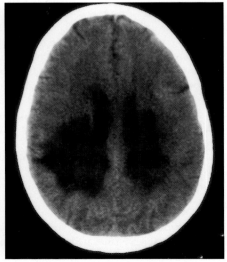

Fig. 10.19 *Magnetic resonance imaging of acute disseminated encephalomyelitis.*

Fig. 10.20 *Computerized tomography in Marburg variant of multiple sclerosis.*

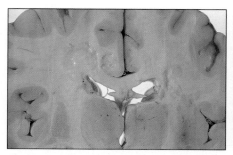

Fig. 10.21 *The macroscopic appearance of the Marburg form of multiple sclerosis.*

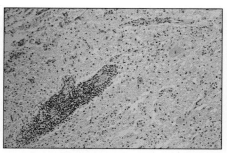

Fig. 10.22 *Devic's disease.* An inflammatory destructive process involving the anterior horn with perivascular lymphocytes but sparing the anterior horn cells.

Neuromyelitis optica – Devic's disease

Strictly, the diagnosis should be limited to patients with bilateral optic neuritis and coincidental transverse myelitis. In some, the illness is monophasic; in others, it is followed by remissions and relapses typical of MS; and, finally, in a third group the pathology is not demyelinating in nature. In typical patients, tissue destruction is prominent and polymorphonuclear leukocytes may be found in the CSF (**Fig. 10.22**).

OTHER DEMYELINATING DISORDERS

ACUTE DISSEMINATED ENCEPHALOMYELITIS

This condition can follow a specific exanthematous illness, vaccination (classically in the past against rabies or smallpox) or an apparently innocuous upper respiratory tract infection. When the condition follows a specific exanthematous illness, 2–20 days elapse from appearance of the rash.

Symptoms appear rapidly and include fever, headache, malaise then depression of the conscious state. Focal neurological signs follow. CSF examination may reveal a slightly elevated protein concentration with a mild lymphocytic pleocytosis but the CSF is normal in approximately one-quarter of patients. Computerized tomography sometimes shows brain-stem oedema together with low-density areas in the basal ganglia and deep white matter along with cortical enhancing lesions. The MRI appearance closely resembles that of MS. Pathological changes include perivascular demyelination together with a monocytic infiltration (**Fig. 10.23**). There is no specific treatment, although dexamethasone is generally used.

ACUTE HAEMORRHAGIC LEUKOENCEPHALITIS

This condition is now regarded as a more fulminant form of postinfectious encephalomyelitis. The brain is markedly swollen and contains multiple petechial haemorrhages (**Fig. 10.24**).

TRANSVERSE MYELITIS

In this disorder, an acutely evolving demyelinating cord lesion typically in the thoracic cord, leads to a paraplegia associated with a truncal sensory level and commonly a disturbance of sphincter function. Progression to MS, at least in Caucasian patients, occurs in less than 10% of individuals. The condition can follow a specific viral illness (e.g. chicken pox) and is encountered in collagen vascular diseases.

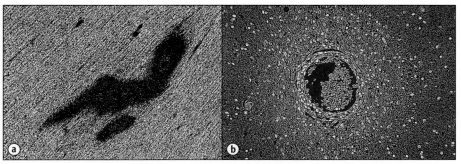

Fig. 10.23 *Acute disseminated encephalomyelitis.* *(a)* Cerebral white matter showing periventricular demyelination (mag X 20) and *(b)* the cellular reaction in the Virchow–Robin space and in the parenchyma around the venule (mag X 200).

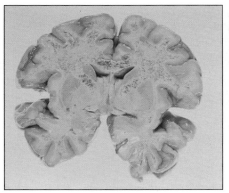

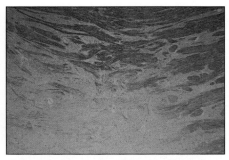

Fig. 10.25 *Central pontine myelinolysis,* showing the central demyelinated zone.

Fig. 10.24 *Acute haemorrhagic leukoencephalitis.* A coronal brain slice showing extensive white matter petechial haemorrhages.

CENTRAL PONTINE MYELINOLYSIS

This condition, which leads to confluent demyelination of the basis pontis (**Fig. 10.25**), was originally described in patients who abused alcohol. It also occurs in other serious medical disorders and in malnourished individuals. In many instances, the condition appears to have been triggered by the overzealous correction of a hyponatraemic state. Clinically, the patient has a depressed conscious level with abnormal horizontal eye movements, anarthria and a tetraparesis. The outcome is often poor, with some patients entering a locked-in state. Imaging can identify the abnormal area (**Fig. 10.26**).

THE LEUKODYSTROPHIES

In the leukodystrophies, diffuse white matter degeneration is found in the centrum ovale and cerebellum, along with axonal loss and degeneration of the cerebral peduncle and pyramidal tracts. There is little inflammatory reaction. Presentation in adult life is rare. Many of the conditions are genetically determined, inherited as X-linked or recessive forms and are the result of a metabolic derangement of myelin.

ADRENOLEUKODYSTROPHY

Usually inherited as a sex-linked, recessive disorder. The neurological features include dementia with pyramidal and cerebellar signs. There is an associated adrenal failure which can precede or coincide with the neurological presentation.

METACHROMATIC LEUKODYSTROPHY

Inherited as a recessive, sex-linked or dominant disorder, the condition is the consequence of a deficiency of the enzyme sulphatase A. In the adult-onset form, there are dementia, ataxia and pyramidal signs. An associated peripheral neuropathy leads to depression of the tendon reflexes.

The enzyme deficiency can be detected in the urine, leukocytes or cultured fibroblasts. Computerized tomography shows symmetrical, nonenhancing, low-density areas in the white matter. In addition to the CNS demyelination, pathological sections reveal an accumulation of extracellular and intracellular metachromatic material (**Fig. 10.27**).

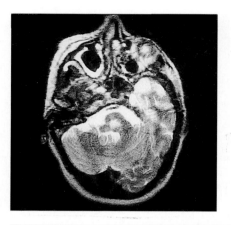

Fig. 10.26 *Magnetic resonance imaging showing an altered pontine signal.*

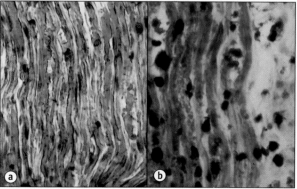

Fig. 10.27 *Metachromatic leukodystrophy. A peripheral nerve showing (**a**) myelin fragmentation with phagocytic infiltration and (**b**) myelin fragmentation with phagocytes containing metachromatic material.*

chapter 11

Central Nervous System Infection

MENINGITIS

Definition of meningitis

Meningitis is an inflammatory reaction of the meninges triggered by an infective agent (viral, bacterial, tuberculous, fungal), a chemical agent or tumour infiltration.

VIRAL MENINGITIS

Viral meningitis produces an acute illness with fever, headache and signs of meningeal irritation. Impairment of the level of consciousness is uncommon.

Symptoms of viral meningitis

- Acute onset
- Fever
- Headache
- Additional symptoms include rash, arthralgia, muscle pain, sore throat and vomiting or diarrhoea

The illness predominantly affects young adults and clusters in the summer and autumn. Computerized tomography (CT) or magnetic resonance imaging (MRI) is unremarkable. Cerebrospinal fluid (CSF) changes include:

- A normal or slightly elevated protein concentration
- A lymphocytic pleocytosis with counts reaching 1000 cells/mm³. Rarely, in the early stages, polymorphonuclear leukocytes predominate
- The glucose concentration is usually normal but sometimes (with mumps, herpes zoster, herpes simplex Type 2 or lymphocytic choriomeningitis) can be moderately depressed
- Attempts to isolate the causative organism or show a significant rise in CSF antibody titre are often unsuccessful
  Treatment is symptomatic. There are no long-term sequelae, although patients may complain of fatigue and malaise for some months after the illness.

MOLLARET'S MENINGITIS

In this condition, recurrent attacks of aseptic meningitis occur, over months or years. CSF shows a lymphocytic pleocytosis with large, endothelial (Mollaret) cells, which are probably monocytes. Herpes simplex virus, particularly Type 2, is responsible for many of the cases.

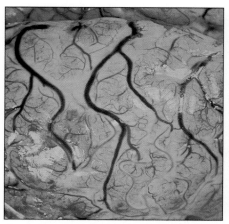

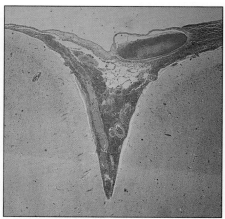

Fig. 11.1 *Bacterial meningitis.* Lateral surface of the cerebral hemisphere showing a purulent exudate.

Fig. 11.2 *Bacterial meningitis.* Section showing exudate in the subarachnoid space of a cerebral sulcus.

BACTERIAL MENINGITIS

PATHOLOGY AND PATHOPHYSIOLOGY

In most patients, the responsible agent reaches the meninges via the blood stream, the portal of entry probably being the choroid plexuses. An intense inflammatory reaction occurs. Macroscopically, there is clouding of the meninges with opalescent streaks surrounding the veins of the cerebral cortex (**Fig. 11.1**). Microscopy reveals polymorphonuclear and mononuclear cells lying between the pia and arachnoid with a fibrinous exudate which extends into the Virchow–Robin spaces (**Fig. 11.2**). Cerebral oedema is particularly common in cases caused by *Haemophilus influenzae*. A vasculitic process affecting both arteries and veins can involve the superficial cortical vessels and those over the base of the brain. Exudate formation can further damage the emergent cranial nerves.

Release of certain cell wall components (endotoxin in the case of meningococci and *H. influenzae*, other components in the case of pneumococci) stimulates release of pro-inflammatory cytokines. These, with other factors, are responsible for the acute inflammatory reaction in the central nervous system (CNS). The prognosis for recovery from the meningitis correlates with CSF levels of endotoxin and pro-inflammatory cytokines.

Cerebral autoregulation is probably preserved in most patients but in more severely ill patients may be lost, perfusion then being dependent on systemic blood pressure.

EPIDEMIOLOGY

Haemophilus influenzae, *Neisseria meningitidis* and *Streptococcus pneumoniae* account for approximately three-quarters of cases of bacterial meningitis in which an organism is isolated.

H. influenzae   Chiefly affects children under 5 years old

N. meningitidis   Predominates in childhood but also affects adolescents and adults. Group B strains are responsible for most cases in the UK

S. pneumoniae   Affects all ages but particularly the very young and the very old Infection may be a manifestation of immune deficiency or due to a congenital skeletal anomaly, allowing access of the organism to the CNS.

Other organisms are uncommon. Their presence (e.g. *Escherichia. coli*, *Klebsiellaspp* or

Listeria monocytogenes) raises the possibility of infection in an immunocompromised individual. Infection with more than one organism occurs in approximately 1% of patients.

Mortality in the UK from meningitis caused by the meningococcus or *Haemophilus* is approximately 5% but approaches 20% for pneumococcal cases.

CLINICAL MANIFESTATIONS

Symptoms

Symptoms of bacterial meningitis

- Fever
- Malaise
- Headache
- Photophobia
- Subjective neck stiffness
- Seizures, particularly in young children
- Mania, in meningococcal meningitis in young adults

The symptoms usually evolve over 24–48 h but sometimes (particularly with the meningococcus) are more fulminant. The clinical picture may be attenuated in elderly people.

Signs

Signs of meningeal irritation (neck stiffness and a positive Kernig) are not inevitable. They are often absent in elderly people, in those in deep coma and in those with immunoparesis.

Rashes are found in approximately one-third of patients. Approximately one-half of the patients with meningococcal meningitis have a maculopapular rash, often with petechial or purpuric elements. Occasionally, a similar (although less florid) rash occurs with other bacterial agents and sometimes with certain enteroviruses.

Focal neurological signs are the consequence of raised intracranial pressure (e.g. a sixth nerve palsy), the result of cerebral vasculitis (e.g. a hemiparesis) or a reaction to basal exudate (e.g. cranial nerve palsies). The level of consciousness correlates with outcome.

INVESTIGATION

Lumbar puncture

CSF examination remains of critical importance in confirming the diagnosis and establishing the organism but is not without hazard. Cerebral oedema is common in meningitis, particularly with *Haemophilus* infection, and evidence of tonsillar herniation after lumbar puncture has been reported in up to 4% of childhood cases. Lumbar puncture is contraindicated if there is papilloedema (a rare finding) and its desirability is questionable if the patient is in coma, if there is a rapidly deteriorating level of consciousness, or if there are focal signs or prolonged seizures.

The pressure is usually elevated. The other findings are summarized in **Figure 11.3**. Gram staining is positive in up to three-quarters of patients. CSF culture is performed both to identify the organism and to obtain data on sensitivities. Various techniques are available for identifying the bacterial antigen, for example, latex particle agglutination and polymerase chain reaction (PCR). Blood as well as CSF culturing should be undertaken.

CSF findings in acute bacterial meningitis

Protein concentration	Usually raised but seldom above 5 g/l
Cell count	Polymorphonuclear leukocytes predominate. The count may reach 100 000 cells/mm^3. Rarely, the cell count is barely elevated or normal
Glucose concentration	Below 2.2 mmol/l in approximately 50% of cases. The concentration is less than one-third of the blood glucose concentration in approximately 75% of patients.

Fig. 11.3 *CSF findings in acute bacterial meningitis.*

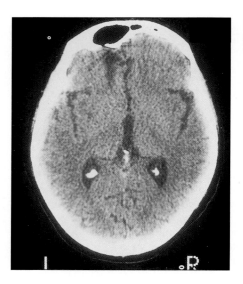

Fig. 11.4 *Recurrent pneumococcal meningitis.* *CT scan showing a defect in the posterior wall of the frontal sinus.*

CT or MRI in the early stages is seldom helpful, although it may reveal gyral enhancement. The performance of these tests should not be a reason for delaying therapy. Scanning is essential if there is papilloedema or focal neurological signs. At a later stage hydrocephalus is encountered in some patients. Patients with recurrent attacks of bacterial meningitis need investigation for a spinal or skull defect that allows access of organisms to the CNS (**Fig. 11.4**).

MANAGEMENT
Management of the common causes of meningitis is complicated in the Western world by the emergence of resistant strains. A summary of the drugs used and their dosages is given in **Figure 11.5**. Treatment is usually given for 10 days, although 7 days suffices for meningococcal meningitis.

Other problems
- Antibiotic treatment before admission lessens the chance of isolating the organism and may induce a lymphocytic picture in the CSF

Drug treatment of acute bacterial meningitis	
Meningoccocal meningitis	High-dose intravenous penicillin, 2.4 g every 4 h High-dose intravenous ampicillin, 2 g every 4 h Intravenous chloramphenicol, 750 mg every 6 h Intravenous cefotaxime, 2.6 g every 8 h (Some infections are penicillin resistant) (7 days, treatment suffices)
Pneumoccocal meningitis	High-dose intravenous penicillin, 2.4 g every 4 h Intravenous chloramphenicol, 750 mg every 6 h Intravenous cefotaxime, 2.6 g every 8 h (Penicillin-resistant organisms are becoming increasingly common)
Haemophilus meningitis	Intravenous cefotaxime, 2.6 mg every 8 h Intravenous ceftriaxone, 4 g every 24 h
Meningitis of unknown cause	Intravenous cefotaxime, 2.6 g every 8 h Intravenous ceftriaxone, 4 g every 24 h

Fig. 11.5 *Drug treatment of acute bacterial meningitis.*

- Meningitis caused by a shunt infection is often the result of coagulase-negative staphylococci and is treated with vancomycin
- Listerial infections respond to ampicillin
- Failure to respond should initiate a review of treatment, fresh scanning to exclude subdural or intracerebral abscess formation and repeat of the CSF examination

Steroid therapy

Dexamethasone treatment, in doses of approximately 0.15 mg/kg every 6 h for 4 days, if initiated early (preferably before starting antibiotics), improves outcome in childhood cases of haemophilus meningitis. The role of the drug in adult patients and in other forms of bacterial meningitis is less certain.

Contact treatment

Used for cases of meningococcal and haemophilus meningitis. Rifampicin is used in both instances, although in differing regimes. Treatment is given to close family and school or nursery contacts, and to the patient before discharge.

Prevention

Most haemophilus meningitis is caused by Group B organisms. Vaccines have been developed for use in young children and have led to a reduction in incidence of haemophilus meningitis. Capsular polysaccharide vaccines against Groups A and C meningococci are available and are used in outbreaks. Vaccine against Group B organisms is still being developed. As yet vaccines do not play a significant role in the prevention of pneumococcal meningitis.

Sequelae

Bacterial meningitis is the most common cause of acquired sensorineural deafness, which appears in approximately 10% of patients. Other neurological sequelae of a serious degree are found in perhaps 5% of patients.

- *H. influenzae, N. meningitidis* and *S. pneumoniae* account for approximately three-quarters of cases of bacterial meningitis
- Lumbar puncture carries a significant risk, particularly in childhood cases of bacterial meningitis
- Steroids, if administered early, improve outcome in childhood cases of haemophilus meningitis infection

TUBERCULOUS MENINGITIS

PATHOLOGY AND PATHOPHYSIOLOGY

After tuberculous bacteraemia, small infective foci (Rich's foci) may appear in the brain, spinal cord or meninges. Expansion of the focus produces a mass lesion (tuberculoma), whereas its rupture into the subarachnoid space or the ventricular system results in meningitis with a gelatinous exudate forming, mainly in the basal cisterns (**Fig. 11.6**). Microscopy reveals an inflammatory cell reaction containing lymphocytes, plasma cells and epithelioid cells. Tubercle bacilli may be sparse or plentiful. An accompanying vasculitis accounts for any focal neurological deficit, although later, with fibrotic change in the meninges, hydrocephalus is common.

Epidemiology

Tuberculous meningitis remains common in economically deprived countries and should be considered in immigrants from areas of high prevalence. It is more common in the Asian community in the UK than in the White population. It figures as one of the opportunistic infections in HIV patients.

CLINICAL MANIFESTATIONS

Symptoms and signs

Initial symptoms of tuberculous meningitis

- Fever
- Headache
- Malaise
- Muscle pain

The initial symptoms are non-specific. Signs of meningeal irritation appear slowly over 1–3 weeks and are accompanied by dulling of the conscious state. Basal exudation with a secondary vasculitis accounts for focal neurological signs (**Fig. 11.7**).

Investigation

An abnormal chest radiograph is found in approximately half of the patients. A tuberculin skin test is often negative. CSF examination is essential. The findings are summarized in **Figure 11.8**. It is common not to find the organism on Ziehl–Neelsen staining but the yield

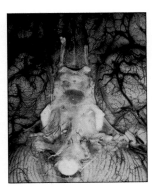

Fig. 11.6
Tuberculous meningitis. Gelatinous exudate occupying the basal cisterns.

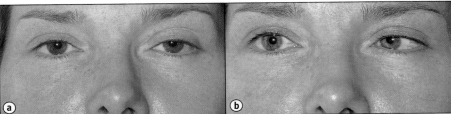

Fig. 11.7 *Tuberculous meningitis.* Right sixth nerve palsy. *(a)* Forward gaze. *(b)* Right lateral gaze.

CSF findings in tuberculous meningitis	
Protein concentration	Usually 1–5 g/l
Cell count	Usually 100–400 lymphocytes/mm³ but, rarely, normal in tuberculin-negative cases. Sometimes up to 1000 cells/mm³ and predominantly polymorphonuclear leukocytes in acutely evolving infections
Glucose concentration	Between 1.7 and 2.5 mmol/l in approximately 50% of cases

Fig. 11.8 *CSF findings in tuberculous meningitis.*

from staining and culture increases if sequential specimens are examined. Mycobacterial antigen can be detected in the CSF. CT shows enhancement of the basal cisterns with low-density areas in the basal ganglia region. Hydrocephalus is common and some patients have concomitant tuberculomas.

MANAGEMENT

Early treatment is essential if long-term complications are to be avoided. The choice of drugs is based largely on their CSF penetrance. Concentrations of pyrazinamide and isoniazid approach those in the serum. Rifampicin concentrations, however, are only approximately one-tenth of serum levels, whereas penetration of streptomycin and ethambutol ceases when the meninges are no longer inflamed.

Initial treatment consists in administration of pyrazinamide, isoniazid and rifampicin, possibly with the addition of streptomycin. If streptomycin is used, it is stopped after 3 months. The other three drugs can be given by mouth or nasogastric tube. Pyridoxine is also given to prevent isoniazid neuropathy. Intrathecal streptomycin is unnecessary. The treatment is continued for 9–12 months. The role of steroids is uncertain. They are frequently used in more severely ill patients or in those with evidence of impending spinal block. Shunting is indicated if hydrocephalus develops.

TUBERCULOMA

Many cases of tuberculoma in the UK occur in the Asian community. The tumours are usually infra-tentorial in children and supra-tentorial in adults. They are multiple in up to one-third of patients.

They consist of a central caseating core surrounded by a collagen capsule containing epithelioid cells, lymphocytes and giant cells. Organisms are found on microscopy in approximately 70% of cases(**Fig. 11.9**).

CLINICAL MANIFESTATIONS
- Typically presents with signs of raised intracranial pressure
- Seizures occur in at least 50% of patients
- Hemiparesis occurs in approximately one-third of patients
- Fever is uncommon

INVESTIGATION
- Chest radiograph is abnormal in approximately 50% of patients
- Skin testing is often negative
- The erythrocyte sedimentation rate is usually normal
- The most common CSF abnormality is a raised protein concentration
- CT identifies low- or high-density areas, often with marked oedema. Enhancement may occur either diffusely or in a ring form

MANAGEMENT
Antituberculous chemotherapy usually suffices, with steroids if there is extensive oedema. Surgery is seldom necessary.

CRYPTOCOCCAL MENINGITIS

Cryptococcus neoformans is an ovaloid body measuring 2–15 μm surrounded by a polysaccharide capsule. The organism, found in the soil of bird colonies, gains access to the body via the respiratory tract. The initial pulmonary infection may be silent. With haematogenous dissemination, infiltration of the leptomeninges occurs, leading to meningeal thickening and proliferation of the organisms within the Virchow–Robin spaces (**Fig. 11.10**). Granuloma may appear in the brain or spinal cord.

In the past, infections have predominated in patients with defects of the immune system, although in some countries, they occur without clear predisposing factors. Cryptococcal meningitis is now one of the most common CNS infections seen in AIDS patients.

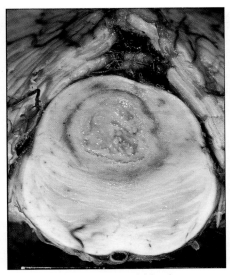

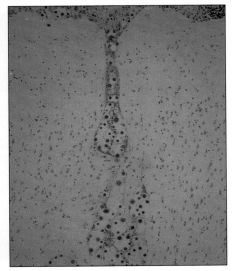

Fig. 11.9 *Tuberculoma within the pons.*

Fig. 11.10 *Cryptococcal meningitis.*
*Cryptococci distending the perivascular space
of a cortical blood vessel.*

CLINICAL MANIFESTATIONS

The features resemble tuberculous meningitis, with malaise, headache and vomiting, followed by the development of focal neurological signs. Optic nerve infiltration by granuloma is common, as is the later appearance of papilloedema.

INVESTIGATION

- The chest radiograph is abnormal in approximately 25% of cases
- The CSF pressure is usually raised with a lymphocytic pleocytosis, a mildly elevated protein concentration and depressed glucose concentration
- India ink staining identifies the encapsulated budding cells in up to 90% of cases
- The polysaccharide capsular antigen can be identified using a latex agglutination test
- CT changes are non-specific. There may be meningeal enhancement

MANAGEMENT

Agents used include amphotericin and fluconazole. The most effective regime and the best dosage and duration of treatment remain unsettled. In patients with immune suppression (including those with AIDS), long-term prophylaxis with fluconazole 200 mg daily is advised.

- Initial treatment of tuberculous meningitis is with pyrazinamide, soniazid and rifampicin, possibly with the addition of streptomycin
- Most cases of tuberculoma in the UK occur in the Asian community
- Cryptococcal meningitis shares many features with tuberculous meningitis

OTHER FUNGAL INFECTIONS

ASPERGILLOSIS

Occurs in immunocompromised patients. The organism invades blood vessels, leading to occlusion or mycotic aneurysm formation. A focal mass lesion sometimes appears. Treatment is by a combination of surgery, amphotericin and 5-fluorocytosine.

MUCORMYCOSIS

Virtually confined to individuals with a predisposing condition, for example, diabetes mellitus. The organism tends to gain access to the CNS through the paranasal sinuses. Features include facial pain, proptosis and ophthalmoplegia followed by arterial or retro-orbital venous occlusion. Treatment combines surgery with amphotericin.

COCCIDIOMYCOSIS

This agent affects the lung then the CNS, producing a granulomatous reaction in the meninges and sometimes the parenchyma, resembling the changes seen in tuberculous meningitis. Treatment is with amphotericin.

CANDIDIASIS

Candida infection is virtually confined to patients with a systemic illness, for example, AIDS, or those who have been treated with antibiotics, steroids or both. It can produce a meningitis or focal encephalitis and is treated with amphotericin, sometimes with the addition of 5-fluorocystosine.

HISTOPLASMOSIS

Infection by *Histoplasma capsulatum* is endemic in the Central and Eastern states of the USA. The infection is usually confined to the lung but can spread to the CNS, causing a meningitis or disseminated parenchymal granulomata.

PARASITIC INFECTION

HYDATID DISEASE

Hydatid disease is caused by infestation by the cystic stage of *Taenia echinococcus* (*Echinococcus granulosus*). The heads of the worms are produced from the inner walls of the cyst capsule (**Fig. 11.11**). Involvement of the brain may be silent or lead to epilepsy.

CYSTICERCOSIS

Cysticercosis is the encysted stage of the pork tapeworm, *Taenia solium*. Ingestion of contaminated food containing the ova allows them to penetrate the gut and develop into the cystic stage of the disease. The CNS is infected in 60–90% of patients with cysticercosis. The cyst formation may be silent or result in epilepsy. Invasion of the arachnoid by the cysticerci leads to meningeal fibrosis and obstructive hydrocephalus. CT shows multiple small foci of cysts, or calcification (**Fig. 11.12**). If the disease is active, an inflammatory reaction, sometimes with eosinophils, is found in the CSF. Cysticercal antigens can be detected in the CSF. Drug therapies include praziquantel and albendazole, often with prior corticosteroid cover.

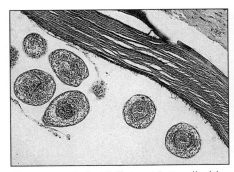

Fig. 11.11 *Hydatid disease.* Cyst wall with laminated chitinous layer and inner germinal layer, surrounding scoleces with invaginated heads.

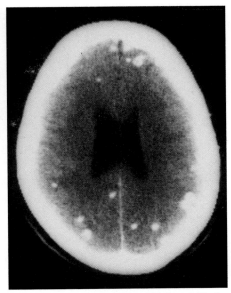

Fig. 11.12 *Cysticercosis.* Multiple calcified cysts on CT.

CEREBRAL ABSCESS

The incidence of cerebral abscess is said to be 1 per 10 000 general hospital admissions.

PATHOLOGY AND PATHOPHYSIOLOGY

Most intracerebral abscesses are secondary to infection in the paranasal sinuses or middle ear, although in up to 20% of patients the source of infection cannot be identified. The initial process is a cerebritis followed by necrosis, capsule formation and adjacent oedema. The site of the abscess is determined by the mode of spread. Local spread from the ears or paranasal sinuses affects primarily the temporal lobes, frontal lobes or cerebellum. Blood-borne infection localizes to the grey–white matter junction and is often multifocal. Cerebral abscess is a recognized hazard in patients with congenital cyanotic heart disease and pulmonary arteriovenous malformations and for intravenous drug abusers. Abscesses can also result from direct trauma of the skull from perforating injuries. The organisms responsible are often mixed and frequently include anaerobes.

CLINICAL MANIFESTATIONS

Presentations include
- Fever, drowsiness and seizures but no focal neurological deficit
- Evidence of an expanding mass lesion without indications of its infective basis

INVESTIGATION

- The electroencephalogram (EEG) frequently shows a focal slow wave disturbance
- The CSF is often abnormal but lumbar puncture is hazardous and should not be performed
- CT or MRI detects all symptomatic intracerebral abscesses. Cerebritis results in a non-homogeneous mass with irregular margins and diffuse enhancement. As abscess

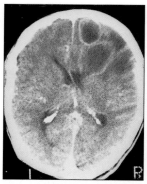

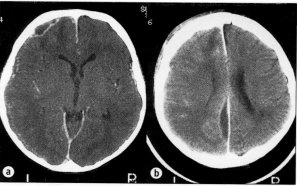

Fig. 11.13 *Cerebral abscess.* *CT scan showing ring enhancement in multiple frontal abscesses.*

Fig. 11.14 *Subdural empyema.* *CT showing (a) a left frontal and (b) an interhemispheric collection.*

formation occurs, ring or dense homogenous enhancement appears, sometimes with ependymal enhancement. A proportion of abscesses are multiple (**Fig. 11.13**)

- Routine haematological and biochemical investigations are performed, along with blood cultures, but these seldom provide diagnostic information

MANAGEMENT

Some abscesses, particularly those that are multiple and inaccessible, are managed with antibiotics alone. The usual drug combination is:

- Intravenous penicillin 24 MIU every 24 h
- Intravenous chloramphenicol 4 g every 24 h
- Metronidazole

Treatment is given for 6 weeks or longer. Dexamethasone is usually added. Additional antibiotics are needed if staphylococcal infection is suspected or confirmed.

Surgery is indicated if there is doubt about the diagnosis or if the abscess is causing significant space occupation. Aspiration under CT stereotactic control provides diagnostic material in the vast majority of patients. Serial CT or MRI is used to assess progress. Prophylactic anticonvulsant therapy is not justified.

SUBDURAL EMPYEMA

Subdural empyema usually follows infection of the paranasal sinuses or as a consequence of bone infection after surgery or trauma. The majority of cases occur in individuals under 20 years of age. The collection of pus is often extensive with a tendency to accumulate along the falx as well as over the convexities. Cortical thrombophlebitis frequently follows. The responsible organism cannot be cultured from the collection in up to 25% of patients.

Typically, signs of sinus infection are followed by focal, then generalized, severe headache. Signs of sepsis are usual, including fever, tachycardia and malaise. Later, focal neurological deficit appears, associated with a decline in the conscious state and seizures, frequently focal and often intractable.

Rarely, the CT scan is negative but, typically, it reveals one or more collections of pus, with enhancement between the inner surface of the collection and the adjacent cortex (**Fig. 11.14**). The EEG is often suggestive with focal δ waves of up to 2 s duration associated with extensive unilateral depression of cortical activity.

Treatment combines antibiotic therapy with craniotomy and removal of pus.

- In a significant number of patients with cerebral abscess, the source of infection cannot be identified
- Some patients with cerebral abscess present with a mass lesion without evidence of infection
- CSF examination should not be performed in patients with suspected cerebral abscess
- Intractable seizures are a common feature of patients with subdural empyema

ENCEPHALITIS

VIRAL ENCEPHALITIS

The agents causing viral encephalitis vary from one part of the globe to another. In the UK, herpes simplex is the most common cause of sporadic encephalitis. In the USA, both sporadic and epidemic forms are caused by the arbor viruses. The illness results from direct invasion of the brain parenchyma via the blood stream. Portals of entry include the skin, through insect bites, and the gastrointestinal or the respiratory tracts. Invasion via neurons is also a recognized mode of entry to the CNS.

Features of viral encephalitis

- A prodromal illness
- Fever
- Headache
- Depression of the conscious state
- Focal or generalized seizures – common
- Focal neurological signs

EEG shows diffuse slow-wave activity. Temporal localization of periodic epileptic discharges is particularly suggestive of herpes simplex infection. The CSF pressure may be raised. Typically, the protein concentration is slightly raised, the glucose concentration normal and the cell count elevated, the majority of cells being lymphocytes. Rarely, the cell count (lymphocytes) is normal or over 100 cells/mm^3. An increased red cell count simply reflects the haemorrhagic component in some patients. Rarely, the CSF is normal. Viral antigen is only infrequently recoverable from the CSF. Delayed diagnosis is achieved on the basis of rising antibody levels in the CSF, with a specificity and sensitivity of approximately 80% respectively.

SPECIFIC AGENTS

Herpes simplex

Most cases are caused by Type 1. The basal frontal and temporal lobes are principally affected. The lesions are often haemorrhagic (**Fig. 11.15**). The condition is treated with acyclovir, 10 mg/kg by intravenous infusion over 1 h, three times a day, for 10 days. Dexamethasone is usually additionally used if there is considerable mass effect.

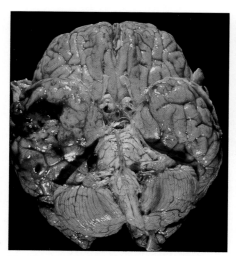

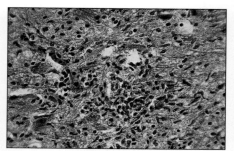

**Fig. 11.16   *Poliomyelitis.* Clusters of
microglia and lymphocytes around anterior
horn neurons.**

Fig. 11.15   *Herpes simplex encephalitis.*
*Basal view showing haemorrhage and necrosis
in the right temporal lobe. There is brain
swelling.*

Other agents associated with sporadic encephalitis include varicella zoster,
cytomegalovirus, mumps, measles and Epstein Barr viruses. Management of these patients
is symptomatic.

Epidemic encephalitides

These are associated with arbor viruses spread by insect bite. Forms encountered in the USA
include Eastern equine encephalitis, Western equine encephalitis, St. Louis encephalitis and
California and La Crosse encephalitis.

Rabies

Rabies is still relatively common worldwide and presents in either an encephalitic or
paralytic form. Retrograde axoplasmic transport is the means by which the virus gains
access to the CNS from the peripheral nerve. Transmission is almost always through the
bite of an infected animal. After local pain, the condition rapidly evolves with agitation and
reflex muscle spasms triggered by minor stimulation. The diagnosis is most rapidly
achieved by detecting viral antigen in skin biopsies taken from the hairline in the neck.
Treatment of the established disease requires sedation, paralysis and artificial ventilation. If
exposure is suspected, administration of a combination of human rabies immunoglobulin
and human vaccine is required.

Poliomyelitis

Poliovirus gains access to the CNS via the gut or respiratory tract. Adults living in temperate
climates who have not acquired immunity and who become exposed to the virus are liable
to develop a more profound illness than children who have been exposed to the virus from
an early age. The major site of pathology is the anterior horn cell but also affected are the
brainstem and the motor cortex. There is a perivascular inflammatory cell infiltration with
petechial haemorrhages. The white matter is relatively spared (**Fig. 11.16**).

Infection is often asymptomatic or results in a non-specific viraemia. If paralysis appears, it does so as the initial fever and signs of meningeal irritation settle; it reaches a maximum in 4–5 days. It is usually asymmetric and predominates in the lower limbs. Residual disability is common in the form of abnormal foot postures, flail joints or kyphoscoliosis. In some patients, muscle wasting appears years after the acute illness (postpolio syndrome). The CSF shows an inflammatory reaction with polymorphonuclear leukocytes predominating initially. There is no specific treatment.

Subacute sclerosing panencephalitis

Subacute sclerosing panencephalitis, an inclusion-body encephalitis, follows measles infection after a mean period of 5 years. There is no relationship between subacute sclerosing panencephalitis and postmeasles acute encephalomyelitis or the subacute measles encephalitis which sometimes occurs in immunocompromised individuals. The condition does not occur after the age of 25 years. The incidence is approximately 1–3 per 1 000 000.

The condition presents with a behavioural disturbance followed by dementia, myoclonus and incoordination. The EEG shows repetitive slow-wave discharges alternating with periods of relative electrical silence. The CSF contains oligoclonal (immunoglobulin G) measles antibody. CT or MRI identifies low-density lesions in the subcortex and periventricular areas.

Generally, the course is progressive and occasionally it appears to arrest or even temporarily improve. There is no specific treatment.

Creutzfeldt–Jakob disease

Creutzfeldt–Jakob disease is the most commonly encountered of the spongiform encephalopathies. All of these conditions are associated with the accumulation of an abnormal prion protein in the brain. They include:

- Scrapie
- Transmissible mink encephalopathy
- Chronic wasting disease of mole, deer and elk
- Bovine spongiform encephalopathy
- Feline spongiform encephalopathy
- Exotic ungulate encephalopathy
- Kuru
- Creutzfeldt–Jakob disease
- Gerstmann–Sträussler–Scheinker disease
- Fatal familial insomnia

Prions are small proteinaceous particles that resist inactivation by procedures that modify nucleic acid. Prion protein is found in normal brain as well as (in a different form) in the spongiform encephalopathies. The function of prion protein is unknown. The prion diseases are transmissible but can also occur by mutations in prion protein. Creutzfeldt–Jakob disease occurs principally as a sporadic disorder, sometimes from accidental inoculation of material from affected patients, as a familial, dominantly inherited disorder caused by mutations in the prion protein gene and perhaps as a consequence of the ingestion of contaminated material.

Genetic factors influence the liability to develop the disease and its clinical expression. Individuals with the E4 allele of apolipoprotein ϵ are at higher risk of developing the condition.

The triad of microscopic features that characterize the spongiform encephalopathies is neuronal spongiform degeneration, severe astrocytic gliosis and amyloid plaque formation. (Fig. 11.17). In the UK, 50–100 cases occur each year approximately.

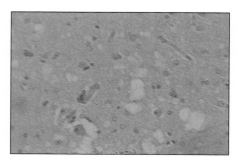

Fig. 11.17 *Creutzfeldt–Jakob disease.*
Section showing neuronal loss with astrocytic proliferation and spongiform vacuolation (mag X 350).

The disease usually presents in older individuals with personality change, seizures, focal neurological deficit and dementia. Myoclonus sensitive to noise or touch emerges in the majority, often showing a characteristic rhythmicity. In the UK, cases in younger individuals have emerged recently, characterized by initial psychiatric symptoms, followed by a cerebellar syndrome leading then to memory failure and akinetic mutism. The familial form (Gerstmann–Sträussler–Scheinker) accounts for approximately 10% of patients and principally affects the cerebellum.

The EEG reveals, at least in older patients, repetitive complexes that coincide with the myoclonus. The CSF protein is sometimes moderately elevated. Atrophy may be apparent in the later stages with CT or MRI. There is no treatment.

- Herpes simplex is the commonest form of sporadic encephalitis in the UK
- Acyclovir significantly improves the outcome in patients with herpes simplex encephalitis
- The EEG is a valuable diagnostic test in suspected Creutzfeldt–Jakob disease
- Transmission of bovine spongiform encephalopathy to humans is possible but unproven

CEREBRAL MALARIA

Cerebral malaria occurs with *Plasmodium falciparum* infection. The mortality rate lies between 25% and 50%. Particularly susceptible are individuals who have travelled to endemic areas and have not taken prophylaxis.

The clinical manifestations result from direct endothelial damage triggered by an immune-mediated inflammatory reaction together with vessel occlusions as the result of sequestration of red cells in small cerebral venules. Hypoglycaemia is common and may contribute to the clinical state.

The level of consciousness is impaired with confusion, hallucinations and psychotic features. Both pyramidal and extrapyramidal features may be found. Seizures are common.

Thick and thin blood films should be examined immediately and blood sugar levels monitored. CSF examination is usually performed to exclude other, infective processes.

Quinine is the drug of choice, given as an intravenous infusion of 5 mg/kg over 2 h and repeated two to three times a day. An antifolate metabolite, for example, doxycycline, is

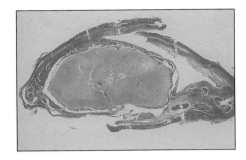

Fig. 11.18 *Syphilitic pachymeningitis.*
Section showing cervical cord with collagenous
thickening of dura and leptomeninges,
particularly around the nerve roots.

given at the same time. Other complications include Gram-negative septicaemia, acute tubular necrosis, anaemia and jaundice.

SPIROCHAETE INFECTIONS

SYPHILIS

Syphilis is caused by the spirochaete treponema pallidum. The organism can reach the CNS early in the course of infection, even in the primary stage. Meningeal involvement, revealed by the presence of a CSF pleocytosis, is present in the majority of patients by the stage of secondary syphilis but is often asymptomatic. The initial pathological event in the nervous system is a meningitis which may be indistinguishable from acute viral meningitis. This stage of infection is often occult but is followed, months or years later, by the tertiary stage of the disease, to which both meningeal and parenchymal pathological changes contribute.

MENINGOVASCULAR SYPHILIS

Endarteritis of cerebral or spinal vessels, sometimes leading to vessel occlusion (Heubner's endarteritis) is accompanied by meningeal thickening and infiltration by lymphocytes and plasma cells (**Fig. 11.18**).

Clinical features include cranial nerve palsies, hydrocephalus and focal deficit associated with the endarteritis.

The CSF is always abnormal with a lymphocytic pleocytosis, a moderately elevated protein concentration and abnormal serology in the vast majority of cases. Angiography shows concentric constriction of large vessels with focal dilation and constriction of smaller vessels. Response to penicillin is usually good.

TABES DORSALIS

Approximately 70% of cases of tabes appear within 20 years of the primary infection. Pathologically, there is dorsal root atrophy with posterior column degeneration and thickening of the overlying meninges.

Clinical features include:
- Root pain, radicular sensory loss, ataxia and areflexia
- Lightening pains (severe, brief, lancinating pains in the limbs or trunk)
- Abnormal pupils
- Optic atrophy
- Autonomic dysfunction affecting the gut, bladder or larynx
- Severe joint dysfunction (Charcot's joints) secondary to loss of pain sensitivity (**Fig. 11.19**)
- Perforating skin ulcers

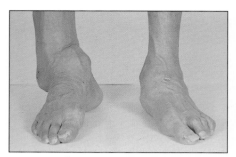

Fig. 11.19 *Tabes dorsalis.* Deformity of the right ankle caused by a Charcot joint.

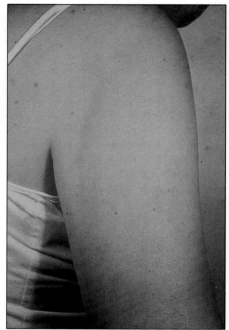

Fig. 11.20 *Lyme disease.* Erythema chronicum migrans.

Approximately 50% of patients have either an elevated cell count (lymphocytes) or protein concentration in the CSF. Positive serology, in the CSF, occurs in approximately three-quarters of patients.

Tegretol is effective in relieving the lightning pains. Procaine penicillin is given, intramuscularly, in a dose of 0.6 MIU daily for 3 weeks. A Jarisch–Herxheimer reaction (including fever, joint pains and exacerbation of the effects of pre-existing lesions) is avoided by giving prednisolone 20–30 mg daily for 24 h before and 48 h after starting treatment. Response is usually limited. CSF cell count should have returned to normal within 1 year of treatment and the protein concentration within 2 years. Erythromycin or tetracycline has been suggested as an alternative in penicillin-sensitive individuals.

GENERAL PARESIS

General paresis is now rare. Pathologically, there is meningeal thickening with cortical atrophy, mainly affecting the frontal and parietal lobes. Spirochaetes invade the brain, resulting in neuronal death, gliosis and patchy subcortical demyelination.

Clinical features include altered judgement, dementia, dysarthria, tremor and seizures. Approximately 50% of patients have small, irregular pupils that are either fixed or minimally reactive to light. The accommodation reaction is preserved (Argyll Robertson pupils). Later, there is pyramidal deficit and incontinence. The CSF serology is almost always positive. Treatment is as for tabes dorsalis.

LYME DISEASE

Lyme disease is caused by the tick-borne spirochaete, *Borrelia burgdorferi*. Deer are the only natural hosts for the adult ticks but the immature ticks are found in other species. The organism can be cultured from brain, CSF, blood and skin. Pathological changes in the nervous system include meningeal inflammation, perivascular inflammatory cell formation and focal demyelination.

The disease follows a three-stage course:

- Initial skin reaction (erythema chronicum migrans) associated with muscle pain, malaise, fever and headache (**Fig. 11.20**)
- Neurological features (in 10–15% of patients). Cranial nerve palsies (mainly fifth and seventh), radicular signs, meningitic and encephalitic features
- Arthritis. Either single or multiple joints, typically remitting–relapsing

Accompanying the meningitic phase is a CSF lymphocytosis with an elevated protein concentration and, in some cases, an elevated immunoglobulin G concentration with oligoclonal IgG. The diagnosis is confirmed by finding elevated serum antibody levels to *B. burgdorferi*. The condition is treated with intravenous ceftrixone.

LEPTOSPIROSIS

Leptospirosis is caused by the spirochaete *Leptospira interrogans*. In addition to hepatic and renal changes, meningitic and encephalitic features are recognized. Aseptic meningitis may be the presenting feature. Virtually any combination of symptoms and signs can occur in the encephalitic stage, including intracerebral or subarachnoid bleeding. Peripheral nervous system involvement is seen. Treatment is with penicillin or tetracycline.

- Hypoglycaemia is an important cause of morbidity in cerebral malaria
- Tertiary syphilis is now rare but meningovascular syphilis occurs more frequently, for example, in AIDS patients
- The neurological complications of Lyme disease are accompanied by a lymphocytic pleocytosis in the CSF

RETROVIRUS INFECTION

Two retroviruses, oncovirus and lentivirus, are pathogenic in humans. The former, as human T cell lymphotrophic virus (HTLV-1), causes adult T cell leukaemia and lymphoma and HTLV-1 associated myelopathy (see Chapter 13). The latter, as human immunodeficiency virus (HIV-1) causes AIDS. The related viruses, HTLV-2 and HIV-2 are of uncertain pathogenicity.

ACQUIRED IMMUNE DEFICIENCY SYNDROME

HIV-1 infects mononuclear phagocytes and CD4+ T lymphocytes. The neurological manifestations of AIDS are caused by:

- Direct invasion of the nervous system
- Secondary infection by opportunistic organisms

Direct effects

Pathological changes in the CNS are associated with HIV-1 infection of microglia and monocyte–macrophages.

AIDS DEMENTIA COMPLEX (ADC)

High levels of unintegrated HIV-1 DNA are found in the brains of ADC patients. Polymerase chain reaction allows the detection of HIV-1-infected cells in the CSF in AIDS dementia complex patients and asymptomatic carriers.

Pathologically, there is cerebral atrophy with white matter degeneration and perivascular and parenchymal infiltration by macrophages and lymphocytes (**Fig. 11.21**).

Symptoms of AIDS dementia complex

- Insidious onset of altered concentration and memory
- Altered personality
- Difficulty in walking and incoordination

Slow verbal and motor responses are slow and eye movement disorders appear, of the type seen in Parkinson's disease. Later, substantial weakness emerges, with seizures, mutism and incontinence.

CT shows cortical and deep atrophy, while MRI identifies the white matter changes. The CSF is often abnormal and may show oligoclonal bands but the changes are not specific.

AIDS dementia complex usually appears in the setting of moderately advanced immunosuppression. Its prevalence is uncertain. A well-established AIDS dementia complex is found in approximately 15% of patients with advanced HIV disease.

Zidovudine is given, in a dose of approximately 800–1000 mg/day. Approximately 50% of patients respond.

HIV MYELOPATHY

This is pathologically distinguishable into two forms, vacuolar myelopathy and multinucleated giant cell encephalitis. The two produce similar clinical features with a spastic paraparesis and impaired proprioception and vibration sense.

The vacuolar myelopathy is possibly caused by an opportunistic infection. Multinucleated cell myelitis is associated with direct viral invasion. The former does not respond to antiviral therapy, the latter may.

HIV NEUROPATHY

Predominantly sensory neuropathy

The most common form of HIV-1-related neuropathy. Limb weakness of a significant degree is uncommon. The condition is liable to worsen with antiretroviral agents. The pathogenesis of the condition is uncertain.

Autonomic neuropathy

Usually occurs in conjunction with the sensory neuropathy.

Mononeuritis multiplex

Occurs rarely in advanced HIV disease.

Guillain–Barré-like syndrome

This or a chronic inflammatory demyelinating neuropathy can occur in the relatively early stages of the disease. Plasmapheresis is effective.

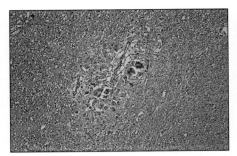

Fig. 11.21 *AIDS dementia complex.* Central area of inflammation and myelin loss around a blood vessel in the deep cerebral white matter. There are several multinucleated cells.

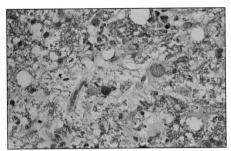

Fig. 11.22 *Progressive multifocal leukoencephalopathy.* Section at edge of lesion. Central infected oligodendrocyte surrounded by reactive astrocytes (mag X 100).

Muscle disease

A primary muscle disorder resembling polymyositis is seen.

OPPORTUNISTIC INFECTION

This is often multiple in nature.

Bacterial infection

Typically caused by unusual organisms, for example, Gram-negative bacilli, *Nocardia asteroides* or *Listeria monocytogenes*.

Fungal infection

Cryptococcal infection is the most common fungal disorder seen, generally as a meningitis.

Progressive multifocal leukoencephalopathy

Progressive multifocal leukoencephalopathy results from reactivation of latent JC virus infection that has reached the brain by the haematogenous route. The primary JC virus infection usually occurs in childhood. The virus causes destruction of oligodendrocytes, with demyelinated lesions principally appearing at the grey–white matter junction (**Fig. 11.22**). Up to 15% of AIDS patients have been found to have the pathological changes of progressive multifocal leukoencephalopathy. The condition is also seen in other conditions in which there is immunoparesis.

The condition is progressive and associated with hemispheric signs including sensory or motor deficits, aphasia and apraxia. Eventually, extensive bilateral signs appear.

Using *in situ* hybridization with specific DNA probes, JC virus has been shown in the kidney and in B cells in the bone marrow. The virus can also be identified in the CSF.

CT may miss the early lesion but MRI readily identifies the areas of white matter demyelination.

Cytosine arabinoside has been used in treatment but with equivocal benefit.

CYTOMEGALOVIRUS INFECTION

Encephalitis

Commonly diagnosed pathologically but seldom in life. Clinical features described include a relatively acute illness with encephalitic features, together with nystagmus and cranial nerve signs. Retinitis is found in at least 50% of patients. There is a CSF pleocytosis with depressed glucose levels. Cytomegalovirus can be found by polymerase chain reaction analysis of the CSF in one-third of the patients.

Radiculomyelitis

Results in back and radicular pain, ascending weakness, saddle sensory loss and altered sphincter function. There is a CSF pleocytosis (including polymorphs), elevated protein and depressed glucose concentrations.

Ganciclovir is sometimes effective in the radiculomyelitis syndrome.

Other viruses

Herpes zoster infection is common, producing a focal cranial neuropathy or a more disseminated infection affecting either the brain, meninges or spinal cord.

PARASITIC INFECTIONS

Toxoplasmosis

Up to one-third of AIDS patients are serum-positive for *Toxoplasma gondii*. Toxoplasmosis is the likeliest cause of a focal neurological deficit developing in an AIDS patient. Multiple small granulomas or large space-occupying abscess-like cavities appear.

Typically, an encephalopathic picture emerges over days or weeks with features suggesting predominant cerebral hemisphere rather than brainstem or cerebellar involvement. The patient is usually febrile and headache is common.

Absence of serum antibodies to *Toxoplasma* is strong evidence against the diagnosis. The patient is usually in the later stages of the illness with a CD4 count of under 100. The finding of *Toxoplasma* DNA by polymerase chain reaction evaluation of the CSF has a very high specificity but low sensitivity for making the diagnosis.

CT shows multiple lesions, typically affecting the cortex or deep grey matter, associated with oedema and accompanied by ring enhancement (**Fig. 11.23**). The main differential diagnosis is multicentric lymphoma.

The condition is usually highly sensitive to a combination of pyrimethamine and sulphadiazine, response being assessed by serial CT or MRI. An alternative regime is pyrimethamine and clindamycin. Failure to improve after 14 days should lead to consideration of brain biopsy. If the patient responds to chemotherapy, it is continued indefinitely.

- AIDS dementia complex usually appears in the setting of moderately advanced disease
- One form of HIV myelopathy is caused by direct virus invasion, the other is probably secondary to an opportunistic infection
- The demyelinating neuropathies occurring in AIDS patients are responsive to plasmapheresis
- Up to 16% of AIDS patients have been found to have the changes of progressive multifocal leukoencephalopathy at postmortem
- Toxoplasmosis is the likeliest cause of a focal neurological deficit in an AIDS patient

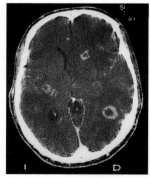

Fig. 11.23　*Toxoplasmosis.* *Multiple enhancing lesions on CT.*

chapter 12

Motor Neuron Disease and Peripheral Nerve Disorders

MOTOR NEURON DISEASE

Motor neuron disease (MND) is known as amyotrophic lateral sclerosis in the USA. It is a progressive disorder of the central nervous system combining degeneration of the cortico-spinal pathways with fall-out of cortical pyramidal cells, brainstem motor nuclei and anterior horn cells. Different subgroups of the condition are defined on the basis of the predominant clinical presentation.

Definitions of motor neuron disease

Progressive muscular atrophy.
Progressive bulbar palsy.
Primary lateral sclerosis.
Amyotrophic lateral sclerosis.

The condition is of unknown aetiology.
Suggested risk factors include:
- Trauma
- Heavy metal exposure
- Previous polio
- Heavy manual labour
- Lymphoma

Criteria for the diagnosis have been established (**Fig. 12.1**).

Fig. 12.1 *Diagnostic criteria for MND.*

Diagnostic criteria for MND

Findings should include:
- Lower motor neuron signs (which may include EMG manifestations in clinically normal muscles)
- Upper motor neuron signs
- Progression
- Absent findings include:
  Sensory changes
  Sphincter disturbances
  Visual disturbances
  Autonomic dysfunction
  Parkinsonism
  Dementia of Alzheimer type

PATHOLOGY
- Loss of pyramidal cells from layer V of the motor cortex, associated with degeneration of corticospinal pathways (**Fig. 12.2**)
- Degeneration of cranial nerve motor nuclei, particularly of V, VII, X and XII
- Anterior horn cell degeneration, maximal in the cervical and lumbar regions
- Sparing of motor neurons in the lateral aspect of the ventral horns of the sacral cord (nucleus of Onufrowicz)
- Ventral root atrophy, with sparing of the dorsal roots (**Fig. 12.3**)
- Chronic partial denervation in skeletal muscle

PATHOPHYSIOLOGY
- Upper motor neuron damage produces weakness, spasticity and hyper-reflexia
- Lower motor neuron damage results in wasting, weakness and fasciculation
- An intact nucleus of Onufrowicz allows sparing of sphincter function

> - Sparing of sensation and sphincter function in MND can be correlated with the distribution of the pathological process

Epidemiology
- Incidence rate is 1–2 per 100 000
- Prevalence rate is 4–6 per 100 000
- Peak incidence lies between 60 and 70 years of age
- Men are more affected than women (1.5:1)
- A rare form, combined with dementia and parkinsonism, clusters in parts of Japan and Guam, in the Western Pacific
- A familial form, inherited as a dominant condition, accounts for 5–10% of cases. Point mutations in the copper–zinc superoxide dismutase (Sod 1) gene on chromosome 21 are responsible

CLINICAL MANIFESTATIONS

symptoms

> **Symptoms of motor neuron disease**
>
> - 75% of patients present with limb symptoms
> - 25% present with bulbar symptoms

Progressive muscular atrophy

The initial complaint is usually of weakness confined to part of one limb. If the hand is affected, the patient notices difficulty with everyday tasks, for example, turning a key in a lock. If the leg is affected, the patient will describe an altered gait pattern or a tendency to trip. Often fasciculation or loss of muscle bulk has been noted before the initial consultation. At this stage, the condition can be confused with a peripheral nerve or root

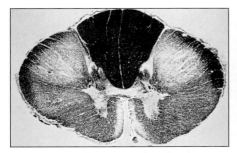

Fig. 12.2 *Myelin preparation showing pallor of the lateral and anterior corticospinal tracts.*

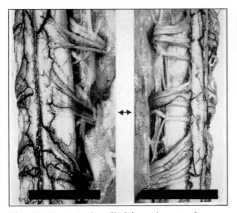

Fig. 12.3 *Anterior (left) and posterior (right) nerve roots from the cervical cord of a patient with MND.*

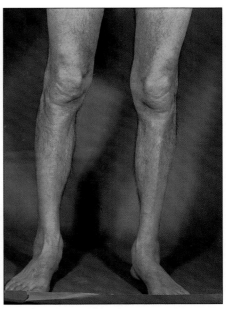

Fig. 12.4 *Predominant wasting of the left lower limb in MND.*

disorder (**Fig. 12.4**). Ill-defined sensory symptoms occur in a minority of patients and, later, limb pain is sometimes prominent.

Progressive bulbar palsy

Here the symptoms reflect bulbar dysfunction. A slurring dysarthria appears, sometimes associated with a reduction of speech volume. A nasal element to the speech reflects palatal weakness. Sometimes the bulbar symptoms appear abruptly. Dysphagia reflects an abnormality of the tongue, palate or upper oesophagus. Eventually, laryngeal penetration occurs during swallowing leading to bouts of coughing and choking. Involvement of cortico-bulbar fibres is associated with emotional lability.

Primary lateral sclerosis

In this variant, which is rare, the patient complains of leg weakness and is found to have a relatively pure spastic paraparesis.

Amyotrophic lateral sclerosis

Here there is a combination of upper and lower motor neuron features. Typically, all patients evolve to this pattern in the later stages of the disease.

- The individual clinical forms of MND converge to a single pattern during the course of the illness
- The majority of patients present with limb symptoms
- The bulbar manifestations sometimes appear abruptly

Signs

- Intellect is spared, although in up to 5% of patients, a dementia of frontal lobe type is seen
- Eye movements are spared unless life is prolonged by assisted respiration
- The lower cranial nerve signs are influenced by the duration of the disease and whether the process is primarily bulbar or pseudo-bulbar. Jaw weakness occurs and the jaw jerk is exaggerated in some patients. Facial weakness appears and can be accompanied by fasciculation. The gag reflex is depressed in some, exaggerated in others. Initially, the tongue appears normal. Eventually, fasciculation appears and motility lessens. Finally, the tongue is shrunken, lying stiff and immobile in the floor of the mouth (**Fig. 12.5**)
- Characteristically, in the limbs, there is a combination of upper motor neuron and lower motor neuron signs. For example, the triceps muscle may be wasted with fasciculation but retains a relatively brisk reflex. Eventually, wasting is profound. Typically, the hands become flexed (**Fig. 12.6**). The lower limbs seldom show substantial spasticity. Fasciculation tends to lessen as the condition progresses
- To a bedside evaluation, sensation is normal
- Involvement of the respiratory muscles is inevitable but not always symptomatic. Orthopnoea can be prominent
- The median survival is approximately 3.5 years. A small proportion of patients (perhaps 10%) live for more than 10 years. Early bulbar involvement worsens prognosis

- Characteristically in MND, upper motor neuron and lower motor neuron signs coincide in the same limb and within the same muscle. Only rarely is the patient's intellect affected

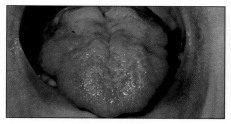

Fig. 12.5 *Wasting of the tongue.*

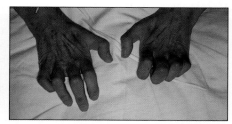

Fig. 12.6 *Severe wasting of the hand muscles.*

INVESTIGATION

Extensive investigation is seldom necessary. In some patients, imaging of the cervical spine and cord is required to exclude a focal basis for the presentation. Creatine kinase levels and cerebrospinal fluid protein concentrations are modestly elevated in the early stages. The essential investigation is electromyography (EMG) (**Fig. 12.7**). The main differential diagnosis is of a multifocal motor neuropathy (see p 237).

Benign fasciculation should not be confused with MND. It is mainly confined to the calves but can affect other upper and lower limb muscles. The muscles are clinically normal and show no evidence of denervation on EMG. The discharge frequency tends to be higher than that seen in MND.

MANAGEMENT

The diagnosis needs to be fully and frankly discussed with the patient as soon as it is established. Contact with the Motor Neuron Disease Association provides valuable support.

SPECIFIC THERAPY

Various approaches have been studied including the use of glutamate inhibition. To date, evidence for benefit has been slight. Riluzole, acting probably through presynaptic inhibition of glutamate release, has a marginal effect on life expectancy.

Fig. 12.7 *EMG criteria.*

EMG criteria
• Fasciculation and fibrillation potentials in both upper and lower limbs
• Reduced number of motor unit action potentials, with increase in their amplitude and duration
• Normal motor conduction velocities (a reduction to 70% of normal allowed in nerves supplying severely affected muscles)
• Normal sensory conduction

SYMPTOM MEASURES

Symptoms management in MND

- Dysphagia
- Excess salivation
- Dysarthria
- Respiratory failure

Dysphagia

Most MND patients develop significant swallowing problems. Assessment in a Swallow Clinic, using video-fluoroscopy allows a more rational approach to management. Myotomy of the cricopharyngeal muscle can overcome the effects of spasm therein, relevant to symptoms in patients with a pseudo-bulbar syndrome. The procedure carries a high mortality. Percutaneous endoscopic gastrostomy should be offered when bulbar involvement is substantial but limb function relatively preserved.

Excess salivation

Drugs usually suffice to control this problem, along with advice about head posture. Amitriptyline has sufficient anticholinergic effect to be helpful. Otherwise, hyoscine skin patches provide relief.

Dysarthria

Referral to a Communication Aids Centre will be necessary eventually. Various devices exist allowing the patient to type in their thoughts, subsequently to be verbalized along with a visual display; these can be invaluable.

Respiratory failure

At least in the early stages, chest infections should be treated vigorously and advice given to try to avoid aspiration. Tracheostomy with intermittent positive pressure ventilation will prolong life but can seldom be justified nor is it something that the patient particularly seeks.

> • The major management issues include a full discussion of the diagnosis and its implications with the patient and active attempts to alleviate the problems of dysarthria and dysphagia

SPINAL MUSCULAR ATROPHY

The spinal muscular atrophies are a group of genetically determined disorders in which the main pathological focus is the anterior horn cell. Classification is based on the clinical phenotype, age of onset and mode of inheritance (**Fig. 12.8**).

Classification of the spinal muscular atrophies

- Type 1 (Werdnig–Hoffman disease)
- Type 2 (Chronic infantile form)
- Type 3 (Kugelberg–Welander disease)
- Chronic distal
- Bulbospinal
- Scapuloperoneal
- Facioscapulohumeral

Fig. 12.8 *Classification of the spinal muscular atrophies.*

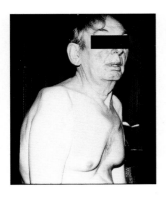

Fig. 12.9 *Proximal wasting in bulbospinal muscular atrophy.*

- In some patients, the bulbar cranial nerve nuclei are affected, leading to potential confusion with motor neuron disease (**Fig. 12.9**). The sensory and pyramidal tract pathways are spared, although the sensory ganglia usually suffer some neuronal loss. Fasciculation is less conspicuous than in MND
- A recessive form of inheritance is usual but dominant and X-linked recessive forms occur
- Nerve conduction is normal but EMG reveals evidence of denervation, with fibrillation and fasciculation potentials
- Creatine kinase levels are sometimes moderately elevated
- There is no specific treatment

PERIPHERAL NERVE DISORDERS

Peripheral nerve disorders can be first classified according to their distribution.

Definitions of peripheral nerve disorders	
Mononeuropathy	A disorder affecting a single peripheral nerve.
Mononeuritis multiplex	A disorder affecting several individual peripheral nerves, not explicable on the basis of a single lesion.
Plexopathy	A disorder of the brachial or lumbar plexus.
Polyneuropathy	A diffuse disorder of the peripheral nerve.
Sensory neuronopathy	A disorder primarily affecting the dorsal root ganglion.

MONONEUROPATHIES

Typically caused by external trauma to the nerve at an exposed site or its compression within a restricted bony or fibrous canal. The damage is related to mechanical derangement of the nerve fibres causing, predominantly, focal demyelination.

CARPAL TUNNEL SYNDROME

- The most common entrapment neuropathy
- Predominates in women
- Usually idiopathic (although those affected have smaller carpal tunnels than control individuals)
- More common in acromegaly, hypothyroidism, rheumatoid arthritis and after wrist fracture. The symptoms can be triggered by pregnancy
- Classically, it causes nocturnal pain, numbness or tingling in the hand or forearm. The

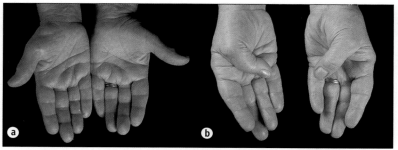

Fig. 12.10 *(a) Wasting of the thenar eminence with (b) failure of opposition.*

patient shakes the hand to relieve the symptoms, which are typically diffuse rather than focal in distribution

- The condition often remits spontaneously but may subsequently relapse
- Signs may be few. Mild weakness in the thumb is detectable in the majority of cases. Wasting is a late feature (**Fig. 12.10**)
- Sensory examination can show a slight alteration of feeling across the ring finger, comparing its radial with its ulnar border
- Tinel's sign is positive in approximately 25% of the patients. Tapping the nerve at the wrist triggers tingling in the median innervated digits
- Phalen's sign is more often positive. With sustained, forced flexion of the wrists, tingling appears in the relevant digits

Investigation
For almost all the entrapment mononeuropathies, EMG is invaluable in diagnosis. Delay in conduction across the compromised section of the nerve is the cardinal feature.

Treatment
Diuretics seldom ease the symptoms. Wearing cock-up splints at night can prevent nocturnal paraesthesiae. Injections of steroid into the carpal tunnel can temporarily relieve symptoms. The definitive treatment is surgical, necessitating adequate decompression of the stenosed section of the nerve (**Fig. 12.11**).

ANTERIOR INTEROSSEOUS PALSY
- Caused by compression of the nerve by the origin of the deep head of pronator teres
- Leads to weakness of pronator quadratus, flexor pollicis longus and flexor digitorum profundus to the second and third digits (**Fig. 12.12**). Sensation is normal

ULNAR NERVE LESIONS
- Most ulnar nerve lesions occur at the level of the elbow. Many are asymptomatic. Distal lesions of the nerve are rare
- Repetitive stretch and compression of the nerve from elbow pressure is the most common aetiological mechanism. Less often the nerve is compressed by the aponeurosis of flexor carpi ulnaris within the cubital tunnel. Patients confined to bed, particularly if the arm is immobilized by an intravenous infusion, are particularly susceptible
- Affected muscles in the hand include the interossei, adductor pollicis and the muscles of the hypothenar eminence (**Fig. 12.13**)
- Involvement of the lumbricals to the fourth and fifth fingers produces hyperextension of the metacarpophalangeal joints with flexion at the interphalangeal joints

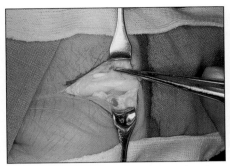

Fig. 12.11 *Operative photograph showing a constricted median nerve within the carpal tunnel.*

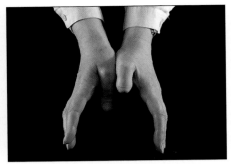

Fig. 12.12 *Right anterior interosseous nerve palsy. There is failure of thumb flexion.*

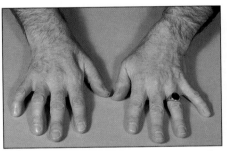

Fig. 12.13 *Ulnar nerve lesion. Wasting of the dorsal interossei on the right.*

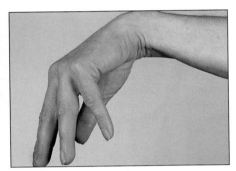

Fig. 12.14 *Left wrist drop*

- Sensory change is confined to the ulnar digits and the ulnar border of the hand
- Long flexors sometimes affected if the lesion is proximal are flexor carpi ulnaris and flexor digitorum profundus to the fourth and fifth digits
- Tinel's sign may be positive at the elbow
- EMG can show slowing across the elbow segment of the nerve when the lesion is proximal
- With distal lesions, sensory loss is absent and the motor deficit more restricted

Treatment

The nerve can be transposed from behind the elbow to prevent further compression. Recovery of any existing deficit is unlikely.

RADIAL NERVE PALSY

The nerve is liable to damage within the spiral groove. Triggering factors include fractures of the humerus and prolonged pressure on the nerve during drug- or alcohol-induced sleep (Saturday night palsy).

- Triceps is usually spared but there is weakness of wrist and finger extensors, supinator and brachioradialis (**Fig. 12.14**)
- Sensory loss is often confined to the anatomical snuff box

Treatment

When conduction block only has occurred, recovery is the rule. The wrist should be splinted to avoid a flexion deformity.

POSTERIOR INTEROSSEOUS PALSY

This branch of the radial nerve is liable to entrapment as it passes through the supinator muscle immediately beyond the tip of the lateral epicondyle. Weakness is confined to the extensors of the wrist, fingers and thumb. Relative sparing of the radial extensors produces radial deviation during attempted wrist extension (**Fig. 12.15**).

SCIATIC NERVE LESIONS

Sciatic nerve injury can occur with pelvic trauma, by direct injection into the nerve or after a period of prolonged recumbency. Weakness affects the hamstrings and all the muscles supplied by the medial and lateral popliteal branches of the nerve, although those supplied by the latter tend to be more affected. Sensation is altered over the lower calf and the lateral aspect of the foot. The ankle jerk is depressed or absent.

FEMORAL NEUROPATHY

During its passage through the psoas muscle, the femoral nerve can be damaged by a localized infection or haematoma or by an infiltrating retroperitoneal tumour. At this level, damage to the nerve causes hip flexion weakness but with a more distal lesion, weakness is confined to the quadriceps muscle, accompanied by depression of the knee jerk and sensory loss over the anterior thigh and the medial aspect of the shin (**Fig. 12.16**). The main distinguishing feature from an L3 root lesion is involvement of the adductors of the thigh with the root but not the nerve lesion.

MERALGIA PARAESTHETICA

The lateral cutaneous nerve of the thigh is liable to compression in the groin. The patient complains of pain, numbness or tingling in the anterolateral thigh. The symptoms are sometimes exacerbated by walking. The only abnormality on examination (and it is often slight) is a sensory change over the distribution of the nerve. Only seldom is decompression of the nerve indicated. The condition tends to remit spontaneously.

LATERAL POPLITEAL NERVE LESIONS

The lateral popliteal nerve is prone to compression as it winds round the neck of the fibula. The damage may be the result of external trauma or the consequence of bed rest in an immobile individual. Weakness affects dorsiflexion of the feet and toes, and eversion (**Fig. 12.17**).

Maximally, sensory loss extends over the dorsum of the foot onto the anterolateral aspect of the calf but is confined to a small area between the first and second toes if only the deep branch of the nerve is affected. There are no reflex changes.

TARSAL TUNNEL SYNDROME

The posterior tibial nerve traverses the tarsal tunnel, an analogous structure to the carpal tunnel in the wrist. Compression of the nerve in the tunnel produces pain, numbness and tingling in the sole of the foot. Selective involvement of the medial or lateral plantar branches of the nerve produces sensory symptoms confined to the medial or lateral aspect of the sole, respectively. The symptoms are usually only prominent when standing or walking. Tinel's sign may be positive behind the medial malleolus. The condition is usually accompanied by specific changes in conduction in the relevant nerve.

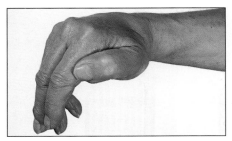

Fig. 12.15 *Posterior interosseous palsy.*
Radial deviation during attempted
dorsiflexion of the wrist.

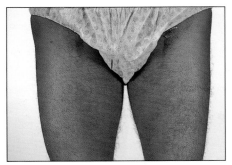

Fig. 12.16 *Left femoral nerve lesion with*
quadriceps wasting after femoral
profundoplasty.

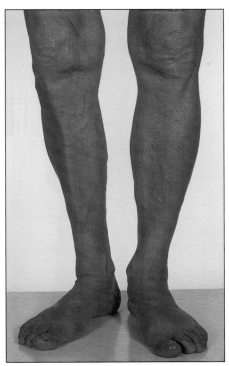

Fig. 12.17 *Severe wasting of the anterior*
tibial compartment in a patient with a
right lateral popliteal palsy.

Treatment

Treatment consists in decompression of the nerve.

- The most common mononeuropathy of the upper limb is carpal tunnel syndrome and of the lower limb, meralgia paraesthetica. Nocturnal, painful paraesthesiae are particularly characteristic of carpal tunnel syndrome
- Many ulnar nerve lesions are asymptomatic
- Many of the mononeuropathies are managed conservatively but carpal tunnel decompression is usually a very effective procedure

MONONEURITIS MULTIPLEX

In mononeuritis multiplex, there is simultaneous or sequential damage to individual peripheral nerves that can not be explained on the basis of a single lesion. Causes include a vasculitis, for example, polyarteritis nodosa, diabetes and infections (e.g. leprosy).

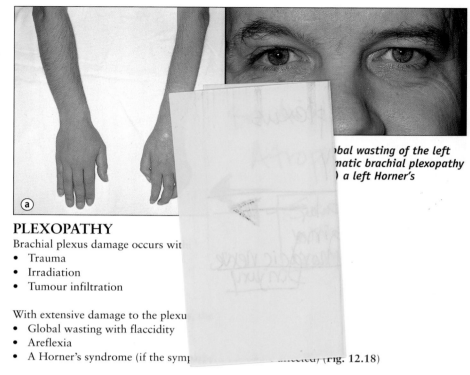

...bal wasting of the left ...matic brachial plexopathy ... a left Horner's

PLEXOPATHY

Brachial plexus damage occurs wit

- Trauma
- Irradiation
- Tumour infiltration

With extensive damage to the plexu

- Global wasting with flaccidity
- Areflexia
- A Horner's syndrome (if the symp .... (**Fig. 12.18**)

Brachial plexopathy (neuralgic amyotrophy)

This condition occurs spontaneously but can also follow an intercurrent infection, trauma or a surgical procedure. A hereditary form exists. Clinical features include:

- Severe pain around the shoulder
- Subsequent weakness and wasting, often concentrating on the deltoid and spinati or isolated to serratus anterior
- Sensory changes tending to be inconspicuous
- Approximately one-third of patients with bilateral but usually asymmetrical involvement
- Treatment symptomatic
- The majority of patients making a good functional recovery, although there may be residual wasting (**Fig. 12.19**)

THORACIC OUTLET SYNDROME

This condition is more usually the result of compression by a fibrous band passing from the transverse process of the seventh cervical vertebra to the first rib, rather than pressure from a formed cervical rib. Either the lower trunk of the brachial plexus or the C8 and T1 roots are affected. Clinical features include:

- Pain, usually in the ulnar aspect of the hand or forearm
- Weakness and wasting in the hand, typically more affecting median than ulnar innervated muscles
- Sensory change along the ulnar aspect of the forearm, extending into the fourth and fifth digits
- Symptoms can sometimes be reproduced by downward traction on the arm as it is held against the back

    Radiological findings include beaking of the C7 transverse process. Electrophysiological

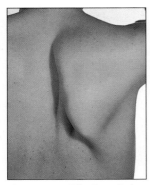

Fig. 12.19 *Winging of the right scapula caused by serratus anterior weakness in a case of neuralgic amyotrophy.*

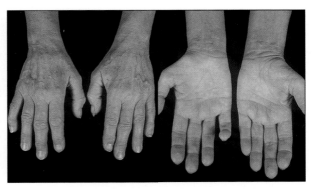

Fig. 12.20 *Right thoracic outlet syndrome.* Wasting of the small muscles of the hand.

abnormalities include delay and depression of the early ulnar somatosensory-evoked potentials. Surgical divison of the band relieves symptoms but does not restore muscle bulk (**Fig. 12.20**).

LUMBOSACRAL PLEXOPATHY

A condition analogous to brachial plexopathy affects the lumbosacral plexus. Pain is followed by weakness, which tends to concentrate in the distribution of the upper part of the plexus. Denervation occurs in affected muscles but a good level of recovery is usually seen.

PERIPHERAL NEUROPATHY

In a peripheral neuropathy, the pathological process diffusely involves the peripheral nerves. The motor, sensory and autonomic fibres can be affected uniformly or in isolation. Classification can be based on:

- The type of nerve fibre affected
- Whether the major change is axonal or demyelinating
- The causative agent

In practice, a classification based on the aetiological mechanism is followed (**Fig. 12.21**). Probably 25% of patients will not have the cause of their neuropathy established.

Classification of peripheral neuropathy
<ul><li>Genetic</li><li>Metabolic or endocrine</li><li>Nutritional deficiencies</li><li>Toxic</li><li>Drug induced</li><li>Connective tissue disease</li><li>Cancer related</li><li>Unknown cause</li></ul>

Fig. 12.21 *Classification of peripheral neuropathy.*

CLINICAL MANIFESTATIONS

Symptoms

The symptoms of a peripheral neuropathy are partly influenced by the pathological process. When axonal degeneration occurs (inevitably accompanied by breakdown of the myelin sheath), the distal part of the nerve is initially affected with subsequent proximal spread (dying-back phenomenon).

Symptoms of a peripheral neuropathy

- Symmetrical, distal motor and sensory deficits
- Initial involvement of the lower limbs

Symptoms of a demyelinating neuropathy

- Proximal as well as distal muscle weakness is encountered
- Sensory complaints tend to be less conspicuous than motor

Signs

With axonal degeneration, the clinical signs include:
- Glove and stocking sensory loss
- Muscle weakness with wasting
- Absent reflexes

With a primary demyelinating neuropathy, certain features may suggest the diagnosis:
- Relative preservation of muscle bulk despite severe weakness
- Sparing of pain and temperature sensation (because of sparing of thinly myelinated and non-myelinated fibres)
- Nerve enlargement (in long-standing cases)

Investigation

Essential tests in a patient with peripheral neuropathy include:
- Haemoglobin
- Full blood count
- Erythrocyte sedimentation rate
- Calcium
- Creatinine
- Fasting glucose or glucose tolerance test
- Protein electrophoresis
- Serum B^{12}
- Urinalysis
- Chest radiograph

Electrodiagnostic tests – These are critical in establishing the diagnosis and determining whether the process is primarily axonal or demyelinating.

- Analysis of sural nerve conduction is the most sensitive guide to the presence of a peripheral neuropathy
- Analysis of H and F waves allows measurement of conduction velocity in proximal nerve segments
- In axonal neuropathies, conduction velocities are near normal
- In demyelinating neuropathies, conduction is slowed by 40% or more of normal values
- The presence of conduction block suggests demyelination

Nerve biopsy – Nerve biopsy is of limited value in diagnosis. It can serve to establish a diagnosis of leprosy, vasculitis or amyloid. When the clinical history does not point to these diagnoses, the yield is extremely low (**Fig. 12.22**).

- Neuropathies are best classified on their aetiological basis
- Cardinal features include distal weakness, distal sensory loss (glove and stocking) and reflex depression
- Nerve conduction studies and EMG are invaluable in diagnosis
- Nerve biopsy is of limited value

THE HEREDITARY NEUROPATHIES

HEREDITARY MOTOR AND SENSORY NEUROPATHY

Hereditary motor and sensory neuropathy was previously called Charcot–Marie–Tooth disease or peroneal muscular atrophy (for Type I and II). Seven distinct types exist. The nomenclature is in a state of flux.

TYPE I (AUTOSOMAL DOMINANT, OCCASIONALLY RECESSIVE)

- Usually onset before 20 years of age
- Produces distal weakness and wasting (**Fig. 12.23**)
- Sensory loss may be slight
- Reflexes depressed
- Enlarged nerves palpable in about one-third of patients
- Associated with segmental demyelination
- Pes cavus usually present

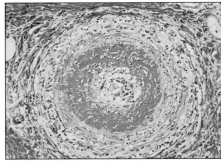

Fig. 12.22 *Sural nerve biopsy in a patient with rheumatoid arthritis. Evidence of fibrinoid arteritis.*

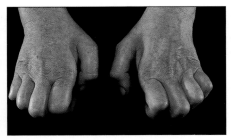

Fig. 12.23 *Wasting of the hands in hereditary motor and sensory neuropathy, Type I.*

TYPE II (AUTOSOMAL DOMINANT, OCCASIONALLY RECESSIVE)

- Similar to Type I but caused by axonal degeneration
- No nerve enlargement
- *Pes cavus* less common

TYPE III (AUTOSOMAL RECESSIVE) DEJERINE–SOTTAS DISEASE

TYPE IV (AUTOSOMAL RECESSIVE) REFSUM'S DISEASE

- Onset before the age of 30 years
- Clinical features include pigmentary retinal degeneration, neuropathy, deafness and skin changes
- Caused by a disorder of phytanic acid metabolism

HEREDITARY SENSORY AND AUTONOMIC NEUROPATHY (FIVE SUBTYPES)

TYPE I (AUTOSOMAL DOMINANT)

- Usually presents in second decade
- Clinical features include sensory loss over the feet, pes cavus and foot ulceration
- Progressive foot mutilation may occur (**Fig. 12.24**)
- Pain and temperature loss predominates, at least initially
- Affected skin shows loss of sweating

INHERITED TENDENCY TO PRESSURE PALSIES (AUTOSOMAL DOMINANT)

- Presents in second or third decade
- Mainly affects nerves susceptible to pressure, for example, ulnar nerve at elbow
- Often evidence of a more generalized neuropathy

PORPHYRIC NEUROPATHY

- Particularly associated with acute intermittent porphyria. Motor deficit predominates, preceded by pain. Sometimes mainly proximal and can present in the upper limbs. Autonomic dysfunction occurs

METACHROMATIC LEUKODYSTROPHY

- Mostly caused by deficiency of arylsulphatase A
- Leads to central and peripheral nervous system demyelination
- Various forms with differing ages of onset
- Lower limb weakness and flaccidity appear, later obscured by pyramidal signs
- Metachromatic granules found in peripheral nerve on light microscopy and inclusion bodies on electron microscopy

AMYLOID NEUROPATHY

Occurs in both the inherited and acquired forms of amyloidosis.

- Familial amyloid polyneuropathy is divided into four types. The majority of cases are related to mutations in the gene for transthyretin
- Type I is the most common. Inherited as a dominant condition, it presents in early adult life with pain and temperature loss, often with lancinating pains. Subsequently, distal weakness and wasting appear. Autonomic symptoms are prominent, with impotence, incontinence, altered sweating and altered bowel habit. Pupillary abnormalities occur and

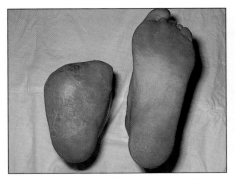

Fig. 12.24 *Foot mutilation in hereditary sensory and autonomic neuropathy, Type I.*

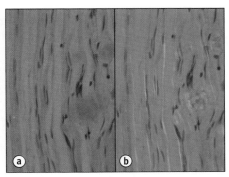

Fig. 12.25 *Amyloid neuropathy. Deposit in peripheral nerve (**a**) with characteristic birefringence (**b**).*

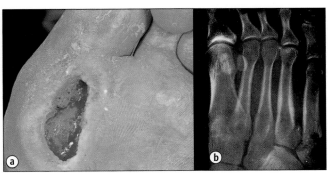

Fig. 12.26 *Diabetes. (**a**) Perforating foot ulcer with (**b**) evidence of metatarsal fractures.*

there is postural hypotension. Amyloid deposits can be identified in peripheral nerve (**Fig. 12.25**).

METABOLIC OR ENDOCRINE NEUROPATHIES

Diabetes is the most common cause of neuropathy in developed countries. Its prevalence, in patients with a history exceeding 20 years, may be as high as 50%. It is more likely in insulin-dependent patients and severity correlates with duration of the condition.

The pathophysiological mechanism for the different clinical types is not uniform. Focal neuropathies and some of the focal proximal limb neuropathies are probably vasculitic. The diffuse sensory and autonomic neuropathy is thought to be metabolic in origin

SENSORY POLYNEUROPATHY
There is insidious onset, with early loss of vibration sense in the feet and loss of the ankle reflexes. If small fibre damage predominates, there is distal pain and paraesthesiae with a liability to foot ulceration or fracture (**Fig. 12.26**).

PROXIMAL MOTOR NEUROPATHY
Usually asymmetrical. Caused by involvement of the lumbosacral plexus. Pain is prominent.

MONONEUROPATHY
Can affect a limb or cranial nerve.

AUTONOMIC NEUROPATHY

Can lead to severe postural hypotension with incontinence, diarrhoea and impotence.

TREATMENT

- Meticulous foot care is mandatory in all diabetic patients
- Prevention of sorbitol and fructose accumulation in nerve; using an aldose reductase inhibitor is of marginal benefit
- Strict diabetic control improves or stabilizes nerve function but at the risk of causing hypoglycaemia
  Neuropathy is also seen in renal and liver failure and in diseases of the thyroid and parathyroid glands.

- Neuropathy occurs in up to 50% of patients with diabetes
- Neuropathy is more likely in insulin-dependent patients
- Both metabolic and vascular components are important in its pathogenesis
- Meticulous diabetic control hinders progression

NUTRITIONAL OR DEFICIENCY-RELATED NEUROPATHIES

Vitamin B^1 deficiency

- The predominant cause of alcoholic neuropathy
- Intense burning paraesthesiae in the feet with muscle tenderness common
- Autonomic features may be seen

Other causes include vitamin B_6 and vitamin B_{12} deficiency

Paraproteinaemias

- Myeloma is associated with clinical evidence of a sensorimotor or motor neuropathy in approximately 10% of patients. The incidence is higher for osteosclerotic myeloma. Neuropathy is also seen with Waldenström's macroglobulinaemia and cryoglobulinaemia
- Approximately 10% of patients with peripheral neuropathy have circulating monoclonal paraproteins. Most are benign and of unknown significance
- The paraprotein may be immunoglobulin M, immunoglobulin G or immunoglobulin A
- Immunoglobulin M patients have more severe sensory deficits and more evidence of demyelination and are more likely to be ataxic
- 50% of the immunoglobulin M patients have antibodies against myelin-associated glycoprotein (**Fig. 12.27**)

Treatment

Plasma exchange, intravenous immunoglobulin, steroids and cytotoxic drugs have all been used. They tend to be more effective in the immunoglobulin A and immunoglobulin G subtypes.

INFECTIOUS AND POSTINFECTIOUS NEUROPATHIES

The most common worldwide cause of neuropathy is leprosy, although the incidence of the disease is falling. Three major forms are described: tuberculoid, lepromatous and borderline (intermediate).

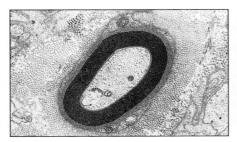

Fig. 12.27 *Immunoglobulin M paraproteinaemic neuropathy. Electron microscopy showing immunoglobulin M deposits in the outer lamellae of myelin.*

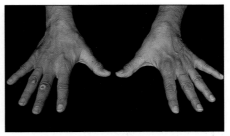

Fig. 12.28 *Wasting of the small hand muscles, with knuckle lesions, in a patient with leprosy.*

In lepromatous leprosy, there is an uncontrolled proliferation of the bacilli, associated with a defect of host cell-mediated immunity. The skin lesions and areas of sensory loss are extensive. In tuberculoid leprosy, dissemination of bacilli is more limited and the number of skin lesions and areas of cutaneous sensory loss fewer. Thickened peripheral nerves are found in both forms (**Fig. 12.28**).

Treatment recommendations are based on the clinical type. Rifampicin and dapsone are used for both, with the addition of clofazimine for the lepromatous form. Sometimes an acute reaction develops during treatment, with swelling and inflammatory infiltration of the skin and nerve lesions. An increasing neurological deficit is likely, requiring the use of corticosteroids.

GUILLAIN–BARRÉ SYNDROME

The Guillain–Barré syndrome is now classified into a number of subtypes:

- Acute inflammatory demyelinating polyradiculoneuropathy
- Acute axonal motor neuropathy
- Acute motor and sensory axonal neuropathy
- Miller Fisher syndrome
- Subacute inflammatory demyelinating polyradiculoneuropathy
- Chronic inflammatory demyelinating polyradiculopathy

The acute syndrome can be triggered by a number of different infections, including *Campylobacter jejuni*. Diagnostic criteria have been devised:

- Progressive neuropathic weakness of more than one limb
- Areflexia
- Duration of progression less than 4 weeks
- Absence of other causes of acute neuropathy (e.g. porphyria)
- Relatively symmetrical weakness
- Mild sensory involvement
- Autonomic dysfunction
- Absent fever
- Raised cerebrospinal fluid protein concentration
- EMG evidence of demyelination

Epidemiology

- Annual incidence is 1–2 per 100 000
- Increased risk in elderly people

235

- Prior infective illness in about two-thirds of patients
- Pain often prominent initially
- Rapidly evolving weakness, sometimes predominating proximally
- Usually symmetrical
- Sensory symptoms and signs relatively slight
- Areflexia
- Facial paralysis in approximately 50% of patients
- Bulbar involvement in approximately one-third of patients
- Artificial ventilation is necessary in approximately 15% of patients
- About two-thirds of patients have reached peak deficit within 2 weeks
- Mortality in up to 10% of patients
- Residual disability in up to 20% of patients (**Fig. 12.29**)

Investigation
Cerebrospinal fluid
- Abnormal protein concentration in the majority of patients (not immediately)
- Mean protein concentration is approximately 1.2 g/l
- Perhaps 10% of patients have a raised lymphocyte count but not above 50 cells/mm^3
- Oligoclonal bands appear in a minority of cases, usually with comparable bands in the serum
Electromyogram
Reveals a demyelinating neuropathy, sometimes predominantly proximal. Maximal change occurs approximately 3–4 weeks after onset.

Treatment
Corticosteroids are unhelpful. Plasma exchange and intravenous immunoglobulin are probably of comparable benefit. Nursing care and recognition of the need for respiratory support are critical.

ACUTE AXONAL MOTOR NEUROPATHY
- Can mimic Guillain–Barré syndrome
- Is sometimes epidemic
- Sensory findings are slight
- May be preceded by *Campylobacter jejuni* infection
- High titres to GM1 ganglioside in 25% of cases
- Treatment entails plasma exchange or intravenous immunoglobulin administration

MILLER FISHER SYNDROME
Consists of ataxia, ophthalmoplegia and areflexia without significant limb weakness. Generally benign, it is often preceded by a viral-like illness. Nearly all patients have immunoglobulin G antibodies to GQ1b ganglioside. The antibody may cause the neurological deficit by triggering neuromuscular block at the motor end plate (**Fig. 12.30**).

CHRONIC INFLAMMATORY DEMYELINATING POLYNEUROPATHY
Diagnostic criteria have been proposed for chronic inflammatory demyelinating polyneuropathy:
- Progressive weakness of two or more limbs caused by polyradiculoneuropathy
- Lost or reduced tendon reflexes
- Progression for more than 4 weeks; recurrence or relapse
- Neurophysiological evidence of demyelination

Others have suggested progression over 2 months is required for the diagnosis.

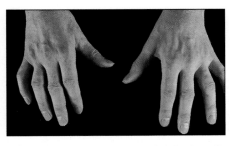

Fig. 12.29 *Residual hand muscle wasting in Guillain–Barré syndrome.*

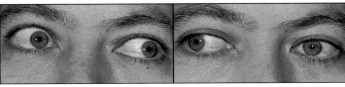

Fig. 12.30 Miller Fisher syndrome. *There is impaired adduction bilaterally.*

- The condition is sometimes preceded by an infectious illness
- The condition is slightly more common in men and can occur at any age
- Motor symptoms again predominate, although positive sensory symptoms, including pain, can occur
- The weakness tends to be both proximal and distal
- The reflexes are depressed
- Cranial nerve involvement is less common than in Guillain–Barré syndrome
- Tremor sometimes occurs

Investigation

Some patients with typical chronic inflammatory demyelinating polyneuropathy are found to have monoclonal gammopathy. Antibodies to tubulin have been found in 50% of patients.

Treatment

The first line of treatment is corticosteroids, with the addition of azathioprine if the response proves unsatisfactory. Plasma exchange, other immunosuppressants and intravenous γ globulin are also effective.

- Guillain–Barré syndrome is an acute inflammatory demyelinating polyradiculoneuropathy. A chronic form occurs in a progressive or in a remitting and relapsing form
- In the Miller Fisher syndrome a specific ganglioside antibody appears to be of pathogenetic significance
- Corticosteroids, immunosuppressants, immunoglobulin or plasma exchange are of value in some of these conditions

MULTIFOCAL MOTOR NEUROPATHY WITH CONDUCTION BLOCK

This condition can be confused with MND. It produces an asymmetrical, progressive, predominantly distal weakness more affecting the arms than the legs. There are no bulbar, sensory or upper motor neuron features.

The cerebrospinal fluid protein is usually normal. EMG shows multifocal conduction block, mainly proximal, with normal sensory conduction.

Some patients have anti-GM1 antibodies.

The condition is usually unresponsive to steroids but may respond to cyclophosphamide.

CONNECTIVE TISSUE DISORDERS

Vasculitis with consequent ischaemic damage to the peripheral nerve is seen in rheumatoid arthritis, polyarteritis nodosa and systemic lupus erythematosus. In rheumatoid arthritis, various forms of neuropathy occur:
- Symmetrical, predominantly sensory
- Digital neuropathy (**Fig. 12.31**)
- Mononeuritis multiplex
- Mononeuropathies secondary to joint deformity

A neuropathy is seen in approximately 50% of polyarteritis nodosa patients. Manifestations include:
- A symmetrical polyneuropathy
- A Guillain–Barré type syndrome
- A cranial or limb mononeuropathy

Central nervous system involvement is more common, however.

TOXIC AND DRUG-INDUCED NEUROPATHIES

Industrial toxins causing neuropathy include organophosphates, acrylamide and N-hexane.

Drugs causing peripheral neuropathies include cisplatin, vincristine, amiodarone, isoniazid, metronidazole, perhexilene and thalidomide. Most of these are axonal. The sensory axonal neuropathy with cisplatin may progress for 1–3 months after stopping the drug.

SENSORY NEUROPATHIES

These result from pathological changes in the dorsal root ganglia:
- They cause symmetrical sensory loss with areflexia
- They may be acute, subacute or chronic
- Motor conduction remains normal
- They are seen with small-cell lung cancer (p 280), as an idiopathic disorder or with Sjogren's disease.

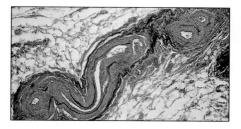

Fig. 12.31 *Digital nerve in rheumatoid arthritis showing thickening of the intima of the vasa nervorum.*

chapter 13

Spinal Cord Disorders

DEGENERATIVE DISORDERS OF THE SPINE

Degenerative changes in the intervertebral disc are inevitable with increasing age. Splits in the annulus fibrosus allow herniation of elements of the nucleus pulposus, whereas shrinkage of the nucleus produces prolapse or folding of the annulus with secondary osteophyte formation at the margins of the adjacent vertebral body. Degenerative changes in the apophyseal joints also predispose to osteophyte formation.

Symptoms arising from these changes are the result of disc or annulus protrusion and narrowing of the spinal canal or intervertebral foramen by osteophytes, often accentuated by a contribution from a congenitally narrow canal or congenitally short pedicles.

Posterior disc protrusions in the cervical and thoracic regions lead to cord compression and in the lumbar region to cauda equina compression. Posterolateral disc protrusions, with or without a contribution from vertebral body or apophyseal joint osteophytes, lead to nerve root compression.

Variations in the relationship between the spinal levels and the pattern of emergence of nerve roots account for different effects of disc protrusions between the cervical and lumbar regions. For example, at the C4/5 level, the C5 nerve root exits above the pedicle of C5 (in the inferior aspect of the C4/5 neural foramen) and is liable to compression by a disc protrusion between C4 and C5. The L5 nerve root, however, emerges from the theca opposite the L4 vertebral body then passes over the posterolateral aspect of the L4/5 disc before coursing along the L5 vertebral body to emerge beneath the L5 pedicle at the next intervertebral foramen. Consequently, a disc protrusion at L4/5 will usually affect the L5 root and only involve the L4 root if it extends sufficiently laterally or distally (**Fig. 13.1**).

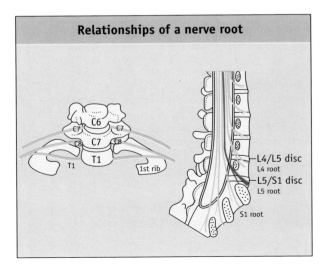

Relationships of a nerve root

C6 — C7 — C7 — C8 — C7 — C8 — T1 — T1 — 1st rib

L4/L5 disc
L4 root
L5/S1 disc
L5 root
S1 root

Fig. 13.1 *Relationship of nerve root to vertebral body, disc and the articular facets in the (a) cervical and (b) lumbar regions.*

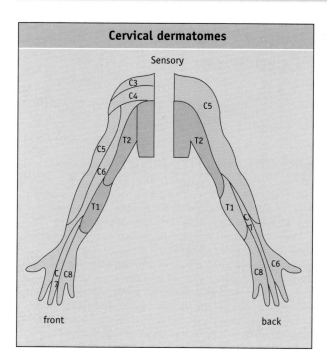

Fig. 13.2 *Distribution of dermatomes in the upper limbs.*

Pain of spinal origin affects over one-half of the population at some point in time. Many patients with back pain do not have a typical disc syndrome and some patients with disc protrusions present with atypical physical findings.

CERVICAL SPONDYLOSIS

Degenerative disease in the cervical spine predominantly affects the C5/6 and the C6/7 levels.

RADICULOPATHY

Symptoms

Symptoms of radiculopathy

- Neck pain
- Pain in the medial aspect of the scapula, the shoulder or arm. The referred pain is myotomal or sclerotomal in distribution
- Sensory symptoms, whether tingling or numbness, are distributed in a dermatomal fashion (**Fig. 13.2**)
- Weakness follows the pattern of innervation of the affected root (**Fig. 13.3**)
- Headache, occipital or suboccipital, has been attributed, in some patients, to cervical spondylosis. The association is uncertain

Third occipital headache describes a condition in which compression of the C3 root by disease of the C2/3 zygapophyseal joint results in occipital pain sometimes referred to the forehead.

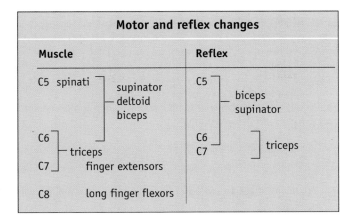

Motor and reflex changes

Muscle	Reflex
C5 spinati ⎤ supinator	C5 ⎤ biceps
⎟ — deltoid	⎟ supinator
⎟ biceps	
C6 ⎤ ⎦	C6 ⎦ ⎤ triceps
⎟— triceps	C7 ⎟
C7 ⎦ finger extensors	
C8 long finger flexors	

Fig. 13.3
Distribution of weakness and reflex changes in cervical root compression.

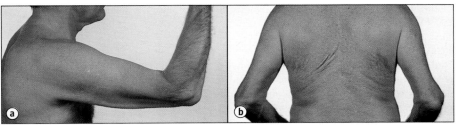

Fig. 13.4 *Wasting of the right triceps associated with a C6/7 disc protrusion.*

Signs

In the presence of pain, neck movements are restricted and may exacerbate the pain. A combination of sensory, motor and reflex abnormalities can serve to localize the relevant level (**Fig. 13.3**). Wasting with fasciculation in triceps, for example, would suggest a C6/7 disc protrusion (**Fig. 13.4**).

CERVICAL MYELOPATHY

SYMPTOMS

The most common levels for cord compression caused by cervical spondylosis are C5/6 and C6/7, although multiple level compression is common, particularly in patients with a congenitally narrow canal.

Symptoms attributable to cord compression

- Difficulty in walking
- Altered sensation in the feet
- Sphincter disturbances (late manifestations)

SIGNS

- The most common findings in extrinsic compression of the spinal cord in the neck are proximal lower limb weakness and loss of vibration sense in the feet

- Glove-like sensory loss with relatively slight motor deficit and relatively mild sensory change in the legs can occur (usually with cord compression between C3 and C5)
- If the compression is above C5, all the upper limb reflexes are exaggerated with a spastic tetraparesis
- If the compression is between C5 and C7, lower motor neuron findings are likely in the upper limbs. The biceps and supinator reflexes may be inverted (see p 21)
- Wasting of the small hand muscles is sometimes seen in high cervical cord compression
- Upper motor neuron signs are found in the lower limbs

INVESTIGATION

Plain radiographs

Degenerative changes in the neck are visualized by radiography in 50% of the population at the age of 50 years and in 75% over the age of 65 years. In most patients, the changes are asymptomatic. Some supportive evidence for a cervical radiculopathy or myelopathy is obtained if there is focal foraminal narrowing or reduction of the diameter of the spinal canal below 13 mm.

Further imaging

High-resolution magnetic resonance imaging (MRI) is the preferred diagnostic technique for most patients, with computerized tomography (CT) myelography as the main alternative. Conventional myelography is no longer performed (**Fig. 13.5**).

MANAGEMENT

Most patients with a radicular syndrome are managed conservatively, with judicious physiotherapy, analgesics and a stiff collar which suffices to inhibit neck movement.

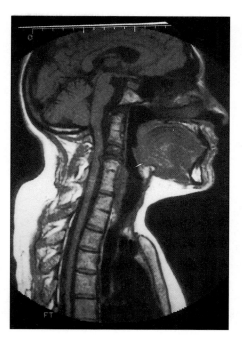

Fig. 13.5 *Cervical myelopathy.* *MRI showing prolapse of the C4/5 disc with cord compression. There is congenital fusion of several cervical vertebrae.*

Occasionally, when the problem is related to a posterolateral disc prolapse, excision of the disc is performed. Patients with cord compression caused by a single level disc prolapse are offered a Cloward procedure, in which the disc material is drilled out and the adjacent vertebrae fused. For multiple level disease or spinal stenosis, cervical laminectomy is performed. However, it must be recognized that radiological evidence of spondylitic myelopathy is clinically silent in some individuals, that some patients with alleged spondylitic myelopathy prove to have other conditions (e.g. multiple sclerosis or ALS) and the exact benefit arising from these procedures remains controversial.

- Cervical spondylosis mainly affects the C5/6 and C6/7 discs
- Cervical radiculopathy is usually managed conservatively
- Cervical myelopathy can present with glove-like sensory loss with relatively minor motor deficit and mild lower limb sensory involvement
- MRI is the investigation of choice for cervical radiculopathy and myelopathy

THORACIC DISC DISEASE

Symptomatic thoracic disc disease is rare, although prolapsed thoracic discs are found in approximately one out of seven scanned dorsal spines. It predominates in the lower thoracic region and is more common in men. Clinical presentations include a progressive spastic paraparesis, a spinal stenosis syndrome with exercise-induced motor or sensory symptoms or both. MRI and CT myelography are the alternative imaging techniques. Various surgical approaches have been advocated, some of which carry a substantial morbidity. A microsurgical posterolateral costotransversectomy is perhaps preferable.

LUMBOSACRAL DISC DISEASE

Degenerative disease of the lumbar spine involves the lower two levels in over 90% of patients. Disc protrusions may be lateral, posterolateral or central (**Fig. 13.6**).

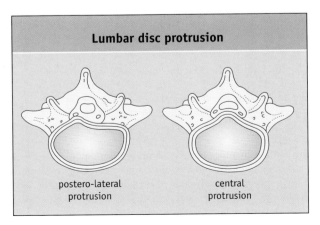

Fig. 13.6 *Patterns of lumbar disc protrusion.*

LATERAL DISC PROTRUSIONS

These represent 10% of all lumbar disc herniations. Pain is referred to the anterior thigh and leg. Plain CT is a sensitive diagnostic technique.

POSTEROLATERAL PROTRUSIONS

SYMPTOMS

Symptoms of posterolateral protrusions

- Pain is common. Areas involved, even without root involvement, include the back, the sacroiliac joint, the medial aspect of the buttock and upper thigh
- Radicular pain is exacerbated by movement and straining. Medial calf pain suggests L5, and lateral calf pain S1, root compression
- Sensory symptoms are common and segmental in distribution

SIGNS

Back examination

Findings include focal tenderness, limitation of movement and a scoliosis secondary to paravertebral spasm.

Stretch tests

Restricted straight-leg raising occurs with irritation of a root at or below the L5 level. A positive femoral stretch test suggests irritation of the roots of L2, 3 or 4.

Focal signs

Focal signs are determined by the root affected (**Fig. 13.7**).

CENTRAL DISC PROTRUSIONS

Central disc prolapses, which can occur spontaneously or after trauma, present with pain, lower limb weakness and impaired sphincter function. Saddle anaesthesia is common.

INVESTIGATION

Plain radiographs are usually unhelpful. High resolution, uncontrasted CT is valuable for investigating both lumbar disc disease and spinal stenosis. MRI is the preferred technique for investigating disc disease. It shows protrusion and sequestration and, by using gadolinium, annular tears. It has largely replaced CT myelography (**Fig. 13.8**).

Other techniques

Sampling of lower limb muscles by EMG sometimes serves to establish the exact level of denervation in the affected limb, although segmental innervation is not necessarily uniform. Discography can identify tears of the annulus. Reproduction of the patient's pain by the procedure and its subsequent relief by the injection of local anaesthetic has been advocated as a valuable diagnostic test but false positive and negative findings occur.

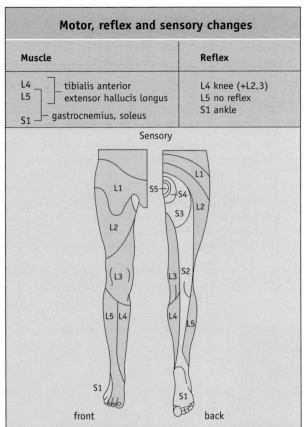

Motor, reflex and sensory changes

Muscle		Reflex
L4 ⎤	tibialis anterior	L4 knee (+L2,3)
L5 ⎦	extensor hallucis longus	L5 no reflex
S1 ⎦	gastrocnemius, soleus	S1 ankle

Sensory

front   back

Fig. 13.7 *Motor, sensory and reflex changes in lumbosacral root disorders.*

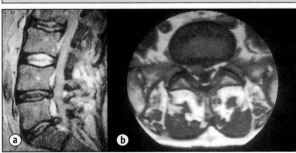

Fig. 13.8 *Posterolateral disc protrusion. MRI scan. (a) Sagittal and (b) axial sections.*

MANAGEMENT

When a specific root syndrome has been identified and root compression confirmed by imaging, removal of disc material produces an excellent outcome in terms of pain control. Increasingly, microsurgical techniques are used, leading to a much shorter hospital stay. Major neurological deficit after lumbar laminectomy occurs in 0.3% of patients and pulmonary embolism in 0.1%.

When there are less clear radicular signs or simply non-specific back pain, surgical results are poor. Patients with a chronic back syndrome are often found to have a previous psychiatric history and frequently have developed symptoms after injury.

Conservative management of back pain includes analgesics, appropriate exercises and periods of bed rest. Active treatment whether given to an in-patient or out-patient leads to a better outcome compared with control groups. Identification of psychological factors is important in patients with a chronic back syndrome.

SPINAL STENOSIS

Spinal stenosis is either congenital (e.g. in achondroplasia) or secondary to a combination, of varying degree, of hypertrophy of the bony elements of the lumbar canal, ligamental hypertrophy and disc degeneration. The stenosis can primarily affect the canal itself, the lateral recess (the area between the thecal sac and the pedicle) or the intervertebral foramen and nerve root canal.

Canal stenosis predominates in middle-aged men. Typically, paroxysmal numbness or paraesthesiae appear in the lower limbs during exercise or when standing in certain postures (neurogenic claudication). The symptoms often march from the distal to the proximal parts of the legs, then on to the buttocks. They are relieved by rest. Physical examination is usually relatively normal.

High-resolution CT defines stenosis of the central canal or the lateral recess (**Fig. 13.9**). MRI is the alternative diagnostic procedure. Decompression of the canal or the foramen is usually curative.

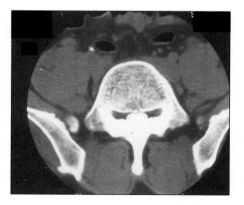

Fig. 13.9 *Lumbar canal stenosis. CT.*

- Lumbar spondylosis involves the lower two spaces in over 90% of patients
- Abnormalities of straight-leg raising or the femoral stretch test are important pointers to the level of root compression
- MRI is the investigation of choice for lumbar spondylosis
- CT is valuable for the investigation of spinal stenosis
- Specific radicular syndromes caused by lumbar disc disease respond well to surgery

PAGET'S DISEASE OF THE SPINE

Overgrowth of part of one or more vertebrae, particularly at the thoracic or lumbar level, can lead to nerve root or cord compression or the syndrome of neurogenic claudication. Pain is common. Involvement of the base of the skull is associated with cranial nerve compression or basilar impression with secondary hydrocephalus. Disease activity correlates with levels of serum alkaline phosphatase activity and urinary excretion of hydroxyproline. MRI or plain CT allows definition of focal changes relating to the neuraxis, whereas bone scanning helps to establish the extent of the disease.

The drugs used in Paget's disease include calcitonin and the bisphosphonates. Disodium etidronate is the initial therapy most often used. A daily dose of 5 mg/kg is given for 6 months. Synthetic salmon calcitonin (salcatonin) is useful for pain control and can reduce some of the neurological complications, for example, deafness. It is given by subcutaneous or intramuscular injection.

RHEUMATOID ARTHRITIS AND THE SPINE

Cervical subluxation is found in up to one-third of rheumatoid patients, although in many, the changes are asymptomatic. The atlanto-axial joint is most often affected (**Fig. 13.10**). Significant subluxation is defined as an atlanto-axial subluxation of 3 cm or more in men and 2.5 cm or more in women.

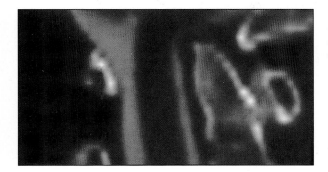

Fig. 13.10 *Rheumatoid arthritis. CT myelogram showing atlanto-axial subluxation with posterior angulation of the cord.*

Focal pain is often prominent and may be referred to the occiput in the distribution of the occipital nerve (C3). Neurological complications of the subluxation include a spastic tetraparesis. Stability of the spine is usually achieved by a posterior fusion of the atlas, axis and occiput.

ANKYLOSING SPONDYLITIS

Ankylosing spondylitis predominates in men (by four times). Typically, it causes low back pain and stiffness. Osteoporotic changes occur with ageing and if fractures of the spine occur, secondary cord compression may follow.

INFECTION

SPINAL EPIDURAL ABSCESS

Infection of the epidural space occurs either by direct spread (e.g. from a vertebral abscess or through some surgical or anaesthetic procedure) or by haematogenous spread from a distant source. Risk factors include chronic medical disorders, immunosuppression and drug abuse. The abscess is found most often in the lumbosacral region. Secondary involvement of the spinal vessels is common.

A typical sequence of clinical events is local back pain, then radicular pain, then a rapidly evolving neurological deficit incorporating motor, sensory and sphincter disturbances. In some patients, the neurological evolution is gradual over several weeks.

Staphylococcus aureus accounts for approximately one-half of the infections. Identification of the organism (which is not always possible) is achieved, in descending order of frequency, from operative tissue, blood culture and cerebrospinal fluid culture. An elevated erythrocyte sedimentation rate is common but the peripheral white cell count may be normal. In the absence of abscess rupture, the cerebrospinal fluid shows features of parameningeal sepsis with an elevated white cell count (polymorphonuclear leukocytes or lymphocytes), an elevated protein concentration but a normal glucose level.

Imaging

The investigations of choice are CT myelography and MRI. Plain CT can show paraspinal soft tissue masses, whereas CT myelography will reveal partial or complete block of the subarachnoid space (**Fig. 13.11**). MRI is abnormal in 95% of patients. The lesion is isodense or hypodense on T1-weighted and hyperdense on T2-weighted images. Both homogeneous and peripheral enhancement occur with gadolinium.

Treatment

Consists in decompression, drainage and any necessary stabilization of the spine. Antibiotic therapy is continued for up to 2 months. Perhaps 80% of patients either fully recover or are ambulant with assistance. Prognosis is closely linked to delay in surgical intervention. Some patients with minimal deficit can be managed with antibiotic therapy alone.

INTRAMEDULLARY ABSCESS

This is a rare condition. The primary source of infection and its nature are often not identified. Clinical features include pyrexia, back pain and a myelopathy. MRI is the imaging procedure of choice, identifying an intramedullary mass with enhancement.

TUBERCULOUS DISEASE OF THE SPINE

Tuberculous disease of the spine predominates in the thoracolumbar region. Multiple level involvement is usual. The disease process starts in the vertebral body adjacent to the cartilage plate with relative sparing of the vertebral interspace. Spread round the anterior or posterior longitudinal ligaments (the latter with posterior vertebral involvement) leads to a paraspinal abscess (**Fig. 13.12**). Anterior spread leads to psoas abscess formation and posterior spread to cord compression. Additional damage to the neuraxis can arise from vertebral collapse.

Initial clinical features include fever, malaise and weight loss, followed by focal pain and tenderness. Later, radicular pain is likely, followed by evidence of cord or root compression.

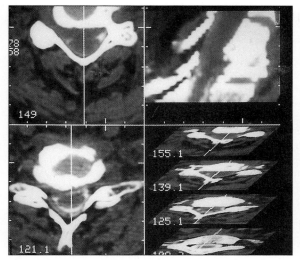

Fig. 13.11 Spinal epidural abscess. CT myelography.

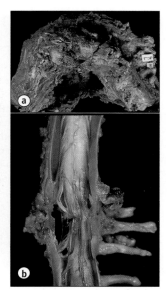

Fig. 13.12 **Spinal tuberculosis. (a)** Severe kyphosis. **(b)** Marked focal atrophy of the cord at the site of compression.

Imaging

Plain radiographs are usually abnormal. Plain CT is highly accurate in diagnosis, the sites for scanning being determined either clinically or by bone scan. MRI identifies multiple level disease, the relative preservation of the disc spaces and the extent of posterior vertebral involvement.

Treatment

Standard antituberculous therapy is given combined with surgery when there is neurological involvement.

BRUCELLOSIS

Brucella spondylitis most often affects the midlumbar region and is readily visible on plain CT. Brucella myelitis can occur in isolation, as part of a meningoencephalitis or secondary to vertebral disease. Back pain is accompanied by signs of spinal cord involvement.

SCHISTOSOMIASIS

Spinal cord disease in patients with schistosomiasis is usually caused by *Schistosoma. mansoni.* Granuloma formation occurs either within or outside the cord or cauda equina. A transverse myelitis appears, sometimes abruptly. The cerebrospinal fluid reveals an elevated protein concentration, a lymphocytic pleocytosis and schistosomal antibodies. Treatment combines corticosteroids with antischistosomal drugs.

HTLV-1 MYELOPATHY (TROPICAL SPASTIC PARAPARESIS)

The HTLV-1 virus causes a spastic paraparesis. The virus is endemic in West and Central Africa, the Caribbean and parts of Japan, the USA and Central America. The virus is transmitted by whole blood transfusion, the use of contaminated needles, breast milk or sexual intercourse. Clinical features include optic atrophy, spastic paraparesis, ataxia and peripheral neuropathy. There may be a mild inflammatory reaction in the cerebrospinal fluid with an elevated protein concentration. An epidemiological study from the UK has suggested that screening for antibodies to the virus in patients with unexplained myelopathy was not justified unless they belong to a high-risk group or originate from a country where the virus is endemic. Immunomodulating drugs have been used in treatment with borderline evidence of success.

TRANSVERSE MYELITIS

An acute transverse myelopathy (transverse myelitis) can result from a variety of pathological mechanisms, some of them non-infective. Non-infective causes include multiple sclerosis, systemic lupus erythematosus and after vaccination. Viruses implicated in the condition include Echo virus, herpes zoster, Epstein Barr virus and cytomegalovirus. Non-viral infective agents causing a transverse myelitis include schistosoma, mycoplasma and toxoplasma. An acutely evolving cord syndrome is seen. The majority of childhood patients make a good recovery but residual deficit is not uncommon in adults. Zoster myelitis follows the rash after approximately 2 weeks and evolves over some 10 days . The major cord involvement is ipsilateral to and at the level of the rash with horizontal and vertical spread. Zoster myelitis is treated with acyclovir.

SUBACUTE MYELOPATHY OF AIDS

See p 213–216

- Although cervical subluxation is found in up to one-third of rheumatoid patients, in many the appearance is asymptomatic
- MRI identifies the vast majority of epidural abscesses and is the initial investigation of choice
- Tuberculous disease of the spine predominates in the thoracolumbar region and is managed, when there is neurological involvement, with a combined medical and surgical approach
- Transverse myelitis occurs with both infective and non-infective processes. Less than 10% of White patients with transverse myelitis progress to multiple sclerosis

VASCULAR DISEASE

SPINAL EXTRADURAL HAEMATOMA

Spinal extradural haematoma can appear spontaneously, follow trauma or result from a bleeding diathesis. Any spinal level can be affected.

The onset is usually abrupt with severe focal pain followed by a rapidly evolving neurological deficit. CT myelography reveals a complete or partial spinal block, although without necessarily localizing the pathology to the extradural space. MRI identifies the lesion, its age and the degree of cord or cauda equina compression (**Fig. 13.13**). Surgical intervention is required.

SPINAL CORD INFARCTION

The spinal cord is supplied by separate anterior and posterior arterial systems. The anterior cord is supplied by the anterior spinal artery (cervical), radicular arteries (at all levels) and the artery of Adamkiewicz, a radicular artery that is a major contributor to the blood supply of the lower thoracic and lumbar cord. The posterior aspect of the cord is supplied by the posterior spinal arteries, supplemented by posterior radicular vessels. Ischaemic events occur in either the anterior or posterior territories or in the watershed areas between or among them.

Involvement of the anterior arterial territory, typically by atheroma or aortic dissection, produces a flaccid weakness, sometimes with wasting. Infarction of the cord in the distribution of the posterior spinal arteries is rare. Generally, the lesion is bilateral and involves the posterior columns. The pyramidal and anterolateral tracts are often involved.

Watershed infarction occurs at the junction of the two arterial territories and can occur after cardiac arrest, acute hypoxia or after aortic surgery and clamping. MRI is the imaging procedure of choice for the investigation of suspected spinal cord ischaemia.

SPINAL ARTERIOVENOUS MALFORMATIONS

Dural arteriovenous malformations lie in the spinal dura and adjacent nerve roots. They are supplied by branches of the intercostal or lumbar arteries. Intradural malformations are either arteriovenous fistulas, in or outside the cord and having a direct arteriovenous connection, or intramedullary malformations in which the nucleus is in the cord or pia.

Dural arteriovenous malformations (**Fig. 13.14**) mainly occur in the thoracolumbar

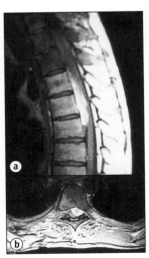

Fig. 13.13 Spinal extradural haematoma. MRI (a) sagittal (b) axial views.

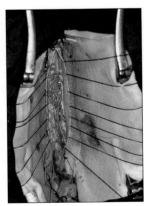

Fig. 13.14 Dural arteriovenous malformation. Operative view illustrating the dilated draining veins.

251

region. They usually present with a gradually evolving mixed sensory, motor and sphincteric deficit with some of the symptoms typically exacerbated by exercise. The motor deficit, in the lower limbs, tends to combine lower and upper motor neuron features. Intradural malformations, which are distributed more evenly along the spinal axis, can also present insidiously but at least 50% of patients have had a subarachnoid haemorrhage by the time of diagnosis.

INVESTIGATION
- Providing supine screening is undertaken, conventional myelography is almost always abnormal
- MRI, in the case of dural fistulas, shows serpiginous low signal intensity lesions over the dorsal aspect of the cord on T2-weighted images together with high signal areas within the cord (which may be expanded) on both T1 and T2
- Spinal angiography shows the feeding vessel or vessels

MANAGEMENT
Alternative approaches include surgery, stereotactic radiosurgery and embolization (**Fig. 13.15**).

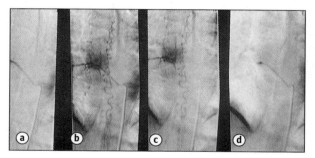

Fig. 13.15 *Spinal arteriovenous malformation.* *Spinal angiogram (**a–c**) before and (**d**) after embolization of the feeding vessel.*

- Most spinal cord infarction occurs in the distribution of the anterior spinal artery
- Dural arteriovenous malformations usually present with a mixed neurological picture in which both upper and lower motor neuron signs occur in the lower limbs
- 50% of intradural malformations have led to subarachnoid haemorrhage by the time of diagnosis

SPINAL TUMOURS

Spinal tumours arise within the spinal cord, from the meninges, the spinal roots or the epidural space (**Fig. 13.16**).

Spinal Tumours

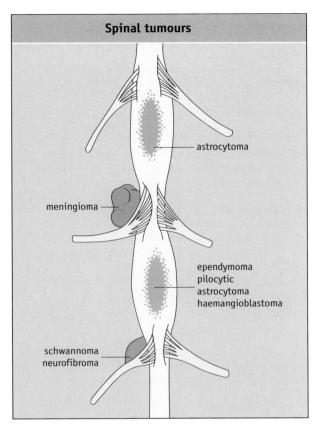

Spinal tumours

- astrocytoma
- meningioma
- ependymoma
  pilocytic
  astrocytoma
  haemangioblastoma
- schwannoma
  neurofibroma

Fig. 13.16
The distribution of some spinal tumours.

FORAMEN MAGNUM TUMOURS

- Pain may be referred to the neck or occiput or to the face if the spinal tract of V is involved
- A tetraparesis is likely, often asymmetrical, sometimes accompanied by wasting of the small hand muscles
- A Horner's syndrome is more likely with intramedullary than extramedullary tumours
- Additional signs include dysfunction of the eleventh and twelfth cranial nerves and downbeat nystagmus

Cervical tumours

- Lower motor neuron findings, including wasting, weakness and fasciculation, appear at the site of the lesion
- Pyramidal deficit is found in the lower limbs if cord compression is present
- The sensory loss is likely to be radicular with extramedullary tumours but a reflection of posterior column or spinothalamic deficit with intrinsic tumours. Sacral sparing of spino-thalamic loss suggests an intramedullary lesion but is sometimes seen with extrinsic compression

Thoracic tumours

- Radicular pain is common with meningioma and neurofibroma
- A spastic paraparesis emerges with a cutaneous sensory level that is usually slightly below the level of compression

253

Conus and cauda equina tumours

- Cauda equina tumours produce a flaccid paraparesis with areflexia, segmental sensory loss and a severe disturbance of sphincter and sexual function
- Conus lesions produce a mixed upper and lower motor neuron syndrome with reflex changes determined by the site of the lesion

Cord compression produces one of three pictures:

Transverse cord

Disrupts all cord function below the level with an appropriate sensory level and motor deficit confined to the lower levels of the lesion or affecting all four limbs, depending on whether the thoracic or cervical cord is compressed.

Hemicord syndrome (Brown–Séquard)

Usually occurs with extrinsic compression. Ipsilaterally, there is pyramidal deficit and posterior column signs and, contralaterally, loss of spinothalamic function.

Central cord syndrome

Intramedullary tumours produce a suspended level of spinothalamic loss with pyramidal signs below the level of the lesion.

SPECIFIC TUMOURS

Astrocytomas

Predominate in the cervical and thoracic segment, and are generally of low malignancy and slow growing. Excellent results are achieved with radical excision, except for patients with anaplastic astrocytoma.

Ependymoma

These account for 60% of intramedullary spinal tumours (**Fig. 13.17**). They predominate in the filum terminale with a liability to spread to the conus or cauda equina. Radical excision is required. Radiotherapy does not confer additional benefit.

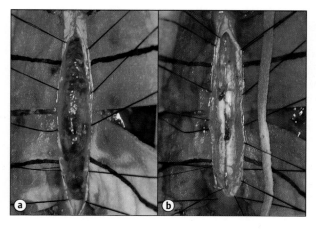

Fig. 13.17 *Ependymoma.* (*a*) *The tumour is seen as a dark sausage-shaped mass fungating out of the midline dorsal myelotomy incision.* (*b*) *After removal.*

Intramedullary metastases

Usually derived from the bronchus. Cerebral metastases often co-exist. The tumour may undergo necrosis and fungate through the dorsal horns into the subarachnoid space. The patient presents with a subacute myelopathy.

Meningioma

Usually occurs in the thoracic region and predominate in women. Spread is principally within the intradural space. Typically symptoms evolve gradually.

Schwannoma

Most schwannomas are isolated tumours arising from the dorsal root. The majority remain confined to the intradural space but some pass through the intervertebral foramen, producing a dumb-bell shaped mass. The vast majority are benign.

EPIDURAL TUMOURS

Metastatic carcinoma

The most common sources for these tumours are the breast, bronchus, prostate and kidney. Approximately two-thirds of tumours occur in the thoracic region. Local or referred pain is the usual initial complaint followed by evidence of spinal cord involvement.

Lymphoma and leukaemia

Lymphoma usually invades the extradural space from a retroperitoneal paraspinal deposit. The midthoracic spine is the favoured site.

Multiple myeloma and plasmacytoma

Either of these disease processes can produce a picture of spinal cord compression similar to that encountered with extradural metastases. Bone scanning is often negative.

Chordoma

Spinal chordomas usually arise in the sacral region. Bone destruction is pronounced and contiguous spread is likely with involvement of the sacral nerve roots.

INVESTIGATION

Plain radiograph

This is of very limited value. It can detect bone erosion caused by neurofibroma or collapse with extradural metastases.

Plain computerized tomography

Allows better definition of bone erosion than achieved by plain radiography.

CT myelography

More accurately shows cord expansion or deformity than can conventional myelography (Fig. 13.18).

Magnetic resonance imaging

MRI reveals the exact extent of any intramedullary tumour and whether it is cystic or solid. Enhancement of any solid component with gadolinium suggests a more aggressive process. Enhancement is also prominent with meningiomas and some neurofibromas (Fig. 13.19).

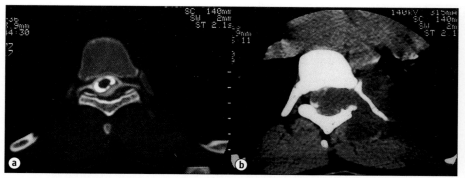

Fig. 13.18 *Thoracic schwannoma.* CT myelogram showing an extradural mass that has extended through the intervertebral foramen into the paravertebral space.

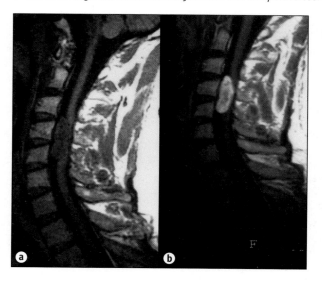

Fig. 13.19 *Spinal schwannoma. (a) Before and (b) after gadolinium. MRI.*

The technique detects multiple site pathology, for example, with extradural metastases; it is the investigation of choice in multiple myeloma.

MANAGEMENT

Aggressive surgery is called for with astrocytomas and ependymomas. In the presence of metastatic spinal cord compression, loss of ambulation is seldom reversed by surgical intervention. Surgical approach, in most instances, is anterior and usually combined with radiotherapy. Surgical excision of benign tumours is usually curative.

- Clinical patterns associated with cord compression include the transverse cord, the hemicord and the central cord syndromes
- Ependymomas account for the majority of intramedullary tumours
- Both astrocytomas and ependymomas of the cord merit a vigorous surgical approach
- MRI is the imaging technique of choice for most spinal tumours

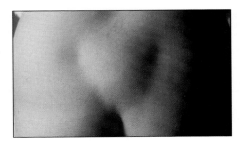

Fig. 13.20 *Spinal dysraphism.* *Lipoma overlying the lumbosacral region.*

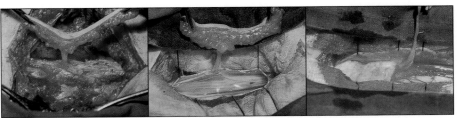

Fig. 13.21 *Extension of a track from the skin to a dermoid lying within the conus*

CONGENITAL DISORDERS

SPINA BIFIDA CYSTICA

Definition of terms describing congenital disorders

Meningocoele	Protrusion of the meninges through a vertebral defect.
Myelomeningocoele	Protrusion of the meninges and the spinal cord or nerve roots.
Myeloschisis	Exposed spinal cord due to a failure of fusion.
Diastematomyelia	Separation of the spinal cord by a bony spur or fibrous band.

Meningocoele and myelomeningocoele are evident in infancy and liable to produce, in the case of the latter, a substantial lower limb disability with wasting. Some disorders of midline fusion may present in adult life and can be associated with tethering of the cord or cauda equina, lipomata and dermoid tumours. The presence of the lesion is sometimes suggested by finding a dimple, tuft of hair, a naevus or a lipoma over the lumbosacral spine (**Fig. 13.20**). Intradural lipomas are likely to be adherent to adjacent structures. Plain radiographs reveal the bony abnormality, whereas MRI defines the true extent of the lesion. Dermoids can often be successfully removed (**Fig. 13.21**).

ARACHNOID CYSTS

Most arachnoid cysts are congenital. They are either extradural or intradural in location. Extradural cysts are single, occur particularly in the thoracic region and consist of a posterior protrusion of arachnoid through the dura. They are usually asymptomatic but sometimes produce nerve root and spinal compression. Intradural cysts can be enclosed or still in communication with the subarachnoid space. They are usually multiple. Plain radiographs can show the bony changes caused by extradural cysts but MRI is the imaging technique of choice. Symptomatic cysts are decompressed.

SYRINGOMYELIA

Causes of syringomyelia include:

- Developmental anomalies at the cervicocranial junction
- Intramedullary tumour
- Trauma

In syringomyelia, cavitation of the spinal cord occurs, principally in the cervical region, sometimes in association with cavitation of the brainstem (syringobulbia). The cavity interrupts decussating spinothalamic fibres in the anterior commissure, later extending into the anterior and posterior horns and finally the lateral and posterior columns.

Clinical features

In the early stages, the clinical features are those of an accompanying Chiari malformation (see p 90–91). In a fully developed case (now rare), there is dissociated sensory loss over the cervical and upper thoracic dermatomes often with spontaneous pain. Self-injury is common. Later, touch and proprioception may be affected. The upper limbs become weak with wasting of the small hand muscles (**Fig. 13.22**), whereas the lower limbs become spastic. The upper limb reflexes are depressed, the lower limb reflexes exaggerated. Autonomic disturbances include altered sweating over the face and arms, sphincter disturbances and a Horner's syndrome. Scoliosis is a recognized feature of a cervical syrinx.

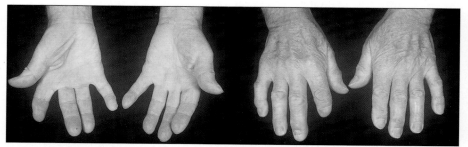

Fig. 13.22 *Syringomyelia.* *Wasting of the small hand muscles and loss of the terminal phalanx of the right index finger.*

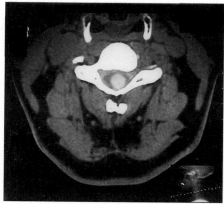

Fig. 13.23 *Post-traumatic syringomyelia.* *CT myelography showing contrast within the cord.*

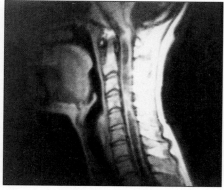

Fig. 13.24 *Syringomyelia.* *MRI showing cord cavitation and a cystic expansion in the posterior fossa.*

Investigation

CT myelography can detect cerebellar ectopia and may, with delayed films, show filling of the cavity (**Fig. 13.23**). MRI is the procedure of choice, defining any abnormality at the foramen magnum together with the extent of the cavity (**Fig. 13.24**).

Treatment

Various forms of surgical treatment have been used, including foramen magnum decompression, plugging of the obex and syringoperitoneal or subarachnoid shunting. Muscle wasting, ataxia and scoliosis are poor prognostic signs for return of normal neurological function.

SUBACUTE COMBINED DEGENERATION OF THE SPINAL CORD

This is secondary to vitamin B^{12} deficiency. Pathological changes include myelin degeneration in the posterolateral columns, principally in the cervicothoracic region, followed by axonal degeneration. Similar changes are found in the optic nerves and, sometimes, in the cerebral white matter and the peripheral nervous system.

> **Symptoms of subacute combined degeneration of the spinal cord include**
>
> - Stiffness and weakness of the legs
> - Mood and behaviour changes
> - Sensory complaints

Peripheral paraesthesiae appear in the feet then the hands with stiffness and weakness of the legs. Sometimes there are changes in mood and behaviour. Findings include Lhermitte's sign (in 20% of cases), posterior column sensory loss and a paraplegia often with depressed or absent ankle reflexes. Recognized non-neurological features include a lemon-yellow colour to the skin, premature greying, vitiligo and glossitis (**Fig. 13.25**).

Abnormalities on investigation include a macrocytic anaemia with a megaloblastic bone marrow (although both may be absent), neutropenia with a right shift, thrombocytopenia and vitamin B^{12} levels usually well below 100 ng/l. Antibodies to intrinsic factor are found in the majority of cases. Abnormal electrophysiological findings include altered peripheral nerve conduction and central delay of somatosensory evoked potentials. The condition, if diagnosed early, responds well to B^{12} therapy, which is continued indefinitely.

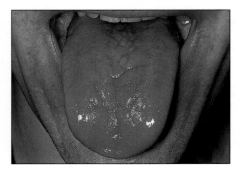

Fig. 13.25 *Subacute combined degeneration.* *Appearance of the tongue.*

ARACHNOIDITIS

Causes of spinal arachnoiditis include:
- Idiopathic
- Trauma
- Myelography with oil-containing media

After an initial inflammatory reaction, fibrosis appears with thickening of the membranes, obliteration of the subarachnoid space, cyst formation and vessel occlusion.

> **Symptoms of arachnoiditis**
>
> - Pain
> - Numbness
> - Paraesthesiae
> - Weakness
> - Usually slowly progressive

MRI is the investigation of choice. Various patterns have been described in the lumbo-sacral region, including nerve root clumping centrally, peripheral adhesion of roots to the theca and an increase in signal intensity within the theca obscuring the differentiation of cerebrospinal fluid from the nerve root (**Fig. 13.26**). There is no specific treatment.

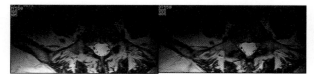

Fig. 13.26 *Arachnoiditis.* *Axial MRI at two levels showing peripheral clumping of nerve roots.*

RADIATION MYELOPATHY

The incidence of radiation myelopathy after spinal cord irradiation has been reported to be between 0.6% and 17.5%.

A transient form, typically associated with a Lhermitte phenomenon when the cervical cord has been irradiated, occurs within a few months of treatment and resolves.

A chronic progressive form occurs when the cumulative dose has exceeded 4000 cGy and can appear from 1 to 5 years after treatment. Concomitant chemotherapy enhances the risk. Insidious sensory symptoms emerge, sometimes in a Brown–Séquard pattern of distribution, followed by paralysis and sphincter impairment. Variants include one in which the anterior horn cells are predominantly affected after retroperitoneal irradiation, leading to a flaccid weakness of the legs without pain or sensory loss.

Pathological changes include grey and white matter necrosis with a prominent vasculopathy. The condition is prevented by limiting cord irradiation.

> - Defects of fusion of the spine are often associated with cutaneous markers
> - Most non-traumatic cases of syringomyelia are associated with an anomaly at the foramen magnum
> - Subacute combined degeneration of the spinal cord can exist in the presence of a normal peripheral blood count
> - Radiation myelopathy can be prevented by limiting the amount of spinal irradiation

chapter 14

Myasthenia Gravis and Muscle Disease

MYASTHENIA GRAVIS

A disease of the neuromuscular junction caused by antibodies against the acetylcholine receptor of the postsynaptic muscle membrane.

> **Definition of types of myasthenia**
>
> Neonatal myasthenia gravis (in infants born to myasthenic mothers)
> Congenital myasthenia gravis (genetically determined)

PATHOLOGY

- Electron microscopy of the motor end plate shows simplification of the postsynaptic region with widening of the synaptic space (**Fig. 14.1**)
- The density of the acetylcholine receptors at the postsynaptic membrane is reduced
- The thymus shows medullary hyperplasia in most young-onset patients
- Thymic medullary cells can synthesize anti-acetylcholine receptor antibodies in culture
- Thymomas occur in 10–15% of myasthenia gravis patients

PATHOPHYSIOLOGY

- 90% of patients with generalized myasthenia have acetylcholine receptor antibodies
- 50% of patients with ocular myasthenia have acetylcholine receptor antibodies
- Another form of antibody is probably present in the acetylcholine receptor antibody-negative group
- The miniature end-plate potentials (the result of on-going, spontaneous release of acetylcholine quanta from the nerve terminal) are reduced in amplitude

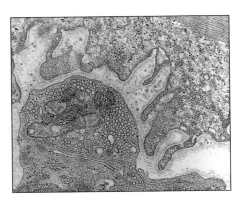

Fig. 14.1 End-plate region in untreated myasthenia gravis. Simplification of the postsynaptic region and widening of the synaptic space (mag X 31,900).

Epidemiology

- Prevalence rate is estimated to be 4 per 100 000 of the population
- Bimodal distribution for age of onset in both sexes (age 20–35 and 70–75 years)
- Association of HLA A1, B8 and DR3 with young-onset myasthenia gravis in the White population
- Associations exist with other conditions, including thyroid disease, rheumatoid arthritis and systemic lupus erythematosus

CLINICAL MANIFESTATIONS

Symptoms of myasthenia gravis

- Usually first affects the ocular muscles
- Initial complaints in two-thirds of patients are diplopia and ptosis (**Fig. 14.2**)
- In the remainder, onset is with bulbar symptoms (dysphagia, dysarthria) or with limb symptoms
- Fatiguability is characteristic. Symptoms worsen during the day, in the course of eating a meal or conversation
- A fluctuating course is characteristic. Symptoms may remain confined to the eyes (ocular myasthenia). If they remain so for 2 years, subsequent generalization is very unlikely

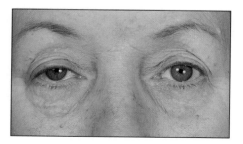

Fig. 14.2 *Unilateral ptosis in myasthenia gravis.*

Signs

- Ocular signs, like the other signs of the disease, can fluctuate wildly. An asymmetrical ptosis is common and can be triggered by prolonged upward gaze. Various eye movement disorders appear and are typically difficult to quantify. A predominant weakness of medial rectus can mimic an internuclear ophthalmoplegia (**Fig. 14.3**)
- Facial weakness is common, with difficulty in closing the eyes tightly and a tendency for the face to sag (**Fig. 14.4**)

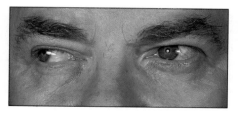

Fig. 14.3 *Pseudo-internuclear ophthalmoplegia in myasthenia gravis.*

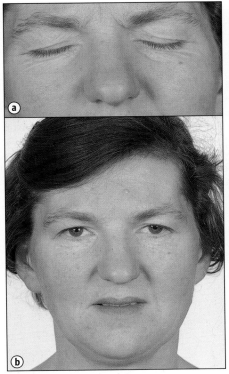

Fig. 14.4 *Failure of complete eye closure (a) with characteristic configuration of the mouth (b).*

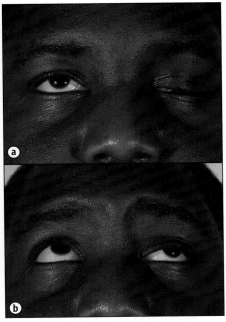

Fig. 14.5 *Appearance of the eyes (a) before and (b) after injection of intravenous Tensilon.*

- Bulbar involvement leads to dysarthria, often with a nasal quality. The palate appears weak and the tongue may display a triple furrow
- Involvement of the axial and limb muscles is notoriously variable and often highly selective. Neck flexion is usually much weaker than extension. Triceps tends to be more affected than other upper limb muscles
- In order to demonstrate fatiguability, the patient is asked to sustain a number of motor tasks: up-gaze, eyelid closure, counting to 50 and prolonged shoulder abduction

INVESTIGATION

Edrophonium

Edrophonium is a short-acting cholinesterase inhibitor. A test dose of 2 mg is given intravenously followed by a bolus of 8 mg if there has been no adverse reaction. In myasthenic patients, subjective and objective improvement in muscle strength appears for 1–2 min (**Fig. 14.5**). The injection must be used with great care in patients with generalized myasthenia, particularly those on oral anticholinesterases. If weakness in those patients is caused by excessive therapy, the injection may exacerbate the existing weakness leading, for example, to respiratory arrest. Minor improvement in muscle strength can occur in other conditions, for example, polymyositis.

Serological tests

Acetylcholine receptor antibodies are found in 90% of patients with generalized myasthenia gravis. Titres correlate rather poorly with clinical severity. Antibodies to striated muscle are found in the vast majority of patients with thymoma. Various auto-antibodies are found more commonly than in the normal population, for example, thyroid antibodies in one-third of patients.

Electrophysiology

Repetitive nerve stimulation at 2–3 Hz produces an abnormal decrement in the amplitude of the evoked potential from the muscle the nerve innervates. With single-fibre techniques, an abnormal variability in the time gap between potentials arising from adjacent muscle fibres belonging to the same motor unit can be detected (jitter) (**Fig. 14.6**). Jitter is found in over 90% of myasthenia gravis patients. The stapedius reflex is measured by assessing the acoustic impedance of the tympanic membrane. Abnormal decrement occurs in over 90% of patients.

Imaging

Computerized tomography shows all thymomas but may also detect thymic abnormalities caused by hyperplasia. A mass detected by computerized tomography but not by mediastinal tomography is probably not a thymoma.

MANAGEMENT

The management of myasthenia gravis is outlined in **Figure 14.7**.

Anticholinesterases

These drugs inhibit acetylcholine breakdown at the neuromuscular junction. The most commonly used is pyridostigmine. Dosage ranges from 90 to 720 mg/day. Side effects are common, including colic, diarrhoea and salivation. Some muscles may be underdosed at the same time that others are overdosed. Increase in dosage can then exacerbate weakness in the latter (cholinergic crisis). The drug is given every 4 h. Neostigmine is a shorter-acting drug.

Corticosteroids

Initial worsening of symptoms can occur with corticosteroids, particularly if treatment is begun with large doses. Eventually, 60–80 mg daily may be needed, later switching to an alternate-day regime. Substantial benefit is seen in at least three-quarters of patients. A long-term maintenance dose of 7.5–10 mg on alternate days often suffices.

Other immunosuppressants

Azathioprine is the most common immunosuppressant used, other than corticosteroids. Dosage is up to 2.5 mg/kg/day. The response may take several months. Regular blood counts and liver function tests are necessary. Cyclophosphamide is sometimes effective when other drugs have failed.

Plasmapheresis

This treatment is almost always effective with a response usually within 48 h of commencing exchange. The response lasts for several weeks before the patient relapses to his or her previous status. The treatment is usually reserved for patients with acute exacerbations or for those being prepared for thymectomy. Side effects, including dizziness, nausea and cardiac arrhythmias, are usually slight.

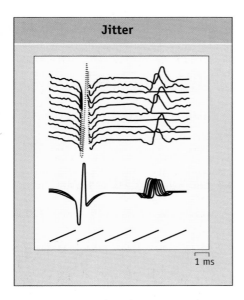

Fig. 14.6 *Jitter recorded with a concentric needle electrode using special filters.* The timing of the second spike varies in relationship to the first because of variable conduction at the motor end plate.

Management options in myasthenia gravis

- Anticholinesterases
- Corticosteroids
- Other immunosuppressants
- Plasmapheresis
- Intravenous immunoglobulin
- Thymectomy

Fig. 14.7 *Management options in myasthenia gravis.*

Immunoglobulin

Intravenous immunoglobulin is effective, given in a dose of 0.4g/kg/day for 5 days. The response is probably comparable with that seen with plasmapheresis.

Thymectomy

Stable remission rates increase in a linear fashion with time after thymectomy. By 5 years, approximately one-third of patients without thymoma are in complete remission, the figure being halved for those with thymoma. A further proportion of patients are improved. The histological appearance of the thymus does not reliably predict outcome. The response is independent of sex and is found in all ages at least until the age of 50 years. All patients with thymoma should have surgery.

PARTICULAR SITUATIONS

Ocular myasthenia

Treatment commences with anticholinesterases. If response is unsatisfactory then alternate-day steroids are used.

Younger, generalized myasthenia

Thymectomy is considered for all these patients. Stabilization before operation is achieved with plasmapheresis or immunoglobulin. If no response occurs, long-term steroid therapy with or without azathioprine is used.

Older, generalized myasthenia

Alternate-day steroids, azathioprine or both are used.

Pregnancy

May be associated with worsening or improvement of myasthenic symptoms. Cytotoxic drugs are avoided in pregnancy.

Other drugs

Certain drugs can produce a blocking effect at the neuromuscular junction and should be avoided in myasthenic patients. They include β blockers, the aminoglycosides, tetracycline, ampicillin, erythromycin and quinidine derivatives. Competitive neuromuscular blocking drugs (e.g. D-tubocurarine) have a prolonged effect in myasthenia gravis.

SYMPTOMATIC MYASTHENIA

Myasthenia is sometimes triggered by treatment with D-penicillamine. Antibodies are present and the condition responds to anticholinesterases. Remission is the rule when the penicillamine is withdrawn. The ocular muscles are those mainly affected (**Fig. 14.8**).

- Myasthenia gravis should always be considered in a patient with fluctuant weakness, even if the signs are not reproducible
- Great caution is needed when using edrophonium, particularly in patients already receiving anticholinesterases
- Thymectomy should be considered in all patients with generalized myasthenia under the age of 50 years
- Certain drugs can exacerbate myasthenia gravis and should be avoided if possible

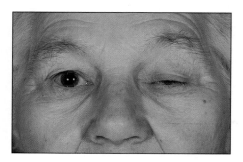

Fig. 14.8   Unilateral ptosis in myasthenia gravis induced by penicillamine.

LAMBERT–EATON MYASTHENIC SYNDROME

This condition is perhaps 30 times less common than myasthenia gravis. Up to 60% of patients have a small cell lung cancer.

- The condition is caused by a deficiency in the number of acetylcholine quanta released at the nerve terminal
- It is associated with antibodies to presynaptic voltage-gated calcium channels
- Electron microscopy studies show an altered appearance of the active zones on the presynaptic membrane
- Clinical features include proximal weakness with pain and autonomic symptoms such as dryness of the mouth. The limb reflexes are depressed but augment after tetanic contraction of the muscle. Ocular and bulbar muscles are usually spared

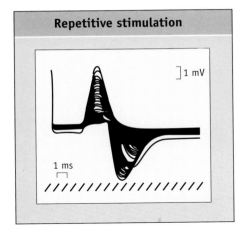

Repetitive stimulation

]1 mV

1 ms

Fig. 14.9 Lambert–Eaton myasthenic syndrome. *EMG showing augmentation of the muscle action potential during repetitive stimulation at 50 Hz.*

- Electromyogram (EMG) shows a characteristic augmentation of the compound muscle action potential after sustained contraction or with rapid (50 Hz) nerve stimulation (**Fig. 14.9**)
- The condition responds positively to 3,4-diaminopyridine, steroids or immunoglobulin
- The condition may remit if the associated cancer is successfully treated

NEUROMYOTONIA (ISAAC'S SYNDROME)

This is a rare disorder associated with continuous muscle fibre activity. The patient complains of muscle cramps, twitches and weakness. Antibodies to potassium channels regulating nerve excitability have been detected and the condition responds positively to phenytoin, tegretol or plasmapheresis.

PRIMARY MUSCLE DISEASE

Definition of the myopathies

The myopathies are primary disorders of muscle. Their characteristics include:
- A tendency to proximal involvement
- Symmetry
- Relative preservation of the reflexes
- Normal sensation
- Normal sphincter function
- Normal intellect (with the exception of Duchenne's muscular dystrophy)
- Pseudo-hypertrophy of muscle, seen in some of the muscular dystrophies; can also occur in spinal muscular atrophy

CLASSIFICATION

- Muscular dystrophies
- The myotonic disorders
- Metabolic myopathies
- Endocrine myopathies
- Alcohol myopathy
- Mitochondrial myopathies
- Inflammatory myopathies
- Parasitic muscle disease
- Periodic paralysis

MUSCULAR DYSTROPHIES

These are genetically determined disorders of muscle. Their classification is based on a combination of genetic features and clinical distribution.

CLASSIFICATION

- **X-linked**   Duchenne's
                 Becker's
                 Scapuloperoneal (Emery–Dreifuss)

- **Recessive** Scapulohumeral
                 Childhood form (pseudo-Duchenne)
                 Distal
                 Congenital

- **Dominant**   Facioscapulohumeral
                 Scapuloperoneal
                 Distal
                 Ocular
                 Oculopharyngeal

DUCHENNE'S MUSCULAR DYSTROPHY

- The most common form of muscular dystrophy
- Virtually confined to males
- Associated with the absence of dystrophin, a cytoskeletal protein encoded by a gene at locus p21 on the short arm of the X chromosome. Dystrophin is found on the inner aspect of the plasma membrane of the skeletal muscle fibre
- Prevalence is approximately 3 per 100 000 of the population
- Approximately one-third of patients have a sporadic form
- Onset in the first decade with weakness of the shoulder and pelvic girdle muscles
- Pseudohypertrophy, particularly of the calf muscles, is almost inevitable
- Walking difficulties are associated with difficulty in climbing stairs and in rising from the floor
- A characteristic manoeuvre (Gowers') is used to rise from a supine position (**Fig. 14.10**)
- Patients are wheelchair bound by approximately 10–12 years old and the majority die before the age of 20
- Cardiomyopathy is the norm and produces cardiac failure in some patients

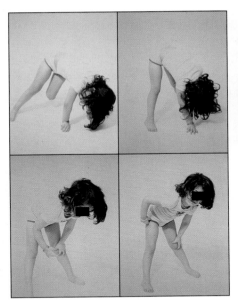

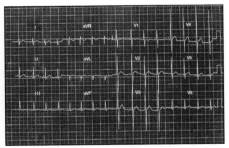

Fig. 14.11 *Electrocardiogram in Duchenne's muscular dystrophy.*

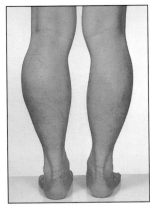

Fig. 14.12 Calf hypertrophy in Becker's muscular dystrophy.

Fig. 14.10 *Gowers' manoeuvre.*

Investigation

- Creatine kinase is elevated, particularly in the early stages
- Muscle biopsy changes are influenced by the duration of disease. There is variation in fibre size, evidence of muscle necrosis and infiltration by fat and connective tissue
- EMG shows myopathic changes with an increased proportion of polyphasic potentials of short duration and reduced amplitude
- Electrocardiogram changes are common with prominent Q waves in the lateral and tall R waves in the septal precordial leads (**Fig. 14.11**)

Management

- Corticosteroids can improve muscle function, although for an uncertain length of time
- Physiotherapy and various surgical procedures are used to improve stability or posture
- Genetic counselling is critical. cDNA probes are used to help to clarify the carrier state

BECKER'S MUSCULAR DYSTROPHY

This condition is allelic with Duchenne's muscular dystrophy. A reduced amount of an abnormally low molecular weight dystrophin is found in most patients.

- The clinical picture is similar to Duchenne's muscular dystrophy but the condition is more benign
- Most patients are still mobile at the age of 40 years
- There is less likelihood of contractures, cardiomyopathy or impaired intelligence compared with Duchenne's muscular dystrophy (**Fig. 14.12**)

269

SCAPULOPERONEAL MYOPATHY (EMERY–DREIFUSS)
- Presents in the first decade and is slowly progressive
- Muscle hypertrophy is absent but contractures of the calf muscles are often prominent
- Cardiomyopathy is common

SCAPULOHUMERAL DYSTROPHY
- Uncommon
- Winging of the scapulae is prominent
- Later proximal lower limb weakness appears

CHILDHOOD, AUTOSOMAL RECESSIVE, MUSCULAR DYSTROPHY
- Produces a pattern similar to Duchenne's muscular dystrophy but with autosomal recessive inheritance
- Muscle dystrophin is normal
- Onset is in the first decade
- The changes on muscle biopsy tend to be patchy, with areas of necrosis bounded by near normal fibres

FACIOSCAPULOHUMERAL DYSTROPHY
- Inherited as an autosomal dominant condition
- Expression of the disease is very variable
- Age of onset varies
- Tends to begin in the facial and shoulder-girdle muscles with later spread to the lower limbs
- Prominent weakness is found in the face, neck flexors, serrati, pectorals, biceps, triceps and wrist extensors
- The scapulae tend to ride up, particularly when the patient abducts the arms at the shoulders
- There is prominent weakness of the anterior tibial muscles
- Associated findings include sensorineural deafness and retinal vascular abnormalities (**Fig. 14.13**)

SCAPULOPERONEAL DYSTROPHY
Appears later than the sex-linked form. Overlap with a similar syndrome caused by spinal muscular atrophy is considerable.

DISTAL MYOPATHY
Rare. Presents with weakness of the small hand muscles, later spreading to the calves and anterior tibial group.

OCULAR MYOPATHY
Rare. Most patients have associated involvement of the peripheral or central nervous system, the condition then being mitochondrial in origin.

OCULOPHARYNGEAL MYOPATHY
Combines external ophthalmoplegia with dysphagia secondary to pharyngeal weakness (**Fig. 14.14**).

LIMB-GIRDLE DYSTROPHY
Many cases are the result of spinal muscular atrophy but true, myopathic cases occur, with both recessive and dominant forms of inheritance.

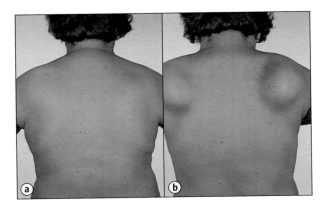

Fig. 14.13 *Facioscapulo-humeral dystrophy.* At rest (a) and (b) with the arms exerting forward pressure.

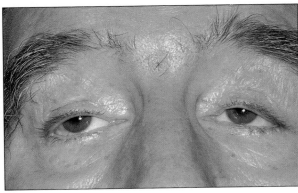

Fig. 14.14 *Oculopharyngeal dystrophy.* Attempted up-gaze.

Although no specific therapy exists for the dystrophies, all patients can be helped by physiotherapy, allied with functional assessment of need by the occupational therapist.

- The muscular dystrophies are inherited disorders
- Classification is based on genetic and clinical characteristics
- Investigations centre on EMG, muscle biopsy and measurement of muscle enzymes
- Absence of a cytoskeletal protein, dystrophin, is the cardinal feature of Duchenne's muscular dystrophy

THE MYOTONIC DISORDERS

CLASSIFICATION
- Myotonic dystrophy
- Congenital myotonia
- Paramyotonia congenita
- Other disorders

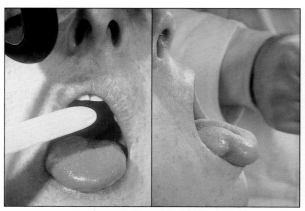

Fig. 14.15 *Myotonia of the tongue, triggered by percussion.*

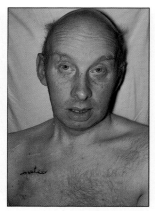

Fig. 14.16 *Myotonic dystrophy. Characteristic facial expression.*

Definition of myotonia

Myotonia is the abnormal persistence of muscle fibre contraction after voluntary effort or in response to a mechanical stimulus (**Fig. 14.15**). It tends to lessen after repeated contraction.

Paramyotonia differs by getting worse during continuous or repeated voluntary muscular contraction.

PATHOPHYSIOLOGY

- The blockade of muscle membrane chloride conductance is the responsible agent in congenital myotonia
- Failure of inactivation of the muscle membrane sodium channel is responsible for the myotonia of paramyotonia congenita
- Myotonic dystrophy is not caused by a genetic defect in an ion channel

CLINICAL FEATURES

Myotonic dystrophy

- The most common form of adult-onset muscular dystrophy
- Inherited as an autosomal dominant condition (chromosome 19)
- The clinical manifestations are extremely variable
- Anticipation occurs, with earlier onset in successive generations
- The muscle weakness is mainly distal with ptosis, facial weakness and striking atrophy of the sternomastoids (**Fig. 14.16**)
- Involvement of the extra-ocular muscles and the muscles of respiration is seen
- Myotonia is often inconspicuous. It can be elicited by percussion or by sustained contraction. It is worse in the cold
- Smooth muscle involvement of the gut leads to dysphagia and constipation
- Cardiac muscle involvement leads to cardiomyopathy along with cardiac conduction defects

Other sytem involvement

- Intellectual impairment
- Cataract
- Premature baldness
- Testicular atrophy
- Pituitary abnormalities
- Diabetes

Congenital myotonia

Thomsen's disease
- Autosomal dominant
- Early onset
- Myotonia resolves with continued activity

Becker's disease
- Autosomal recessive
- Childhood onset
- Muscle hypertrophy common, particularly in males

Paramyotonia congenita
- Autosomal dominant
- Onset in first decade
- The myotonia is cold-induced and may be followed by attacks of flaccid paralysis lasting for several hours
- There is substantial overlap with hyperkalaemic periodic paralysis

- Myotonic dystrophy is the most common form of adult-onset muscular dystrophy
- Anticipation occurs in myotonic dystrophy
- Abnormalities of chloride and sodium conductance are responsible for congenital myotonia and paramyotonia congenita, respectively

METABOLIC AND ENDOCRINE MYOPATHIES

Most of the metabolic myopathies present in childhood. They take the form of progressive muscle weakness or episodic paralysis triggered by exercise.

ACID MALTASE DEFICIENCY (RECESSIVE)

- Associated with accumulation of glycogen in skeletal muscle and other organs
- Presents as a slowly-progressive proximal weakness resembling limb-girdle dystrophy
- Involvement of respiratory muscle is common
- Creatine kinase levels are elevated and EMG shows a myopathic pattern
- Muscle biopsy shows vacuoles (containing glycogen) (**Fig. 14.17**)
- Acid maltase levels are depressed in muscle and cultured fibroblasts

MYOPHOSPHORYLASE DEFICIENCY (RECESSIVE) (McARDLE'S DISEASE)

- Presents with attacks of muscle pain and weakness triggered by exercise
- In one-third of patients, proximal weakness appears

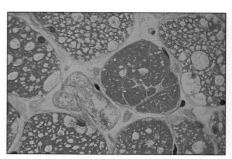

Fig. 14.17 *Acid maltase deficiency.*
Vacuolation of muscle fibres.

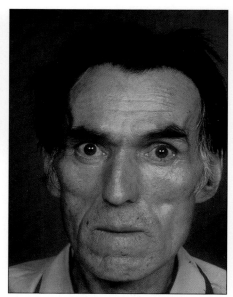

Fig. 14.18 *Thyrotoxic myopathy.*

- Lactate levels fail to rise in venous blood taken from a limb that has undergone ischaemic exercise
- Muscle biopsy shows accumulation of glycogen under the sarcolemma

PHOSPHOFRUCTOKINASE DEFICIENCY (RECESSIVE) (TARUI'S DISEASE)
- Similar to myophosphorylase deficiency

CARNITINE PALMITYL TRANSFERASE DEFICIENCY
- This causes a similar picture to McCardle's disease
- Lactate levels rise normally after ischaemic exercise

  Thyrotoxicosis is the most common endocrinological disorder associated with muscle disease (Fig. 14.18). Other conditions affecting muscle include:
- Hypothyroidism (the combination of pain, muscle weakness and increased muscle bulk is called Hoffmann's syndrome)
- Primary and secondary hyperparathyroidism
- Cushing's disease (perhaps 50%)
- Acromegaly

  In general, the muscle disorders related to endocrinological disease are associated with normal creatine kinase levels and non-specific EMG and muscle biopsy changes. These changes are reversible if the endocrinological disorder is treated.

- Thyrotoxicosis is the most common trigger for an endocrine-related myopathy
- The endocrine myopathies are usually reversible
- A limb-girdle picture with prominent respiratory involvement should suggest acid maltase deficiency.

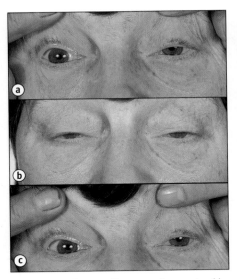

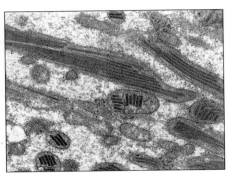

Fig. 14.20 *Mitochondrial respiratory chain disease.* *Abnormal subsarcolemmal mitochondria (mag X 8,800).*

Fig. 14.19 *Kearns–Sayre syndrome.* *Looking (a) to the right, (b) ahead and to the (c) left.*

ALCOHOL MYOPATHY

One form of alcoholic myopathy results in a rapidly developing proximal weakness with pain, tenderness, high serum creatine kinase levels and myoglobinuria. A chronic form exists resulting in a proximal myopathy but with fewer prominent creatine kinase changes.

MITOCHONDRIAL MYOPATHIES

Disorders of the mitochondrial respiratory chain lead to a confusing plethora of neurological diseases, in which proximal weakness is a prominent feature. The diseases are associated with mutations or deletions of mitochondrial DNA.

Classification of the mitochondrial respiratory chain diseases

- Chronic progressive external ophthalmoplegia (CPEO)
- Kearns–Sayre syndrome (KSS) (**Fig. 14.19**)
- Mitochondrial encephalopathy, lactic acidosis and stroke-like episodes (MELAS)
- Myoclonus, epilepsy and ragged red fibres (MERRF)

In addition to the well-recognized syndromes, the disorders can present with less-specific features. Overall characteristics include:

- Large-scale deletions in mitochondrial DNA in CPEO and KSS
- Point mutations in mitochondrial DNA in MELAS and MERRF
- Maternal inheritance is very common for MELAS and MERRF
- Lactic acidosis (perhaps in 50% of patients)
- Normal or only mildly elevated creatine kinase levels in the majority of patients
- Non-specific EMG and EEG changes
- Basal ganglia calcification or low densities on imaging
- Morphological changes on muscle biopsy, a mixture of cytochrome oxidase positive and negative fibres and subsarcolemmal mitochondrial accumulations (**Fig. 14.20**)
- There is no specific treatment

INFLAMMATORY MYOPATHIES

Inflammatory muscle disease is uncommon. The condition can be triggered by a specific infectious agent or be of unknown aetiology. The most common idiopathic forms are polymyositis and dermatomyositis (**Fig. 14.21**). The onset of polymyositis may be acute, subacute or chronic. Polymyositis is associated with invasion of muscle fibres by CD8+ cytotoxic T cells and can be regarded as a cell-mediated autoimmune disease. Dermatomyositis is thought to be initiated by a complement-mediated damage of muscle capillaries.

POLYMYOSITIS AND DERMATOMYOSITIS

- Proximal limb weakness is typical
- Muscle pain and tenderness are inconstant
- Dysphagia is common secondary to pharyngeal involvement
- Weakness of neck flexion is often prominent
- Sometimes the weakness is confined to one limb or follows a myopathic distribution (e.g. facioscapulohumeral)
- Skin changes include an erythematous rash over the face (particularly cheeks and around the eyes), upper limbs and chest and dilated capillaries with haemorrhages in the skin around the nail beds (**Fig. 14.22**)
- Cardiac involvement is common (elevated creatine kinase MB isoenzyme)
- Incidence of malignancy is 10% (20% in patients over 50 years of age)
- The association with malignancy is probably confined to dermatomyositis
- 20% of patients have evidence of a connective tissue disorder, for example, systemic lupus erythematosus or systemic sclerosis

Investigation

- Erythrocyte sedimentation rate elevation is inconstant and does not correlate with disease activity
- Creatine kinase levels are strikingly elevated in the acute form. Levels fall with treatment and may rise before clinical relapse. Normal levels throughout in 1% of patients
- EMG shows myopathic features together with fibrillation potentials, sharp waves and high-frequency discharges
- Biopsy abnormalities in 90% of patients, with inflammatory change in 75%. Multisite biopsies are recommended (**Fig. 14.23**)

Treatment

Objective measurement of muscle power coupled with serial creatine kinase measurements are the best criteria for assessing any treatment response.

- Corticosteroids are the mainstay of treatment. Up to 100 mg daily of prednisolone may be needed to achieve control. Thereafter, the dose is slowly reduced and converted to an alternate-day regime
- Azathioprine can be given as an alternative or in combination with corticosteroids. The dosage is approximately 1.5–2 mg/kg/day
- Other agents sometimes used include cyclophosphamide, whole-body irradiation and intravenous immunoglobulin

INCLUSION-BODY MYOSITIS

- Exists in sporadic and familial forms
- The sporadic form is the most common muscle disease that begins beyond the age of 50
- Predominates in men

Diagnostic criteria for the inflammatory myopathies

1. Predominantly or exclusively proximal weakness
   With or without myalgia
   With or without skin changes
2. Biopsy evidence of muscle necrosis, regeneration and cell infiltration
3. Raised creatine kinase (MM isoenzyme), aldolase or myoglobin
4. Multifocal EMG myopathic change
   4 out of 4 is definite
   3 out of 4 is probable

Fig. 14.21 *Diagnostic criteria for the inflammatory myopathies.*

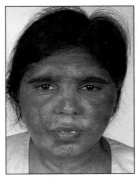

Fig. 14.22 *Facial rash in dermatomyositis.*

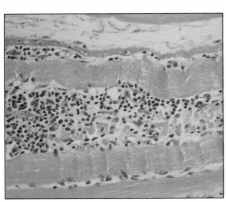

Fig. 14.23 *Muscle biopsy in polymyositis.*

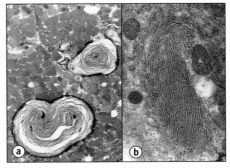

Fig. 14.24 *Inclusion body myositis.* Intranuclear filaments on electron microscopy (a) mag x 12 000, (b) mag x 33 000.

- Produces both distal and proximal weakness with prominent involvement of the forearms and the quadriceps
- Dysphagia is common
- Often, poor response to corticosteroids
- Biopsy reveals a mononuclear infiltration with atrophic fibres. Electron microscopy reveals characteristic cytoplasmic twisted tubulofilaments (**Fig. 14.24**)

An inflammatory myopathy has been described in AIDS.

GRANULOMATOUS MYOSITIS

Symptomatic muscle disease resembling chronic polymyositis is sometimes seen in sarcoidosis. In other patients with sarcoid but without muscle symptoms, blind muscle biopsy can sometimes identify the presence of granuloma.

PARASITIC MUSCLE DISEASE

Cysticercosis

- Caused by dissemination of the ova of *Taenia solium* into muscle and other organs after ingestion of contaminated pork or beef

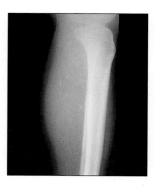

Fig. 14.25 *Radiograph of the calf showing calcified cysticerci.*

- Muscle involvement leads to hypertrophy, sometimes with weakness and, eventually, calcific deposits
- Pain and muscle tenderness are usually lacking (**Fig. 14.25**) (see p 204)

Hydatid disease
- Primarily affects the liver, lung and skeletal muscle
- Caused by dissemination of the ova of echinococcus
- Brain involvement is associated with focal deficit or epilepsy
- Serological tests for echinococcal antigens are available but the yield of positive results varies according to the site of the lesions
- Surgical removal of symptomatic brain cysts is recommended. Of the medical treatments, mebendazole is the one most used

Periodic paralysis
In these conditions, attacks of flaccid paralysis occur, often triggered by exercise. They are dominantly inherited.

Hyperkalaemic periodic paralysis
- Serum potassium levels are usually elevated in attacks but can be normal
- Onset is in the first decade of life, with attacks lasting from minutes to hours, at varying intervals
- Myotonia is found in some patients
- Attacks are triggered by rest after exercise or by ingestion of potassium
- Cold exposure can lead to mild weakness
- Sometimes the attack can be frustrated by mild exercise
- Treatment includes use of a thiazide diuretic or acetazolamide on a long-term basis

Hypokalaemic periodic paralysis
- Begins in the first or second decade
- Myotonia is absent
- Caused by a disorder of a calcium channel in skeletal muscle
- Potassium levels are low in attacks
- Attacks of weakness affect proximal muscles, predominantly with areflexia
- Duration of an attack is usually hours
- Provocative factors include exercise followed by rest and a large carbohydrate load
- Attacks are treated by oral potassium. Prophylaxis against attacks is achieved with acetazolamide

Attacks of periodic paralysis can be associated with thyrotoxicosis, particularly in Asians.

chapter 15

The Neurology of Cancer, Systemic Disease and Psychiatry

THE NON-METASTATIC (PARANEOPLASTIC) SYNDROMES

The paraneoplastic syndromes are disorders of the nervous system related to a systemic malignancy that is not caused by direct invasion of the relevant tissue.

CORTICAL CEREBELLAR DEGENERATION

- Group one – pure cerebellar degeneration
- Group two – cerebellar syndrome with inflammatory reaction I encephalomyelitis
- Associated neoplasms: lung, ovary, breast, Hodgkin's disease
- Pathological changes, loss of Purkinje cells (**Fig. 15.1**)
- May precede malignancy by 3 years or appear up to 2 years after the malignancy has been diagnosed
- Progressive cerebellar syndrome affecting speech, limbs and trunk. Vertigo is common at the onset. Nystagmus is found in 50% of patients
- The cerebrospinal fluid may contain lymphocytes
- Imaging reveals little cerebellar atrophy
- Usually progressive. Occasional arrest or reversal of disease after excision of associated neoplasm
- Auto-antibodies to Purkinje cells are relevant to the pathogenesis (anti-Yo)

ENCEPHALOMYELITIS

This affects cerebral hemispheres (limbic encephalitis), brainstem, cerebellum, spinal cord and dorsal root ganglia. The pathological changes include the appearance of perivascular inflammatory cells, neuronal loss, white matter degeneration and increased microglial activity (**Fig. 15.2**). Three-quarters of patients have an associated carcinoma of the bronchus. Less commonly, associations may be with ovary, stomach, uterus or Hodgkin's disease. Features of limbic encephalitis include agitation, depression, memory disorder,

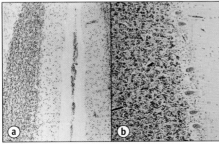

Fig. 15.1 Subacute cerebellar degeneration. (a) An almost total absence of Purkinje cells (mag X 80) compared with **(b)** a normal control individual (mag x 70).

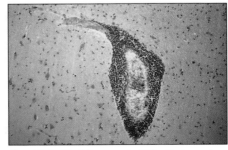

Fig. 15.2 Limbic encephalitis. Perivascular lymphocytic cuffing at the junction of cortex and white matter in the right temporal lobe (mag X 150).

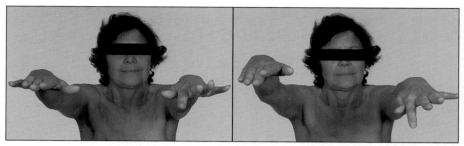

Fig. 15.3 *Subacute sensory neuropathy. Involuntary movements of the fingers appear after eye closure.*

dementia and seizures. Other features are determined the by distribution of the pathological process. The cerebrospinal fluid contains inflammatory cells and a raised protein concentration. The electroencephalogram may contain slow waves, sometimes with temporal spikes in the limbic cases. The course is generally progressive to death within 2 years, although occasionally the condition arrests.

PERIPHERAL NEUROPATHY
- Sensory
- Sensorimotor
- Motor (?)

Incidence, clinically, is 1–5%, electrophysiologically 20–50% (the figure is debated). Subacute sensory neuropathy is closely linked with small-cell carcinoma of the lung. It is associated with the presence of an antineural antibody (anti-Hu) which reacts with neuronal nucleoprotein antigens. It produces progressive peripheral sensory loss, with pain and dysaesthesiae. Loss of proprioception is associated with ataxia and pseudo-athetosis of the upper limbs. The reflexes are absent (**Fig. 15.3**). Dorsal roots show cell loss and lymphocytic infiltration. Other neuropathies are mixed, with a Guillain-Barré or slowly progressive type of presentation.

MYASTHENIC SYNDROME
See Chapter 14.

- Some of the paraneoplastic neurological syndromes are caused by organ-specific auto-antibodies
- The syndromes are mainly seen with small cell-carcinoma of the bronchus. The neurological syndrome can antedate discovery of the malignancy

RADIATION DAMAGE

After irradiation of the brain or spinal cord, necrosis appears after an interval of approximately 2–3 years in a proportion of patients, the incidence determined by the dose

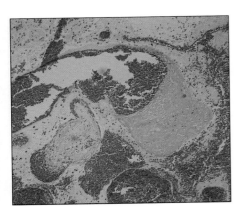

Fig. 15.4 Radionecrosis. *A necrotic vessel with extensive fibrinoid necrosis of its wall.*

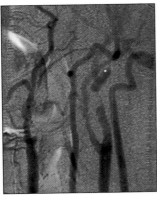

Fig. 15.5 *An occluded right internal carotid artery and distally stenosed left, after irradiation for carcinoma of the thyroid.*

and duration of irradiation. The blood vessels are particularly affected with secondary vascular proliferation and occlusion (**Fig. 15.4**). Imaging reveals mass effect, oedema and patchy enhancement with computerized tomography. Irradiation of the brachial plexus can lead to a progressive brachial plexopathy with reflex loss and motor and sensory deficit. Radiation damage to the extracranial vessels of the neck (e.g. after irradiation of the thyroid) can result in occlusion or stenosis of the carotid or vertebral vessels (**Fig. 15.5**).

DRUG-INDUCED DAMAGE

The drugs associated with a peripheral neuropathy are referred to in Chapter 12. Central nervous system adverse effects are recorded with several drugs, mainly those used for the treatment of malignant disease.

Methotrexate
Causes a leukoencephalopathy with similar features to those of irradiation necrosis. The complication is more likely if concomitant radiotherapy is given.

Cyclosporin
Can provoke seizures, coma and pryamidal signs. Pathological studies show areas of cerebral oedema associated with breakdown of the blood–brain barrier. Imaging reveals altered white matter signal.

Asparaginase and procarbazine
Both produce an encephalopathy with lethargy and confusion.

5-fluorouracil and cytosine arabinoside
Both produce a reversible cerebellar syndrome.

ALCOHOL AND THE NERVOUS SYSTEM

CLASSIFICATION
- Acute intoxication
- Alcohol-withdrawal seizures
- Delirium tremens
- Cerebellar degeneration
- Wernicke–Korsakoff psychosis
- Cerebral atrophy
- Central pontine myelinolysis
- Marchiafava–Bignami disease
- Peripheral neuropathy
- Muscle disease

CEREBELLAR DEGENERATION
Depletion of Purkinje cells, predominantly in the anterior and superior vermis (**Fig. 15.6**). Gait ataxia predominates with relatively normal upper limb co-ordination. Essentially irreversible.

WERNICKE–KORSAKOFF PSYCHOSIS
The acute, haemorrhagic lesions are found in the mammillary bodies, the peri-aqueductal grey matter of the midbrain, the floor of the fourth ventricle and in the paraventricular parts of the thalamus and hypothalamus (**Fig. 15.7**). Clinical features combine ophthalmoplegia, ataxia and a disturbance of orientation. The ophthalmoplegia is accompanied by nystagmus. The ataxia principally affects gait. The patient is drowsy, confused and amnesic. As recovery appears, a Korsakoff syndrome is likely, with profound short-term memory impairment

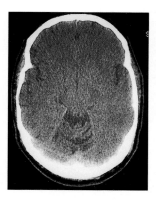

Fig. 15.6 *Computerized tomography showing superior vermian atrophy in an alcoholic patient.*

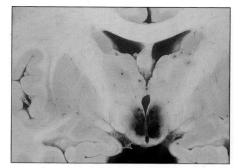

Fig. 15.7 *Wernicke–Korsakoff syndrome. A coronal brain section showing haemorrhages extending upwards from the mammillary bodies alongside the third ventricle.*

associated with confabulation. Defects of frontal lobe function have also been identified. Vigorous treatment with intravenous thiamine (vitamin B^1) reverses the ophthalmoplegia but is less successful in returning cognition to normal.

CEREBRAL ATROPHY

Brain atrophy occurs in alcoholic patients and is mainly caused by white matter shrinkage. The shrinkage is reversible with prolonged abstinence. It is not clear whether a specific dementia occurs with alcoholism. In many such patients, there are complicating factors such as recurrent head injury.

CENTRAL PONTINE MYELINOLYSIS

See Chapter 10.

MARCHIAFAVA–BIGNAMI DISEASE

A rare disorder in which demyelination of the corpus callosum occurs as a result of alcoholism.

PERIPHERAL NEUROPATHY

See Chapter 12.

MUSCLE DISEASE

See Chapter 14.

- The neuropathy associated with alcoholism can be arrested and partly reversed by vitamin B^1
- Patients suspected of having Wernicke–Korsakoff psychosis should not be given intravenous glucose until they have started on vitamin B^1
- Most of the adverse neurological effects of a cytotoxic agent are reversed when the agent is withdrawn

THE NEUROLOGY OF ENDOCRINE DISEASE

PITUITARY DISORDERS

Pituitary tumours are considered in Chapter 9.

Patients with acromegaly are liable to develop muscle weakness and wasting. Creatine kinase levels may be slightly elevated. Entrapment neuropathies are seen (e.g. the carpal tunnel syndrome) and a diffuse hypertrophic demyelinating neuropathy.

The syndrome of inappropriate antidiuretic hormone secretion (SIADH)

This is associated with hyponatremia, normal renal function and normal or increased blood volume. Occurs with various intracranial disorders, including subarachnoid haemorrhage and head injury but also with bronchial carcinoma. The patient becomes drowsy then comatose, eventually with seizures and focal neurological signs. Treatment is by fluid restriction or, in more severe cases, by infusion of hypertonic saline together with a diuretic. Demeclocycline blocks the action of antidiuretic hormone on the renal tubule and is used in more persistent cases.

In other patients with cerebral disease who have hyponatraemia and a similar clinical picture, there is hypovolaemia, the hyponatraemia being secondary to arginine vasopressin secretion, in turn, triggered by the hypovolaemia. These patients have an inappropriately

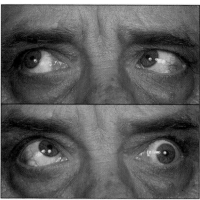

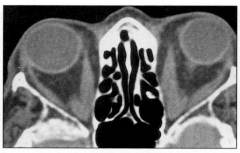

Fig. 15.9 Dysthyroid eye disease. Axial computerized tomography showing expanded medial recti.

Fig. 15.8 Dysthyroid eye disease. Depressed laevo-elevation of the left eye with concomitant lid retraction.

high level of atrial natriuretic peptide and require fluid replacement. The two types can be separated by measuring central venous pressure.

ADRENAL DISEASE

Cushing's disease
At least 50% of patients have proximal weakness. The onset is usually gradual but an acute variant with muscle pain is recognized.

Addison's disease
Muscle weakness is a prominent complaint but not accompanied by evidence of a specific myopathy.

THYROID DISEASE

Thyrotoxicosis
This is ssociated with muscle weakness in approximately three-quarters of patients. There is sometimes pain and stiffness. Bulbar symptoms appear in a small proportion of patients. Creatine kinase levels are usually normal and electromyogram changes non-specific. The muscle problem responds positively to control of the thyroid disorder. Myasthenia is more common in thyrotoxic individuals.

Dysthyroid eye disease
Dysthyroid eye disease occurs in hypothyroid, hyperthyroid and euthyroid patients. Swelling and lymphocytic infiltration of the orbital muscles occur. The condition is said to be the most common cause of spontaneous diplopia in middle-aged people. Lid retraction is common with an apparent failure of elevation caused by fibrotic shortening of the inferior rectus (**Fig. 15.8**). The problem can be confirmed by showing that there is resistance to mechanical elevation of the globe (a positive forced duction test). An abduction failure is similarly caused by fibrotic contraction of medial rectus. The abnormal muscle can be shown by computerized tomography or magnetic resonance imaging (**Fig. 15.9**). When the muscle swelling is severe, the optic nerve may be secondarily compressed. Steroid treatment is used, particularly if the function of the optic nerve is threatened. Surgical decompression of the orbit is only rarely required.

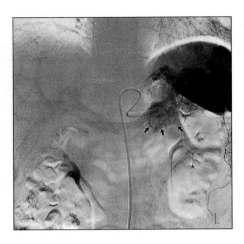

Fig. 15.10 *Insulinoma. Coeliac axis angiography showing a tumour blush (arrows).*

Hypothyroidism

This is associated with:

- Peripheral neuropathy
- Proximal myopathy
- Muscle pain and stiffness (Hoffman's syndrome)
- Deafness
- Cerebellar ataxia
- Encephalopathy, leading, rarely, to dementia

Parathyroid disease

There is proximal, sometimes painful, muscle weakness that is associated with both primary hyperparathyroidism and osteomalacia with secondary hyperparathyroidism. Hypercalcaemia can occur with metastatic bone disease and as an endocrinological manifestation of cancer. Patients become drowsy and confused, eventually lapsing into coma. Hypocalcaemia, usually the consequence of hypoparathyroidism, is associated with tetany, paraesthesiae in the peripheries and around the mouth, and seizures.

PANCREATIC DISEASE

Diabetes

The various peripheral nerve complications are considered in Chapter 12. Cranial neuropathies are encountered. The third and sixth nerves are most frequently involved. An acute optic neuropathy is probably the result of ischaemia of the anterior part of the nerve.

Insulinoma

The incidence of insulinoma is approximately 1 per 100 000 of the population. Symptoms are likely to appear when plasma glucose levels fall below 2.5 mmol/l. Episodic symptoms include drowsiness, altered behaviour, dysarthria, brainstem syndromes, fits and focal deficits mimicking the effect of cerebrovascular disease (similar symptoms can occur as part of a hypoglycaemic reaction in diabetic patients). Many patients develop symptoms after an overnight fast and virtually all become symptomatic during a 72-h fast. The hypoglycaemia is accompanied by inappropriately high insulin levels. The tumour is best localized using coeliac axis angiography (**Fig. 15.10**). Distal pancreatectomy is performed if the tumour is in the tail of the gland.

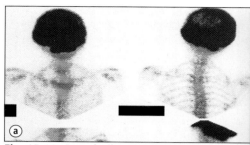
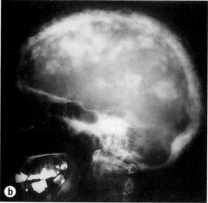

Fig. 15.11 *Paget's disease. (a)* Abnormal
isotope bone scan. *(b)* Skull radiograph.

- Proximal muscle weakness is common in thyrotoxicosis
- The myopathic complications of the endocrine disorders generally improve when the underlying condition is treated
- Dysthyroid eye disease is a common cause of spontaneous diplopia in middle-aged people
- Not all patients with cerebral disease and hyponatraemia have inappropriate antidiuretic hormone secretion

PAGET'S DISEASE

Abnormal osteoclastic activity leads to increased bone resorption and secondary increased new bone formation. The biochemical consequences of this activity include an increased serum alkaline phosphatase activity and increased urinary excretion of hydroxyproline. Bones most affected are the skull, vertebrae, pelvis and the long bones of the lower limbs. Neurological complications are the result of fracture or direct compression of neural tissue by bone altered structurally or undergoing malignant transformation. In addition to various changes on plain radiograph, bone scanning identifies areas of abnormal bone activity (**Fig. 15.11**). Cranial nerve palsies result from compression within the exit foramina. The eighth nerve is most commonly involved. Deformity of the base of the skull with softening leads to invagination of the odontoid process and secondary compression of the brainstem and cerebellum. Spinal involvement is usually multifocal (see Chapter 13). Treatment is predominantly medical and is based on the use of agents that inhibit osteoclast-mediated bone resorption. The drugs used are calcitonin, the diphosphonates and mithramycin. Surgery may be indicated for patients with brainstem or cerebellar compression.

NEUROLOGICAL COMPLICATIONS OF VASCULITIS

Vasculitic disorders show histological evidence of inflammation and necrosis of blood vessels.

CLASSIFICATION
- Polyarteritis nodosa and related conditions
- Hypersensitivity vasculitis

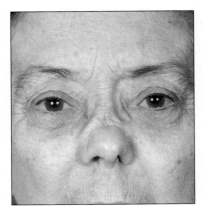

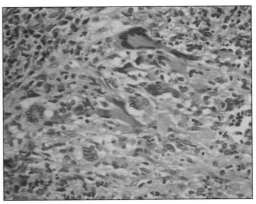

Fig. 15.12 *Wegener's granulomatosis.* Saddle-nose deformity.

Fig. 15.13 *Wegener's granulomatosis.* Nasal septal biopsy showing histiocytic giant cells, lymphocytes and plasma cells (mag X 100).

- Wegener's granulomatosis
- Giant-cell arteritis
- Takayasu's disease
- Behçet's disease
- Granulomatous angiitis

POLYARTERITIS NODOSA

- Inflammation of small- and medium-sized arteries
- Neurological complications in at least 50% of patients
- Neurological features include mononeuritis multiplex, sensorimotor neuropathy, radiculopathy and brachial plexopathy
- Central nervous system involvement includes infarction of the brain or spinal cord or an encephalopathy with altered cognition and seizures. Ischaemic optic neuropathy is common
- Churg–Strauss syndrome (allergic angiitis with granulomatosis) has similar neurological features
- Corticosteroids improve survival but a combination of corticosteroids and cyclophosphamide improves prognosis further

HYPERSENSITIVITY VASCULITIS

Conditions in this group include serum sickness and some cases of essential mixed cryoglobulinaemia. Neurological complications of serum sickness include peripheral and brachial neuropathy, seizures and encephalopathy. Peripheral neuropathy is a recognized complication of cryoglobulinaemia.

WEGENER'S GRANULOMATOSIS

- Granuloma formation with arteritis occurs in various organs, including the brain
- Typically, the condition begins in the upper respiratory tract with a non-specific granulomatous rhinitis or sinusitis
- Subsequent bony destruction affects the nose, sinuses and sometimes the orbits. Saddle-nose deformity is common (**Fig. 15.12**)
- Extension of the granulomas into the orbit, middle or posterior cranial fossae account for many of the neurological complications that appear in up to 50% of the patients. Remote granulomas can arise in individual cranial nerves or within the cerebrum (**Fig. 15.13**)

287

- Vasculitis accounts for the other neurological complications: mononeuritis multiplex, polyneuritis or radiculitis
- Cyclophosphamide is the drug of choice

GIANT-CELL ARTERITIS
See Chapter 2

TAKAYASU'S DISEASE
- A large-vessel arteritis principally affecting the aortic arch and its branches
- Predominates in young women
- Progresses through an acute, inflammatory phase to a later stage of complications secondary to vascular occlusion
- Neurological complications occur secondary to carotid or, less commonly, vertebral occlusion
- The erythrocyte sedimentation rate is elevated in some patients
- Steroids probably reduce the incidence of late vascular complications

BEHÇET'S DISEASE

Symptoms of Behçet's disease

- Recurrent orogenital ulceration associated with relapsing ocular lesions
- Arthritis
- Headache

- Other features include thrombophlebitis and skin lesions
- Neurological complications occur in up to 40% of patients
- Focal neurological features include meningoencephalitis, pyramidal signs, pseudo-tumour cerebri, brainstem or cerebellar signs and paraplegia (**Fig. 15.14**)
- Headache is common and most patients with neurological complications have a cerebrospinal fluid pleocytosis associated with an elevated protein concentration
- Computerized tomography shows areas of low density with cerebral and cerebellar atrophy
- T2-weighted magnetic resonance imaging shows venous sinus thrombosis in about one-third of the patients and multiple small high signal areas (mimicking multiple sclerosis) in approximately 40% of patients
- Combined steroid and immunosuppressive therapy improves outcome in patients with neurological complications

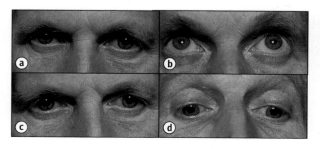

Fig. 15.14 Behçet's disease. Failure of horizontal gaze (**a and c**) associated with preservation of vertical gaze (**b and d**).

GRANULOMATOUS ANGIITIS

- A rare condition characterized by inflammation and necrosis of small leptomeningeal and parenchymal vessels in the central nervous system. Granulomas are contained in the infiltrate (**Fig. 15.15**)
- Headache is almost universal, combined with intellectual impairment and focal neurological signs
- The erythrocyte sedimentation rate is usually normal but the cerebrospinal fluid may show a modest lymphocytosis and elevated protein concentration
- Angiography in some patients shows beading of the affected vessels
- Steroid therapy may arrest the course of the disease

SYSTEMIC LUPUS ERYTHEMATOSUS

Of all the connective tissue disorders, systemic lupus erythematosus is the one most frequently associated with neurological complications. Perhaps up to 50% of systemic lupus erythematosus patients are affected. Vasculitis is not a feature of the pathological state. The high risk of stroke appears related to a thrombotic tendency linked with the presence of antiphospholipid antibodies and cardiac embolism. Antineuronal antibodies are present in the sera; their relationship to neurological disease is uncertain.

Symptoms of systemic lupus erythematosus

- Headache is common and can show migraine characteristics
- Seizures are reported in up to 70% of patients and, in some, appear stroke related
- Psychosis and depression, and spinal cord, peripheral nerve and movement disorders occur

---

Chorea is seen and correlates with the presence of antiphospholipid antibodies. Cerebrospinal fluid abnormalities include an elevated cell count and protein concentration, abnormal Ig G indices, oligoclonal Ig G and decreased C4 levels. Scattered periventricular ischaemic lesions on magnetic resonance imaging bear a superficial resemblance to those seen in multiple sclerosis. Corticosteroids with or without immunosuppressants are used for the more severe neurological complications. Steroids do not influence the occurrence of stroke and for patients with a stroke tendency warfarin is recommended.

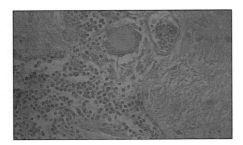

Fig. 15.15 *Granulomatous angiitis.* *White matter containing a dilated perivascular space filled with lymphocytes and a multinucleated giant cell (mag x 100).*

ANTIPHOSPHOLIPID ANTIBODY SYNDROME

Characterized by the presence of abnormal levels of circulating antiphospholipid antibodies and associated with retinal or optic nerve ischaemia, a migraine-like condition, brain infarction and an ischaemic encephalopathy. In addition, patients often have recurrent venous or arterial thromboses with multiple spontaneous abortions secondary to placental infarction. Additional blood findings include a prolonged partial thromboplastin time and a positive flocculation test for syphilis (in 25% of cases). Anticoagulants are the recommended treatment.

SJOGREN'S DISEASE

- Characterized by a mononuclear infiltration of the lacrimal and salivary glands, leading to xerophthalmia and xerostomia
- Peripheral nervous system involvement results in a sensory neuropathy, mononeuritis multiplex and trigeminal sensory neuropathy
- Central nervous system involvement leads to hemiparesis, seizures, cerebellar signs and internuclear ophthalmoplegia. At least part of the pathological process is vasculitic in origin
- A diffuse meningo-encephalitic syndrome is associated with a cerebrospinal fluid pleocytosis including polymorphonuclear leukocytes
- Computerized tomography shows lucent areas in patient with central nervous system involvement
- Vasculitic complications correlate with the presence of anti-Ro antibodies
- Steroid therapy is of uncertain value in management

SCLERODERMA

- There is a close association between progressive systemic sclerosis and the CREST syndrome (calcinosis, Raynaud's phenomenon, oesophageal motility disorder, sclerodactyly and telangiectasiae [**Fig. 15.16**])
- A vasculitic process affecting the central nervous system can occur in both conditions leading to infarction (**Fig. 15.17**)

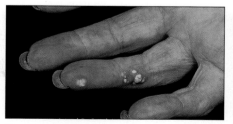

Fig. 15.16 *CREST syndrome. Appearance of the fingers.*

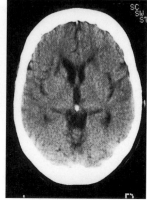

Fig. 15.17
CREST syndrome. Computerized tomography showing bilateral caudate infarcts.

- Other complications include carpal tunnel syndrome, trigeminal neuralgia and muscle weakness associated with abnormal creatine kinase levels

---

- Neurological complications are particularly common in systemic lupus erythematosus
- Different pathological processes contribute to neurological disease in the collagen vascular diseases, including vasculitis, an abnormal thrombotic state and antineuronal antibodies
- Corticosteroids are mainly of value where there is a vasculitic component to the pathological process

---

SARCOIDOSIS

This is a multiorgan, chronic disease of unknown aetiology, characterized by the presence of non-caseating granulomas. In some patients, the disease is confined to the central nervous system. Neurological features reflect either peripheral or central nervous system involvement or primary muscle pathology. Peripheral nervous system manifestations include cranial neuropathies (principally the seventh) and either a mononeuritis multiplex or a diffuse sensorimotor neuropathy. Thoracic neuropathy leads to segmental truncal pain and sensory loss.

Central nervous system features include single or multiple sarcoid granulomas. The hypothalamus is commonly affected, with resulting diabetes insipidus. Diffuse meningeal inflammation can occur with the possibility of obstructive hydrocephalus.

Various forms of ocular inflammatory disease occur, including uveitis, choroido-retinitis and retinal vasculitis. An iridoplegia is recognized, sometimes evolving to a tonic pupil syndrome (**Fig. 15.18**).

Cerebrospinal fluid changes are common. The protein concentration is slightly elevated, accompanied by a lymphocytic pleocytosis. The Ig G ratios may be abnormal, and oligoclonal Ig G is a recognized finding.

Angiotensin-converting enzyme levels are sometimes elevated in both serum and cerebrospinal fluid.

Computerized tomography shows any hydrocephalus and most mass lesions. Magnetic resonance imaging is the preferred imaging technique. An abnormal periventricular signal can be

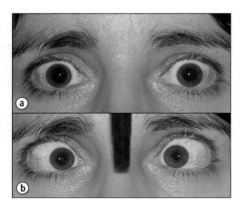

Fig. 15.18 Sarcoidosis. *Partial right iridoplegia with (a) dilated pupil and (b) incomplete near response*

seen, resembling the changes of multiple sclerosis, whereas focal meningeal enhancement with gadolinium is a striking, although non-specific, finding (**Fig. 15.19**). Gallium scanning can identify abnormal activity in other organs, including lymph nodes and salivary glands.

Central nervous system involvement is liable to produce neurological deficit showing little response to corticosteroid therapy. The peripheral nervous system complications are usually self-limiting and more likely to be steroid responsive.

NEUROLOGY AND PSYCHIATRY

Patients with psychiatric disorders are encountered frequently in neurological practice. The patients most likely to be referred for a neurological opinion have one of the following:
- An anxiety state (typically with features of the hyperventilation syndrome)
- Depression
- Conversion hysteria

HYPERVENTILATION SYNDROME

Can occur in the setting of an overt anxiety state or in isolation. Hyperventilation is associated with hypocapnoea and secondary cerebral vasoconstriction. This is the probable basis for symptoms such as faintness, dizziness and syncope. Alteration of ionized calcium concentration can trigger peripheral paraesthesiae or even tetany. Exaggerated autonomic activity can account for tremulousness, sweating and palpitations.

Common symptoms of hyperventilation syndrome

- Dizziness
- Dyspnoea
- Paraesthesiae
- Palpitations
- Visual blurring
- Faintness
- Headaches
- Altered awareness

The condition predominates in younger women. Initially, attacks tend to be triggered in certain environments, for example, on the Tube, on escalators and in supermarkets. Later, attacks are more spontaneous and the symptoms tend to be less paroxysmal. Attacks can be reproduced by asking the patient to hyperventilate while confirming a tendency for low pCO_2 levels to emerge. Counselling, anxiolytics and retraining of the patient's breathing pattern provide relief in the majorit of cases.

DEPRESSION

Somatic complaints often figure prominently in the history of a depressed individual. Chronic headaches are common, whereas difficulty in concentrating and memorizing can suggest the possibility of a dementing illness (pseudo-dementia). To complicate matters further, depression is a recognized feature of many neurological diseases, including dementia. Formal psychometry may be needed to distinguish a true dementia from pseudo-dementia. If uncertainty remains, the patient should be given antidepressants and the psychometry repeated after a period of several months.

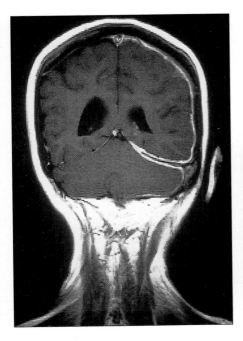

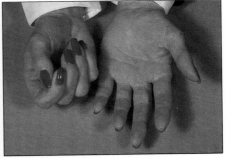

Fig. 15.19 *Sarcoidosis.* Coronal gadolinium-enhanced, T1-weighted magnetic resonance imaging. Meningeal enhancement is seen over the left hemisphere and the tentorium cerebelli.

Fig. 15.20 *Conversion hysteria.* Fixed posture of the fingers of the right hand.

CONVERSION HYSTERIA

Defined as a condition in which mental and physical symptoms, not of organic origin, are produced and maintained by motives never fully conscious, directed at some real or fancied gain to be derived from such symptoms.

Classification

- Conversion reactions superimposed on a physical illness (e.g. pseudo-seizures in a patient with epilepsy)
- Conversion reactions associated with depression
- Conversion reactions of a recurrent nature in a patient with multiple bodily complaints but without evidence of significant organic disease (Briquet's syndrome)

In the vast majority of patients, the tendency to a conversion reaction is established in adolescence or early adult life. Neurological complaints are prominent and include movement disorders, motor symptoms, balance disorders, altered awareness, sensory complaints and visual loss

Movement disorders

Many movement disorders, once classified as being psychological, are now considered to be organic in origin. Non-organic movement disorders are recognized but difficult to distinguish from the 'real thing'.

Motor symptoms

These are commonly found. There may be global involvement of just one limb or one side of the body. The distribution does not follow the pattern of known neurological disease and is typically erratic and not reproducible. Rarely, a fixed limb deformity may emerge with oedema, cyanosis and coldness of the affected part leading sometimes to trophic changes (**Fig. 15.20**).

293

Balance disorders

Ataxia is sometimes a prominent complaint. The patient is liable to lurch violently when being observed. Self-injury does not exclude the possibility of a conversion reaction.

Altered awareness

Pseudo-seizures are not uncommon in epileptic patients but are a rare manifestation in other individuals (see Chapter 3).

Sensory complaints

Sensory symptoms, including pain, numbness or paraesthesiae are a common feature. Typically, on examination, the sensory loss fails to follow anatomical boundaries (**Fig. 15.21**).

Visual loss

Blindness is a rare manifestation of conversion hysteria. A complaint of restricted vision is common, however. Visual field analysis tends to reveal constricted fields to confrontation, whereas formal testing sometimes shows spiralling, a process in which the field apparently shrinks during the process of testing.

Conversion hysteria is a difficult problem to manage. Any causative depressive illness should be treated vigorously. It is seldom helpful to expose the patient either to him- or herselfor to members of his or her family. Insight in these individuals is severely limited and their capacity to benefit from a psychotherapeutic approach correspondingly poor.

- In younger patients with paroxysmal giddiness, unsteadiness or paraesthesiae, hyperventilation should be considered in the differential diagnosis
- Patients with an apparent dementia need careful appraisal for a possible underlying depressive illness
- Great caution should be taken in diagnosing a conversion reaction, particularly in middle-aged and older patients

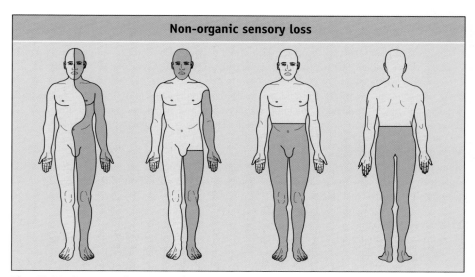

Non-organic sensory loss

Fig. 15.21 *Patterns of non-organic sensory loss.*